THYROID DISORDERS - FOCUS ON HYPERTHYROIDISM

Edited by **Gonzalo Díaz-Soto**

Thyroid Disorders - Focus on Hyperthyroidism
http://dx.doi.org/10.5772/57001
Edited by Gonzalo Díaz-Soto

Contributors
Bogusław Machaliński, Miłosz Kawa, Shi Lam, Brian Hung-Hin Lang, Magnus R. Dias Da Silva, Ana Luiza R. Rolim, Grażyna Wilk, Javier Pou Ucha, Tao Yang, Xiaoyun Liu, Madhuri Kurdi, Mustafa Cesur, Sibel Ertek, Irmak Sayin, Ruth Prichard

Published by InTech
Janeza Trdine 9, 51000 Rijeka, Croatia

Publishing Process Manager Iva Lipovic
Technical Editor InTech DTP team
Cover InTech Design team

First published May, 2014
Printed in Croatia

Additional hard copies can be obtained from orders@intechopen.com

Thyroid Disorders - Focus on Hyperthyroidism, Edited by Gonzalo Díaz-Soto
p. cm.
ISBN 978-953-51-1384-3

For EU product safety concerns:
IN TECH d.o.o., Prolaz Marije Krucifikse Kozulić 3, 51000 Rijeka, Croatia,
info@intechopen.com or visit our website at intechopen.com.

Meet the editor

Gonzalo Díaz-Soto is an Associate Professor of Endocrinology and Nutrition in Medical School of Valladolid University and a researcher at Endocrinology and Nutrition Institute (IEN). He received his MD and Master in Bioscience in experimental Endocrinology on Calcium Sensing Receptor. He finished his specialization on Endocrinology and Nutrition in Hospital Clinic of Barcelona. His PhD was focused on Normocalcemic Hyperparathyroidism. He has completed his PhD program with clinical internship in the Endocrinology Services of the Hôpital Bicêtre and the Institute Gustave Roussy in Paris.
He currently works at Clinical University Hospital of Valladolid in Endocrinology, Diabetes and Nutrition Department. His research areas and published articles are focused on endocrinology, especially thyroid, parathyroid and diabetes disorders.

Contents

Preface

The thyroid disorders are one of the most common and exciting areas of endocrinology. Hypothyroidism, multinodular goiter, hyperthyroidism and thyroid cancer are only few of the several implications that the thyroid disorders have in health. In fact, thyroid hormones regulate not only metabolism process, but also many other molecular and physiological systems. From this point of view, hyperthyroidism complications are a good example of the significance of thyroid hormone actions.

In the last decade the progress and development of biochemical assays of thyroid hormones and related peptides, new conventional or nuclear imaging techniques and a deeper knowledge in thyroid nodule and cancer physiopathology have changed the comprehension, diagnosis and treatment of thyroid disorders.

This book aims to provide a general view of thyroid disorders from different but complementary points of view: historical, physiopathology, diagnosis and treatment. Furthermore, it is focused on hyperthyroidism and its complications and impact in health and disease due to its severe consequences.

This book is the result of collaboration between worldwide authorities of different backgrounds. I am grateful to them for the quality of their contributions.

We hope that the medical and paramedical researchers will find this book helpful and stimulating. We look forward to sharing the state of the art in thyroid disorders with a wider audience.

Dr. Gonzalo Díaz-Soto
University of Valladolid Medical School,
Clinic University Hospital, Valladolid,
Spain

Section 1

Hashimoto Thyroiditis

Chapter 1

Hashimoto's Thyroiditis

Tao Yang and Xiaoyun Liu

Additional information is available at the end of the chapter

http://dx.doi.org/10.5772/57522

1. Introduction

1.1. The centennial history of Hashimoto's thyroiditis

One hundred years ago, a 31-year old Japanese surgeon called Hakaru Hashimoto at Kyoto Imperial University published the description of four cases of goiter in the thyroid resection specimens from four women in a German journal Archiv für Klinische Chirurgie in 1912 just before World War I. This paper contained two Latin words in the title (struma lymphomatosa) and five microphotographs. The histological appearance of these goiters characterized by a lymphoplasmocytic infiltrate with diffuse inflammatory alterations of the thyroid parenchyma and fibrosis was very different from the colloid goiters that he was familiar with, as well as those from Grave's disease, infectious thyroiditis (especially related to tuberculosis or syphilis) and the fibrous thyroiditis described by Riedel in 1896. He emphasized similarity with the histological data observed with lacrimal, salivary, lymph node and splenic involvement of Mikulicz's disease (now Sjögren's syndrome). Mickulicz was the teacher of Hayari Miyake, the head of Hashimoto's department.

The four observed cases involved female patients over the age of 40 years who had formed very firm diffuse goiters, to the extent that the diagnoses were suggestive of fibrous thyroid or cancer at that time. But these were isolated, with hardly any severe signs of compression and no adenopathy. The postoperative course of these goiters seemed more complicated than usual. One case was complicated by recurrence, soon followed by spontaneous reduction of the hypertrophy.

Hashimoto decided to continue his training in Göttingen, Germany and then in England. He was forced to return home after the outbreak of World War I. He continued to practice as a general practitioner in rural Midai in 1916 and died in 1934 at the age of 52 years from typhoid contracted from a patient, without achieving the recognition he deserved.

Hashimoto's discovery was not exactly ignored for the next few decades, but recognition of its existence was certainly slow, possibly related in part to the publication of the paper in German. In 1931, Graham and McCullagh used the term "Hashimoto" for the first time in the title of an article, strongly arguing that struma lymphomatosa was indeed distinct from Riedel's thyroiditis. The description of lymphocytic thyroiditis was rediscovered in the United States in 1936, and the disease was labeled Hashimoto's thyroiditis (chronic lymphocytic thyroiditis) in medical textbooks. In 1939, the prominent British thyroid surgeon Cecil Joll coined the term "Hashimoto disease" and used it in the title of a review he wrote about this condition. Since then, Hashimoto's thyroiditis has gone from being a rarity to one of the most common autoimmune diseases, as well as the most common endocrine disease.

An essential step was the characterization in 1956 by Noel Rose and Ernest Witebsky of experimental thyroiditis created by the injection of thyroid extracts and Freund adjuvant in rabbits, which showed histological aspects similar to those described by Hashimoto. In the same year, Ivan Roitt and Deborah Doniach reported the presence of autoantibodies directed against thyroglobulin in the Lancet. Until then it had seemed inconceivable that an individual would develop antibodies directed against his own body ("horror autotoxicus"). This was the first time that the possibility of autoimmune diseases had been suggested, and Hashimoto's disease established itself as the model of organ-specific autoimmune diseases. It is a good example of a situation in which a brilliant clinician provided the clinical and anatomopathological description of a disease, leaving it to future generations to understand the mechanism and, in the current case, to establish the far-reaching concept of autoimmune diseases, sometimes organ-specific, polyglandular or general.

With regard to history, there is agreement that the hypertrophic forms of lymphocytic thyroiditis, which can progress to atrophy although not inevitable, would be labeled Hashimoto's thyroiditis. In terms of the pathogenic, histologic and biologic perspectives, these forms did not differ greatly from atrophic lymphocytic thyroiditis causing myxoedema, or asymptomatic autoimmune thyroiditis or thyroiditis occurring with nodules or cancer. These aspects are the subject of the article by Orgiazzi. Even before the description of lymphocytic thyroiditis by Hashimoto, the simultaneous occurrence of hypothyroidism with other endocrinopathies had been demonstrated in Germany in 1904 by Erhlich, and in 1908 in France by Claude and Gougerot. In 1980 these conditions of polyglandular failure were divided into four types by Neufeld, and then grouped into two varieties. Childhood-onset type 1 autoimmune polyendocrine syndrome has autosomal recessive transmission linked to a mutation of the AIRE gene, which controls the production of antibodies at the thymic and peripheral levels. This can be differentiated from type 2 (or 2/3), which is much more frequent, starts in adulthood, and is polygenic and multifactorial, the characteristics of which are presented by Kahaly. Whether isolated or occurring with polyendocrinopathies, autoimmune involvement of the adrenal glands alters the quality of life and is life-threatening; it is explained and its care are described in the article by Napier and Pearce. The pathogenic access and assessment of autoimmune involvement in parathyroid and pituitary are still in the early stages, while the immunologic and pathogenic data and management perspectives are better understood in diabetes mellitus, as confirmed in the article by Boitard. The description of the histological changes of Hashimoto's thyroiditis, only just a century ago, gained credibility over several decades. Hashimoto's thyroiditis is now considered the most prevalent autoimmune disease.

2. Prevalence over time

Its incidence is about 1 case per 1000 persons per year. The prevalence is 8 cases per 1000 when estimated from a review of published articles, and 46 cases per 1000 when estimated from the biochemical evidence of hypothyroidism and thyroid autoantibodies in subjects participating to the Third National Health and Nutrition Examination Survey. Caturegli(Caturegli, De Remigis et al. 2013) and colleagues have marked the centenary of Hashimoto's seminal paper by reviewing the extensive surgical pathology archives of the Johns Hopkins Hospital for cases of Hashimoto thyroiditis, spanning an extremely long period from 1889 to 2012. The results are fascinating and a fitting way to mark this important anniversary. The study reveals a remarkable change in incidence, with very few cases for the first half of the period, and then a significant increase between 1943 and 1967, a constant incidence up to 1992 and then another significant increase over the last two decades.

Of course this retrospective pathological analysis can take little account of the clinical reasons for thyroid surgery, which will have a fundamental impact on the incidence, but the results are so striking that a rapid increase in the frequency of Hashimoto's thyroiditis in the second half of the 20th century seems an unavoidable conclusion. Another review supported this by reviewing of 1050 Austrians patients who had surgery for benign goiter between 1979 and 2009; there was a significant increase in the incidence of both lymphocytic thyroiditis and Hashimoto's thyroiditis in resection specimens over this time. In addition, a striking rise in Hashimoto's thyroiditis has been reported recently in Italy. Between 1975 and 2005, there was a 10-fold rise in incidence: patients have become relatively younger, are more likely to be male, and have lower autoantibody responses. While some of this change in incidence could be the result of increased thyroid function testing and earlier detection of disease, the overwhelming conclusion is that environmental factors must be responsible. Increased iodine intake is certainly one possible influence: a recent study in China showing increases in subclinical hypothyroidism and autoimmune thyroiditis in an area of more than adequate iodine intake is the latest among many such reports. But not all studies have shown an adverse effect of excess dietary iodine (possibly related to genetic factors and the rate of the increase in iodine intake in a population) and when it does occur, the effect of iodine may be transient. Nor is thyroid autoimmunity alone in this regard; celiac disease, type 1 diabetes, and multiple sclerosis have all increased in incidence over the last three decades. It is likely that aspects of urbanized living, such as higher standards of hygiene, increased prosperity, and increased exposure to environmental toxins, are responsible for this generalized trend, perhaps by altering the balance between T helper cell subtypes.

3. Pathogenesis and etiology

The pathogenesis of Hashimoto's thyroiditis has elicited interest since it was first reported. Dr. Hashimoto himself speculated on possible explanations of what he saw under the microscope, eventually concluding "at present we cannot say anything definite about the cause". Initial theories postulated this disease was due to infection, understandably, since infections were quite common and a large focus of clinical investigation, but no clear link with microorganisms was ever found. Other theories considered the Hashimoto goiter a premalignant condition. Some scholars believed the thyroid itself possessed a lymphogenic secretory capability that became hyperactive in these patients. Others viewed the goiter as secondary to constant anxiety and emotional unrest. In 1951, Hellwig proposed the colloidophagy theory, based on rodent studies performed in the late 1920s and his own observations in humans that macrophages exist in the thyroid gland and are capable of ingesting colloid. He postulated that thyroid macrophages that have engulfed colloid degenerate and release colloid, which then attracts lymphocytes into the thyroid. Finally, in the early 1950s, the field of autoimmunity began to take shape; animal models were being developed in which injection of a tissue extract was capable of reproducing a lymphocytic infiltration of that particular organ. This experimental approach was applied to the thyroid when, in 1956, lymphocytic infiltration of the rabbit thyroid was induced by injection of rabbit thyroid extracts. The horror autotoxicus dogma was dismantled and autoimmunity became recognized as an important mechanism of disease. In the ensuing five decades, numerous studies have greatly expanded our understanding of the pathogenesis of Hashimoto's thyroiditis and helped translating research findings into clinical practice. We have known since the mid-1980s that thyroperoxidase is a dominant protein antigen targeted by the patient's immune system in Hashimoto's thyroiditis, and, as a result, antibodies to thyroperoxidase are now considered the most sensitive and specific biomarkers to establish this diagnosis. They also have a predictive value since their presence precedes a clinical diagnosis of Hashimoto's thyroiditis by at least 7 years. We have also known since 1971 that Hashimoto's thyroiditis, like other autoimmune diseases, has a genetic basis. Substantial efforts have been devoted to identify the genes that predispose to Hashimoto's thyroiditis, but results have been less fruitful than expected. Genome-wide association studies and candidate gene approaches have identified a handful of confirmed susceptibility genes (MHC class II region, CTLA-4, PTPN22, and ARID5B), each making, however, only a small contribution to the disease phenotype and through mechanisms that remain to be discovered.

4. Susceptibility genes

4.1. Human leukocyte antigen (HLA) genes

The first gene locus identified in association with the autoimmune thyroid disease was major histocompatibility complex (MHC) region on the chromosome 6p21 which encodes human leukocyte antigens (HLAs). HLA region, which is highly polymorphic, comprises several immune response genes. HLA molecule, located on antigen presenting cell (APC), binds and presents an antigenic peptide and in this way enables T cell recognition and response to an antigen. Presumably, specific HLA alleles have a higher affinity for autoantigenic thyroidal peptides and are thus likely to contribute to the development of the autoimmune thyroid disease. Nevertheless, in order to initiate the thyroid autoimmunity autoantigen occurrence within thyroid or thyroid draining lymph nodes is needed, being followed by HLA presentation. In HT, aberrant expression of HLA class II molecules on thyrocytes has been demonstrated. Presumably, such thyrocytes may act as APCs capable of presenting the thyroid autoantigens and initiating autoimmune thyroid disease. In Caucasians, associations of different forms of HT with various HLA alleles were reported, including DR3, DR5, DQ7, DQB1*03, DQw7 or DRB1*04-DQB1*0301 haplotype. In Japanese, associations with DRB4*0101, HLA-A2 and DRw53 were demonstrated, while in Chinese patients association with DRw9 was observed (Hawkins, Lam et al. 1987, Honda, Tamai et al. 1989, Badenhoop, Schwarz et al. 1990, Tandon, Zhang et al. 1991, Bogner, Badenhoop et al. 1992, Wan, Kimura et al. 1995, Hunt, Marshall et al. 2001, Petrone, Giorgi et al. 2001, Jacobson, Huber et al. 2008, Zaletel and Gaberscek 2011).

4.2. Cytotoxic t lymphocyte antigen-4 (CTLA-4) gene

CTLA-4 gene, which is the second major immuneregulatory gene related to autoimmune thyroid disease, lies on chromosome 2q33. The expression of CTLA-4 on the surface of T cells induced by the activation of the T-cell receptor results in suppression of T-cell activation. CTLA-4 gene polymorphisms may reduce expression or function of the CTLA-4 antigen and may therefore contribute to the reduced inhibition of T-cell proliferation and subsequently increase susceptibility to autoimmune response. In the past, several polymorphisms of the CTLA-4 gene in HT patients were studied. Among them, the initially reported (AT)n microsatellite CTLA-4 polymorphism in the 3′ untranslated region (UTR) was found to be associated with HT in Caucasian and Japanese patients, but not in Italian population. In the exon 1 located 49A/G single nucleotide polymorphism (SNP), resulting in threonine to alanine substitution, was associated with HT, however, certain other studies have not confirmed this observation. A large meta-analysis, including both published and unpublished data of 866 HT patients, indicated a significant association with 49A/G (summary OR 1.29; 95% CI, 1.11-1.50). Another CTLA-4 polymorphism is 6230A/G SNP which is located at 3′-UTR and designated CT60. Initial observation of the association with HT was not confirmed by later studies, however, the results of the meta-analysis, based on six published and unpublished studies of 839 HT patients, indicated a significant association with CT60 SNP (summary OR 1.64; 95% CI, 1.18-2.28). Nevertheless, the exact mechanism conferring the susceptibility to HT has not been elucidated yet and further studies are needed to determine which CTLA-4 polymorphism is causative.

4.3. Protein tyrosine phosphatase nonreceptor-type 22 (PTPN22) gene

PTPN22 is the most recently identified immuneregulatory gene associated with the autoimmune thyroid disease, which is located on chromosome 1p13. PTPN22, which is predominantly expressed in lymphocytes, acts as a negative regulator of T-cell activation, much like CTLA-4. 1858C/T SNP of the PTPN22 gene, resulting in arginine to tryptophan substitution at codon 620 (R620W), was demonstrated to be a risk factor for many autoimmune diseases. The mechanism is not clear since the disease predisposing T allele has been demonstrated to enable even more efficient inhibition of T-cell activation. Presumably, weaker T-cell signalling may lead to impaired thymic deletion of autoreactive T cells or an increased PTPN22 function may result in inhibition of regulatory T cells (Tregs), which protect against autoimmunity. An early study in HT patients demonstrated a significant association with 1858C/T SNP (OR 1.77; 95% CI, 1.56-3.97). Afterwards, this observation was neither confirmed in German, Tunisian and Japanese populations nor in Slovenian patients. In a small group of patients with both HT and autoimmune diabetes, T allele was determined in 50% compared with only 14% in healthy controls (OR 6.14; CI, 2.62-14.38), however, in a yet another study estimating the same polymorphism this association was not confirmed. Recently, 5 other PTPN22 SNPs have been tested in Japanese patients, showing no relation with HT, but a novel protective haplotype containing those SNPs has been observed (Ban, Tozaki et al. 2005, Kahles, Ramos-Lopez et al. 2005, Chabchoub, Teixiera et al. 2009, Dultz, Matheis et al. 2009, Ban, Tozaki et al. 2010, Kordonouri, Hartmann et al. 2010, Zaletel and Gaberscek 2011).

4.4. Thyroglobulin gene

Tg is an important thyroid specific antigen, also present in the circulation, which makes it an easy target of the autoimmune response. Gene for Tg is located on the chromosome 8q24 and linkage of this region with HT and autoimmune thyroid disease was first identified by a Japanese and an American whole genome studies. A subsequent fine mapping of this region exposed Tg gene as one of the major thyroid specific susceptibility genes, linked and associated with the autoimmune thyroid disease. Later, different alleles of various microsatellite markers and different SNPs of Tg gene were related to HT, possibly affecting its expression, antigenicity, iodination, or binding to HLA. The association of Tgms2 microsatellite marker in intron 27 with HT was confirmed in Japanese as well as in Caucasian population. Sequencing of human Tg revealed 14 SNPs among which four SNPs, including exon 10-12 SNP cluster and exon 33 SNP, were associated with HT. However, this observation was neither confirmed in a larger data set of the United Kingdom Caucasian patients nor in Chinese population.

4.5. Vitamin D receptor gene

Vitamin D, which acts via vitamin D receptor (VDR), possesses immunomodulatory properties and its deficiency has been implicated in the development of autoimmune diseases. Many immune cells express VDR, dendritic cells in particular, where VDR stimulation has been shown to enhance their tolerogenicity. Tolerogenic dendritic cells promote development of Tregs with suppressive activity and therefore peripheral tolerance. VDR gene is located on the chromosome 12q12 and its polymorphisms have been related to different autoimmune disorders such as type 1 diabetes or Addison's disease. A decade ago, the association between VDR-FokI SNP in exon 2 and HT has been identified which was later confirmed in the observation of Taiwanese Chinese patients. In the Croatian population VDR gene 3′ region polymorphisms were related to HT, possibly affecting VDR mRNA expression. A significant relation has also been discovered between HT and both promoter and intron 6 gene polymorphisms of CYP27B1 hydroxylase, which is located on chromosome 12q13, catalysing the conversion of 25 hydroxyvitamin D3 to its active form.

4.6. Cytokine genes and other immune-related genes

Lately, several genes encoding different inflammatory cytokines have been studied in HT, some of them also influencing the severity of the disease. Interferon (IFN)-γ, produced by T-helper type 1 (Th1) cells, promotes cell mediated cytotoxicity which underlies thyroid destruction in HT. T allele of the+874A/T IFN-SNP, causing the increased production of IFN-γ, was associated with severity of hypothyroidism in HT patients. Higher frequency of severe hypothyroidism was also observed in patients carrying CC genotype of-590C/T interleukin 4 (IL-4) SNP, leading to a lower production of IL-4, one of the key Th2 cytokines which suppresses cell-mediated autoimmunity. Gene polymorphism of transforming growth factor(TGF)-β, inhibitor of cytokine production, was also associated with HT. T allele of+369T/C SNP, leading to a lower secretion of TGF-β, was more frequent in severe hypothyroidism than in mild hypothyroidism. Similarly, more severe form of HT was associated with-2383C/T SNP of gene for forkhead box P3 (FoxP3), an essential regulatory factor for the Tregs development. Unlike the severity of hypothyroidism, the development of HT itself was associated with C allele of tumor necrosis factor (TNF)--1031T/C SNP. Namely, C-allele carriers present with higher concentration of TNF-which acts as the stimulator of the IFN-production.

5. Risk factors

5.1. Role of female sex and reproduction

5.1.1. Female sex

As indicated by numerous epidemiological studies, females present with positive thyroid autoantibodies (TAbs) up to three times more often than males. The largest NHANES III study has shown that females were positive for TPOAbs and TgAbs in 17% and 15.2%, respectively, while males only in 8.7% and 7.6%, respectively. According to the estimation provided by the study of Danish twins, the genetic contribution to TPOAb and TgAb susceptibility in females was 72% and 75%, respectively, while in males it was only 61% and 39%, respectively. The possible explanation for high female predominance in thyroid autoimmunity might be associated with the X chromosome containing a number of sex and immune-related genes which are of key importance in the preservation of immune tolerance. Increased immunoreactivity might therefore be related to genetic defects of the X chromosome, such as structural abnormalities or monosomy. Accordingly, a higher incidence of thyroid autoimmunity was reported in patients with a higher rate of X chromosome monosomy in peripheral white blood cells or in patients with Turner's syndrome. Another potential mechanism of impaired immunotolerance in females is skewed X-chromosome inactivation (XCI) leading to the escape of X-linked self-antigens from presentation in thymus with subsequent loss of T-cell tolerance. Skewed XCI was associated with a higher risk of developing autoimmune thyroid diseases. Recently reported frequencies of skewed XCI in HT were 31%, 34.3%, 25.6% and 20%, respectively, which is significantly higher than in healthy controls, where the prevalences were only 8%, 8%, 8.6% and 11.2%, respectively. Furthermore, a study of Danish twins demonstrated a significant association of skewed XCI with TPOAb serum concentrations in dizygotic but not in monozygotic twin pairs, indicating that shared genetic determinants of XCI pattern and TPOAb production are more likely than causal relationship.

5.1.2. Pregnancy and postpartum period

The tolerance of the fetal semi-allograft during pregnancy is enabled by the state of immunosuppression which is a result of hormonal changes and trophoblast expression of key immunomodulatory molecules. The pivotal players in regulation of the immune response are Tregs, which rapidly increase during pregnancy. Consequently, both cell-mediated and humoral immune responses are attenuated with a shift towards humoral immune response, resulting in immune tolerance of the conceptus tissues and suppression of autoimmunity. Accordingly, the decrease of both TPOAb and TgAb concentrations during pregnancy has been reported, reaching the lowest values in the third trimester. Postpartum rapid decrease of Tregs and re-establishment of the immune response to the pre-pregnancy state may lead to the occurrence or aggravation of the autoimmune thyroid disease. The increase of TPOAb concentrations occurred as soon as 6 weeks after delivery, reaching the baseline level at approximately 12 weeks and the maximum level at about 20 weeks after delivery. In up to 50% of females with positive TPOAbs in the early pregnancy, thyroid autoimmunity in the postpartum period exacerbates in the form of postpartum thyroiditis. It may occur within the first year after delivery, usually clinically presented with transient thyrotoxicosis and/or transient hypothyroidism, while in about a third of females permanent hypothyroidism may even develop.

5.1.3. Fetal microchimerism

The term fetal microchimerism is defined by the presence of fetal cells in maternal tissues which are transferred in the maternal circulation during pregnancy. Several years after the delivery, the chimeric male cells can be detected in the maternal peripheral blood as well as in maternal tissues, such as thyroid, lung, skin, or lymph nodes. The fetal immune cells, settled in the maternal thyroid gland, may become activated in the postpartum period when the immunotolerance ceases, representing a possible trigger that may initiate or exaggerate the autoimmune thyroid disease. In HT, fetal microchimeric cells were detected in thyroid in 28% to 83% which means that their occurrence is significantly higher than in the absence of autoimmune thyroid disease. Furthermore, a recent study of twins supported the putative role of microchimerism in triggering thyroid autoimmunity, showing a significantly higher prevalence of TAbs in opposite sex twins compared to monozygotic twins. Additionally, euthyroid females having been pregnant presented significantly more often with positive TPOAb compared to females with no history of being pregnant. However, the relation between parity and autoimmune thyroid disease was not confirmed by large population-based studies, advocating

http://dx.doi.org/10.5772/57522

against the essential contribution of fetal microchimerism to the pathogenesis of autoimmune thyroid disease.

6. Environmental triggers

6.1. Iodine intake

Excessive iodine intake is well-established environmental factor for triggering thyroid autoimmunity. Several large population-based studies demonstrated higher prevalence of TAbs in the areas with higher iodine supply since the estimated prevalence was approximately 13% in iodine deficiency, 18% in circumstances of sufficient iodine intake and about 25% in areas with excessive iodine intake. Moreover, up to four-fold increase in prevalence of TAbs was demonstrated after the exposure to higher iodine intake due to the improvement of iodine prophylaxis in previously iodine deficient areas. According to the intervention study, deliberate exposure to 500 μg of iodine provoked thyroid autoimmunity in 20% of previously healthy individuals. Valuable evidence was also provided by using experimental animal models of autoimmune thyroiditis, where the prevalence and severity of thyroid autoimmunity significantly increased when the dietary iodine was added (Kahaly, Dienes et al. 1998, Rose, Bonita et al. 2002, Fountoulakis, Philippou et al. 2007, Golkowski, Buziak-Bereza et al. 2007, Heydarian, Ordookhani et al. 2007).

Several putative mechanisms by which iodine may promote thyroid autoimmunity have been proposed. Firstly, iodine exposure leads to higher iodination of Tg and thus increases its immunogenicity by creating novel iodinecontaining epitopes or exposing cryptic epitopes. This may facilitate presentation by APC and enhance the binding affinity of the T-cell receptor which may lead to specific T cell activation. Secondly, iodine exposure has been shown to increase the level of reactive oxygen species in the thyrocyte which is generated during TPO oxidation of excessive amounts of iodine. They enhance the expression of the intracellular adhesion molecule-1 (ICAM-1) on the thyroid follicular cells which could attract the immunocompetent cells into the thyroid gland. Thirdly, iodine toxicity to thyrocytes has been reported, since highly reactive oxygen species may bind to membrane lipids and proteins, causing thyrocyte damage and release of autoantigens. Fourthly, iodine excess has been shown to promote follicular cell apoptosis by inducing an abnormal expression of tumor necrosis factor-related apoptosis inducing ligand (TRAIL) and its death receptor (DR)-5 in thyroid. Fifthly, in vitro evidence also suggests an enhancing influence of iodine on the cells of the immune system, including augmented maturation of dendritic cells, increased number of T cells and stimulated B-cell immunoglobulin production.

6.2. Drugs

Furthermore, certain drugs were reported to trigger or exacerbate thyroid autoimmunity in susceptible individuals (Barbesino 2010, Hamnvik, Larsen et al. 2011). Interferon-α (IFN-α) is extensively used to treat chronic hepatitis and is frequently associated with thyroid autoimmunity since TAbs were observed in up to 40% and clinical disease in 5-10% of patients treated with IFN-α. Presumably, IFN-α has both thyroid toxic effects with consequent autoantigen presentation and immune effects, such as switching to Th1 immune response, suppression of Treg function, activation of immune cells, stimulation of cytokine release and expression of MHC class I on thyroid cells. Similarly, IL-2 treatment, used for melanoma and renal carcinoma, seems to act via immune and toxic mechanisms, leading to both TAb positivity and hypothyroidism.

In patients with known autoimmune thyroid disease lithium may increase the risk of hypothyroidism. According to some studies, treatment with lithium has also been shown to increase TAb titres and the prevalence of thyroid autoimmunity. Among putative mechanisms direct toxicity of lithium on thyroid or toxicity of increased intrathyroidal iodine resulting from lithium treatment were discussed. Similarly, amiodarone alone as well as its high iodine content may act cytotoxically which may lead to thyroid autoantigen presentation and provoke thyroid autoimmunity.

More recently, some small molecule tyrosine kinase inhibitors (TKIs) used for the treatment of metastatic renal cell carcinoma (Muriel, Esteban et al. 2010, Kollmannsberger, Bjarnason et al. 2011, Eisen, Sternberg et al. 2012, Mendez-Vidal, Martinez Ortega et al. 2012, Bianchi, Rossi et al. 2013), gastrointestinal stromal tumours (Joensuu, Trent et al. 2011), thyroid carcinoma and pancreatic neuroendocrine tumours have been shown to cause hypothyroidism related symptoms to a variable extent, which can reduce a patient's quality of life (Torino, Corsello et al. 2009, Zygulska, Krzemieniecki et al. 2012). Sunitinib and sorafenib are multitargeted TKIs that have been demonstrated to induce hypothyroidism and thyroid dysfunction. The reported incidence of sunitinib-induced hypothyroidism is 53-85% and 36-46% in retrospective or prospective studies, respectively, and 18% in patients treated with sorafenib (Torino, Corsello et al. 2009). Mechanisms of hypothyroidism induced by TKIs include drug-induced atrophy of the thyroid through inhibition of its vascularization, drug-induced thyroiditis, reduced synthesis of thyroid hormones, progressive depletion of the thyroid's functional reserve and inhibition of the thyroidal iodine uptake (Torino, Corsello et al. 2009). Makita *et al* (Makita and Iiri 2013) and Bianchi *et al* (Bianchi, Rossi et al. 2013) thought that sunitinib may exert these effects via multiple receptor tyrosine kinases, including vascular endothelial growth factor receptor (VEGFR) and the platelet-derived growth factor receptor (PDGFR). In patients treated with sunitinib or sorafenib, routine thyroid function testing at baseline and measurement of TSH on day 1 at the start of every new treatment cycle is recommended. Levothyroxine is the standard treatment for overt hypothyroidism and is recommended in some patients with subclinical hypothyroidism; overt or subclinical hypothyroidism *per se* does not justify the withdrawal of TKI therapy. Thyroid function test should be included in routine toxicity assessment of TKIs under clinical evaluation (Torino, Corsello et al. 2009, Hamnvik, Larsen et al. 2011, Eisen, Sternberg et al. 2012); however, the clinical relevance of early diagnosis of hypothyroidism in patients with TKIs is still controversial.

6.3. Infections

Not only the IFN-α treatment but also hepatitis C infection itself has been reportedly associated with thyroid autoimmunity and hypothyroidism. Among possible mechanisms, the molecular mimicry between viral and selfantigens has been suggested, whereas the release of proinflammatory mediators caused by viral infection may lead to activation of autoreactive T-cells. Besides, in HT several other putative triggering viruses have been implicated such as parvovirus, rubella, herpes simplex virus, Epstein Barr virus, and human T-lymphotropic virus type 1. A recent study of sera in pregnant women has also indicated an association between a prior infection with Toxoplasma gondii and an increase of TPOAbs. Nevertheless, the evidences are scarce and further studies are required in order to confirm the role of infections as causative agents.

6.4. Chemicals

The exposure to environmental toxicants such as polyaromatic hydrocarbons or polyhalogenated biphenyls, both commonly used in a variety of industrial applications, has been shown to provoke thyroid autoimmunity not only in experimental animals but also in humans. Recently, a significantly higher prevalence of HT and TAb (9.3% and 17.6%, respectively) has been demonstrated in residents living in the area of petrochemical complex of Sao Paolo compared to the control area (3.9% and 10.3%, respectively). In Slovakia, the exposure to polychlorinated biphenyls was associated with TAb and hypothyroidism. Although there is strong evidence attesting the contribution of chemicals to thyroid autoimmunity, the exact mechanisms of their action are yet to be established (Langer, Tajtakova et al. 2007, de Freitas, Grimaldi Campos et al. 2010).

7. Hashimoto's thyroiditis and papillary thyroid carcinoma

There has long been a controversy in the literature about a possible link between HT and PTC. Conflicting reports continue to emerge. Some suggest a positive correlation between the two, and even a cause-and-effect relationship, whereby the activated inflammatory response present in HT creates a favorable setting for malignant transformation. The inflammatory response may cause DNA damage through formation of reactive oxygen species, resulting in mutations that eventually lead to the development of PTC. Nevertheless, it remains unclear whether: (1) HT predisposes patients to develop PTC, (2) HT is an incidental finding with concurrent PTC, or (3)HT is a part of the host tumor response system. A meta-analysis done by Jankovic (McLeod, Watters et al. 2012, Jankovic, Le et al. 2013) revealed significant differences in the prevalence and the risk ratio of PTC in HT specimens obtained via FNAB vs thyroidectomy.

In population based studies where the specimens were obtained from FNAB, the average prevalence of PTC in patients with HT was 1.20%, with an average risk ratio of 0.69. Conversely, in studies from archival thyroidectomy specimens, the average prevalence and risk ratio were as high as 27.56% and 1.59, respectively. This variability could be a result of different methods of obtaining specimens and heterogeneity in the population under investigation in terms of ethnic, geographic, and gender differences.

The prevalence and the risk ratio of PTC in patients with HT compared to those without HT are significantly higher in studies of thyroidectomy specimens, compared to studies of patients undergoing FNAB. In studies that mentioned the indications, thyroidectomy was reserved for patients not responding to thyroid suppression therapy, those with symptoms of compression, worrisome or inconclusive FNA cytology, and historic or physical findings warranting further workup and treatment (e.g., irradiation, nerve paralysis, pain, or cervical lymph node enlargement). It should be noted that the vast majority of patients with HT do not require surgery. Hence, the patients who require thyroidectomy are already at higher risk for malignancy compared to the general population with HT.

There have been a number of proposed hypotheses to explain the linkage between the two diseases. From a histological perspective, Tamimi (Tamimi 2002) assessed the prevalence and severity of thyroiditis among three types of surgically resected thyroid tumors and found a significantly higher rate of lymphocytic infiltrate in patients with PTC. However, PTC with concurrent HT is associated with female gender, young age, less aggressive disease such as small tumor size, less frequent capsular invasion and nodal metastasis, and better prognosis. Furthermore, these patients are also less likely to develop recurrence and have a higher survival rate In the study by Eisenberg et al(Eisenberg and Hensley 1989), none of the patients with a thyroid carcinoma and HT developed relapse or metastases after 74 months of follow-up. Kebebew (Kebebew, Treseler et al. 2001) demonstrated that CLT correlates with improved survival in patients with PTC but is not an independent prognostic factor. Boi et al investigated the relationship between thyroid autoimmunity and thyroid cancer in a series of FNAB of unselected and consecutive thyroid nodules. This study revealed that the positive predictive values for thyroid carcinoma in antithyroid antibody-positive and –negative nodules are not statistically significant for class III (indeterminate risk) and class IV (suspected malignancy) cytology. It should be noted that it is important to distinguish between diffuse vs focal lymphocytic infiltration around the tumor. In the studies that described the histological findings, HT was defined as diffuse lymphocytic infiltration, rather than peritumoral lymphocytic infiltration alone. The significance of this is that HT does not represent a reaction to tumor alone but is an independent chronic process. In chronic inflammation, there are reactive alterations of stroma brought on by injury from chemokines, cytokines, and growth factors that cause damage to stromal cells. This in turn may cause malignant transformation in epithelial cells, thereby resulting in tumor development. In contrast, the lymphocytic infiltrate of HT may be an immunological response with a cancer-retarding effect, contributing to a favorable outcome of PTC compared to other thyroid cancers. Moreover, the relatively high prevalence of PTC in autopsy series may represent host immune control. Interestingly, lymphocytic infiltration within or surrounding the tumor was found to correlate with the existence of CLT. This may explain the "protective" effect of CLT in PTC.

Another hypothesis for the causal relationship between HT and PTC is that elevated levels of TSH found in hypothyroid patients with HT stimulate follicular epithelial proliferation, thereby promoting the development of papillary carcinoma (Jankovic, Le et al. 2013). McLeod *et al* (McLeod, Watters et al. 2012) conducted a systemic review that included 5786 thyroid cancer cases in 43 032 subjects and found that serum TSH confers a greater likelihood of development of thyroid cancer (odds ratio 1.87–2.83, depending on the level of TSH). A subset of studies that was adjusted for autoimmune thyroiditis did not find this relationship between TSH and heightened odds ratio for thyroid cancer. Conversely, several authors identified a few biomolecular markers, including RET/PTC rearrangements, p63 protein, and loss of heterozygosity of hOGG1, that are potentially involved in neoplastic transformation from HT to PTC. So far, no causal genetic linkage has been confirmed.

In conclusion, the existing data provide inconsistent evidence favoring a causal relationship between HT and PTC. Population-based studies using FNAC show no significant increase of PTC in patients with HT, whereas surgical series using thyroidectomy show a heightened risk for coexistent PTC, possibly related to selection bias. Prospective studies involving a large number of subjects and long-term follow-up are needed to further elucidate the relationship. Several studies also suggest that HT appears to confer a better prognosis in patients with PTC, but more research is necessary to further investigate this. At the present time, there is no valid established criterion to identify those patients with HT at a higher risk of developing PTC. Careful observation and follow-up of HT patients is recommended, especially those with nodular variants.

8. Laboratory tests

Elevated anti-TPO or anti-Tg antibody titers are the most specific laboratory findings to establish the diagnosis of autoimmune thyroid disease (AITD) or HT, typically making biopsy unnecessary. The 24-hours thyroid radioactive iodine-123 or-131 (^{123}I or ^{131}I) uptake (RIU) is also helpful to distinguish Hashitoxicosis from Graves' disease (GD); the RIU is low in patients with Hashitoxicosis, whereas it is elevated in those with GD. ^{123}I is preferred than ^{131}I because it has a shorter half-life (13 hours for ^{123}I, 8 days for ^{131}I) allowing quicker dissipation of background radiation. Since radioactive iodine is secreted in breast milk, and ^{123}I has a short half-life, it is recommended for diagnostic thyroid studies in nursing mothers. Breast milk must be pumped and discarded for 2 days after the intake of ^{123}I either used for thyroid uptake or for thyroid scanning.

Scintigraphy reveals in-homogeneous activity throughout the gland in 50% and a pattern suggestive of either hot or cold nodules or a combination of both in 30% of patients. Twenty percent of patient with HT have normal findings at the scintigraphic thyroid imaging.

9. Clinical pictures

Clinical manifestations of HT are variable and commonly include diffuse or nodular goiter with euthyroidism, subclinical hypothyroidism which shows a combination of elevated serum TSH concentrations and normal free T4 and T3 concentrations and permanent hypothyroidism. Not often, HT causes acute destruction of thyroid tissue and release in blood of stored thyroid hormones, causing transient thyrotoxicosis. This condition has been termed "Hashitoxicosis" or "painless sporadic thyroiditis", or "painless postpartum thyroiditis" when occurs in women after delivery. In Hashitoxicosis serum TSH is suppressed, and total and free T3 and T4 are elevated. Also, serum T4 is proportionally higher than T3, reflecting the ratio of stored hormones in the thyroid gland, whereas in GD and in toxic nodular goiter, T3 is preferentially elevated. Rarely, a hypofunctioning gland in HT may become hyperfunctioning with the onset of coexistent GD. In patients with GD, HT is usually present concurrently.

10. Treatment

If overt hypothyroidism is present, the treatment of choice for HT is the administration of L-thyroxine (L-T4) in the usual replacement doses. We also use L-T4 to treat patients with HT subclinical hypothyroidism and high serum thyroid antibody concentrations, because in these cases a progression to overt hypothyroidism is common and hyperlipidemia and atherosclerotic heart disease may develop. L-T4 may mildly and indirectly suppress serum concentrations of autoantibodies due to decreased stimulation of thyroid tissue by TSH and causing reduction of antigenic production. The goal of treatment is to restore clinically and biochemically an euthyroid state. For that, free T4 levels must be within the reference range and TSH at the lower half of the reference range. The usual dose of L-T4 is 1.6-1.8 μg/kg per day and is patient dependent. Elderly patients usually require a smaller dose of L-T4, sometimes less than 1μg/kg per day. The initial dose and the optimal time needed to establish the full replacement dose as above should be individualised relative to age, weight and cardiac status.

In HT patients with a large goiter and normal or elevated serum TSH, we think, L-T4 may be given in doses sufficient to suppress serum TSH in an effort to shrink the thyroid theoretically, although randomized studies are needed to verify the long term safety of this method concerning the potential cardiovascular and skeletal side effects. Suppressive doses of L-T4 tend to shrink the goiter by average of 30% over 6 months. If the goiter does not regress, the L-T4 doses are lowered. Goiters that are hard and fibrotic do not respond to L-T4 treatment. If the thyroid gland is only minimally enlarged, the patient is euthyroid and TSH levels are normal, the patient should remain under medical supervision, since hypothyroidism may often develop years later. Also, patients should be informed about the importance of compliance with replacement treatment and instructed to report any symptoms suggesting hyperthyroidism that could be due to an overdosage of L-T4. The intake of L-T4 should be apart by at least 4 hours from other drugs like calcium carbonate, ferrous sulfate, cholestyramine, sucralfate, iron-containing multivitamins, antacids containing aluminum hydroxide, phenytoin sodium, carbamazepine and amiodarone HCL, all of which impair the absorption/metabolism of L-T4.

Selenium (Se) supplementation in patients with AITD, including HT, seems to modify the inflammatory and immune responses, probably by enhancing plasma glutathione peroxidase (GPX) and thioredoxin reductase (TR) activity and by decreasing toxic concentrations of hydrogen peroxide (H_2O_2) and lipid hydroperoxides, resulting from thyroid hormone synthesis. When Se intake is adequate the intracellular GPX and TR systems protect the

http://dx.doi.org/10.5772/57522

thyrocyte from these peroxides, considering that oxidative stress induces TR1 and GPX. The current recommended dietary intake of selenium in humans to achieve the maximal activity of GPX in plasma or in erythrocytes is between 55 and 75μg per day. It must be considered that organic forms of Se such as Se-methionine and yeast-bound Se, have a much lower toxicity and a much higher effectiveness and safety than inorganic Se like sodium selenate. Several studies have revealed a significant reduction of anti-TPO concentrations in patients with AITD treated with 200 μg Se per day for three, six, or nine months (Gartner, Gasnier et al. 2002, Duntas, Mantzou et al. 2003, Gartner and Gasnier 2003, Turker, Kumanlioglu et al. 2006, Mazokopakis and Chatzipavlidou 2007). Duntas et al. found an overall decrease of 46% of AITD at 3 months ($P<0.0001$) and of 55.5% at 6 months ($P<0.05$) of treatment with L-seleno-methionine plus L-T4. Others found a decrease of 26.2% at 3 months ($P<0.001$) and an additional 23.7% at 6 months ($P<0.01$) after L-Se-methionine treatment. A significant decrease in the mean serum anti-TPO levels was also noted after the daily intake of 200 μg sodium selenite for 3 months. This decrease amounted to 36.4% in the selenium-taking group of patients versus 12% in the control group ($P=0.013$) (Gartner, Gasnier et al. 2002). A recent study in 80 Greek women with HT showed a significant reduction of serum anti-TPO levels during the first 6 months of L-Se-methionine treatment ($P<0.0001$). Anti-TPO decreased by 5.6% and by 9.9% after 3 and 6 months of L-Se-methionine treatment, respectively. The extension of L-Se-methionine supplementation for 6 more months resulted in an additional 8% decrease, while cessation of treatment resulted to a 4.8% increase, in the anti-TPO concentrations.

A systematic review and meta-analysis done by Toulis (Toulis, Anastasilakis et al. 2010) provided evidence that selenomethionine at a dose of 200 mg once per day is effective in reducing TPOAb titers in patients with HT after a 3-month period, compared with placebo. In absolute numbers, this reduction equals ~300 IU/mL. Efficacy of Se supplementation for >3 months could not be supported, because of lack of evidence from randomized, placebo controlled trials. Patients assigned to Se supplementation had also a threefold higher chance of reporting an improvement in well-being and/or mood, compared with controls. No serious adverse effects were recorded after Se supplementation, with the exception of a limited number of gastric discomfort complaints associated with selenomethionine use. In general, there are no data demonstrating that Se treatment had any impact on the natural course of the disease.

Further controlled and extensive studies are needed to clarify the exact mechanisms by which Se exerts effects on anti-TPO production, and investigate the long-term clinical effects of Se treatment.

In a study involving 21 patients with HT and subclinical hypothyroidism, simvastatin in a daily dose of 20 mg orally for a period of eight weeks improved thyroid function inducing an increase in serum free T3 and free T4 levels and a decrease in TSH levels. Decreases in anti-TPO and anti-Tg antibodies were not statistically significant, possibly by stimulating apoptosis of certain types of lymphocytes. Further controlled and extensive studies are needed to investigate the effectiveness of statins treatment on the course of HT.

Patients with Hashitoxicosis may have only mild thyrotoxicosis and may not require treatment. Antithyroid drug treatment with thiourea drugs is contraindicated, because there is no excess of thyroid hormone production. Patients who have more symptoms should have a 24-

hours thyroid RIU test and a radioiodine scan to determine whether GD may be present and may be treated with beta-blockers. In symptomatically thyrotoxic patients with low thyroid ^{123}I uptake test, propranolol treatment is continued and sodium ipodate or iopanoic acid may also be given in doses of 500 mg daily orally, until the patient is euthyroid. Sodium ipodate and iopanoic acid are known iodinated contrast oral cholecystographic agents that inhibit peripheral 5′-monodeiodination of thyroxine, thereby blocking its conversion to active T_3. Patients having low thyroid RIU do not respond to thiourea medication.

Patients with HT and a large goiter with pressure symptoms such as dysphagia, voice hoarseness, stridor and respiratory distress, may require surgical care. Also, in HT the presence of a malignant nodule or of a thyroid lymphoma diagnosed by histology after a fine-needle aspiration is an absolute indication for thyroidectomy.

Author details

Tao Yang* and Xiaoyun Liu

*Address all correspondence to: yangt@njmu.edu.cn

Department of Endocrinology & Metabolism The First Affiliated Hospital of Nanjing Medical University, China

References

[1] Badenhoop, K., et al. (1990). "Susceptibility to thyroid autoimmune disease: molecular analysis of HLA-D region genes identifies new markers for goitrous Hashimoto's thyroiditis." *J Clin Endocrinol Metab* 71(5): 1131-1137.

[2] Ban, Y., et al. (2010). "Association of the protein tyrosine phosphatase nonreceptor 22 haplotypes with autoimmune thyroid disease in the Japanese population." *Thyroid* 20(8): 893-899.

[3] Ban, Y., et al. (2005). "The codon 620 single nucleotide polymorphism of the protein tyrosine phosphatase-22 gene does not contribute to autoimmune thyroid disease susceptibility in the Japanese." *Thyroid* 15(10): 1115-1118.

[4] Barbesino, G. (2010). "Drugs affecting thyroid function." *Thyroid* 20(7): 763-770.

[5] Bianchi, L., et al. (2013). "Thyroid dysfunction and tyrosine kinase inhibitors in renal cell carcinoma." *Endocr Relat Cancer* 20(5): R233-245.

[6] Bogner, U., et al. (1992). "HLA-DR/DQ gene variation in nongoitrous autoimmune thyroiditis at the serological and molecular level." *Autoimmunity* 14(2): 155-158.

[7] Caturegli, P., et al. (2013). "Hashimoto's thyroiditis: celebrating the centennial through the lens of the Johns Hopkins hospital surgical pathology records." *Thyroid* 23(2): 142-150.

[8] Chabchoub, G., et al. (2009). "The R620W polymorphism of the protein tyrosine phosphatase 22 gene in autoimmune thyroid diseases and rheumatoid arthritis in the Tunisian population." *Ann Hum Biol* 36(3): 342-349.

[9] de Freitas, C. U., et al. (2010). "Can living in the surroundings of a petrochemical complex be a risk factor for autoimmune thyroid disease?" *Environ Res* 110(1): 112-117.

[10] Dultz, G., et al. (2009). "The protein tyrosine phosphatase non-receptor type 22 C1858T polymorphism is a joint susceptibility locus for immunthyroiditis and autoimmune diabetes." *Thyroid* 19(2): 143-148.

[11] Duntas, L. H., et al. (2003). "Effects of a six month treatment with selenomethionine in patients with autoimmune thyroiditis." *Eur J Endocrinol* 148(4): 389-393.

[12] Eisen, T., et al. (2012). "Targeted therapies for renal cell carcinoma: review of adverse event management strategies." *J Natl Cancer Inst* 104(2): 93-113.

[13] Eisenberg, B. L. and S. D. Hensley (1989). "Thyroid cancer with coexistent Hashimoto's thyroiditis. Clinical assessment and management." *Arch Surg* 124(9): 1045-1047.

[14] Fountoulakis, S., et al. (2007). "The role of iodine in the evolution of thyroid disease in Greece: from endemic goiter to thyroid autoimmunity." *Hormones (Athens)* 6(1): 25-35.

[15] Gartner, R. and B. C. Gasnier (2003). "Selenium in the treatment of autoimmune thyroiditis." *Biofactors* 19(3-4): 165-170.

[16] Gartner, R., et al. (2002). "Selenium supplementation in patients with autoimmune thyroiditis decreases thyroid peroxidase antibodies concentrations." *J Clin Endocrinol Metab* 87(4): 1687-1691.

[17] Golkowski, F., et al. (2007). "Increased prevalence of hyperthyroidism as an early and transient side-effect of implementing iodine prophylaxis." *Public Health Nutr* 10(8): 799-802.

[18] Hamnvik, O. P., et al. (2011). "Thyroid dysfunction from antineoplastic agents." *J Natl Cancer Inst* 103(21): 1572-1587.

[19] Hawkins, B. R., et al. (1987). "Strong association between HLA DRw9 and Hashimoto's thyroiditis in southern Chinese." *Acta Endocrinol (Copenh)* 114(4): 543-546.

[20] Heydarian, P., et al. (2007). "Goiter rate, serum thyrotropin, thyroid autoantibodies and urinary iodine concentration in Tehranian adults before and after national salt iodization." *J Endocrinol Invest* 30(5): 404-410.

[21] Honda, K., et al. (1989). "Hashimoto's thyroiditis and HLA in Japanese." *J Clin Endocrinol Metab* 69(6): 1268-1273.

[22] Hunt, P. J., et al. (2001). "Histocompatibility leucocyte antigens and closely linked immunomodulatory genes in autoimmune thyroid disease." *Clin Endocrinol (Oxf)* 55(4): 491-499.

[23] Jacobson, E. M., et al. (2008). "The HLA gene complex in thyroid autoimmunity: from epidemiology to etiology." *J Autoimmun* 30(1-2): 58-62.

[24] Jankovic, B., et al. (2013). "Clinical Review: Hashimoto's thyroiditis and papillary thyroid carcinoma: is there a correlation?" *J Clin Endocrinol Metab* 98(2): 474-482.

[25] Joensuu, H., et al. (2011). "Practical management of tyrosine kinase inhibitor-associated side effects in GIST." *Cancer Treat Rev* 37(1): 75-88.

[26] Kahaly, G. J., et al. (1998). "Iodide induces thyroid autoimmunity in patients with endemic goitre: a randomised, double-blind, placebo-controlled trial." *Eur J Endocrinol* 139(3): 290-297.

[27] Kahles, H., et al. (2005). "Sex-specific association of PTPN22 1858T with type 1 diabetes but not with Hashimoto's thyroiditis or Addison's disease in the German population." *Eur J Endocrinol* 153(6): 895-899.

[28] Kebebew, E., et al. (2001). "Coexisting chronic lymphocytic thyroiditis and papillary thyroid cancer revisited." *World J Surg* 25(5): 632-637.

[29] Kollmannsberger, C., et al. (2011). "Sunitinib in metastatic renal cell carcinoma: recommendations for management of noncardiovascular toxicities." *Oncologist* 16(5): 543-553.

[30] Kordonouri, O., et al. (2010). "PTPN22 1858T allele is associated with younger age at onset of type 1 diabetes and is not related to subsequent thyroid autoimmunity." *Hum Immunol* 71(7): 731-732.

[31] Langer, P., et al. (2007). "Thyroid ultrasound volume, structure and function after long-term high exposure of large population to polychlorinated biphenyls, pesticides and dioxin." *Chemosphere* 69(1): 118-127.

[32] Makita, N. and T. Iiri (2013). "Tyrosine kinase inhibitor-induced thyroid disorders: a review and hypothesis." *Thyroid* 23(2): 151-159.

[33] Mazokopakis, E. E. and V. Chatzipavlidou (2007). "Hashimoto's thyroiditis and the role of selenium. Current concepts." *Hell J Nucl Med* 10(1): 6-8.

[34] McLeod, D. S., et al. (2012). "Thyrotropin and thyroid cancer diagnosis: a systematic review and dose-response meta-analysis." *J Clin Endocrinol Metab* 97(8): 2682-2692.

[35] Mendez-Vidal, M. J., et al. (2012). "Management of adverse events of targeted therapies in normal and special patients with metastatic renal cell carcinoma." *Cancer Metastasis Rev* 31 Suppl 1: S19-27.

[36] Muriel, C., et al. (2010). "Impact of the incorporation of tyrosine kinase inhibitor agents on the treatment of patients with a diagnosis of advanced renal cell carcinoma: study based on experience at the Hospital Universitario Central de Asturias." *Clin Transl Oncol* 12(8): 562-567.

[37] Petrone, A., et al. (2001). "Association of DRB1*04-DQB1*0301 haplotype and lack of association of two polymorphic sites at CTLA-4 gene with Hashimoto's thyroiditis in an Italian population." *Thyroid* 11(2): 171-175.

[38] Rose, N. R., et al. (2002). "Iodine: an environmental trigger of thyroiditis." *Autoimmun Rev* 1(1-2): 97-103.

[39] Tamimi, D. M. (2002). "The association between chronic lymphocytic thyroiditis and thyroid tumors." *Int J Surg Pathol* 10(2): 141-146.

[40] Tandon, N., et al. (1991). "HLA associations with Hashimoto's thyroiditis." *Clin Endocrinol (Oxf)* 34(5): 383-386.

[41] Torino, F., et al. (2009). "Hypothyroidism related to tyrosine kinase inhibitors: an emerging toxic effect of targeted therapy." *Nat Rev Clin Oncol* 6(4): 219-228.

[42] Toulis, K. A., et al. (2010). "Selenium supplementation in the treatment of Hashimoto's thyroiditis: a systematic review and a meta-analysis." *Thyroid* 20(10): 1163-1173.

[43] Turker, O., et al. (2006). "Selenium treatment in autoimmune thyroiditis: 9-month follow-up with variable doses." *J Endocrinol* 190(1): 151-156.

[44] Wan, X. L., et al. (1995). "HLA-A and -DRB4 genes in controlling the susceptibility to Hashimoto's thyroiditis." *Hum Immunol* 42(2): 131-136.

[45] Zaletel, K. and S. Gaberscek (2011). "Hashimoto's Thyroiditis: From Genes to the Disease." *Curr Genomics* 12(8): 576-588.

[46] Zygulska, A. L., et al. (2012). "Hypothyroidism during treatment with tyrosine kinase inhibitors." Endokrynol Pol 63(4): 302-306.

Section 2

Multinodular Goiter

Chapter 2

A Review of the Pathogenesis and Management of Multinodular Goiter

Shi Lam and Brian Hung-Hin Lang

Additional information is available at the end of the chapter

http://dx.doi.org/10.5772/57547

1. Introduction

1.1. Definition and gross pathology

Multinodular goiter (MNG) is a clinicopathological entity characterized by an increased volume of the thyroid gland with formation of nodules. Goiter is defined as a thyroid gland weighing over 20-25g or with a volume of over 19ml in women and 25ml in men. [1-2] Gross examination of a MNG specimen with full-blown features would reveal a heterogeneous formation of solid and cystic nodules. A solid nodule can be adenoma, as defined by possession of a well-formed capsule, or more commonly a hyperplastic nodule, which lacks a complete encapsulation. Cystic lesions can be colloid cysts or hemorrhagic cyst from a degenerated nodule. Lymphocytic infiltration and fibrous deposition among the follicular parenchyma is a common microscopic observation seen in about 10% of cases. [3, 4]

2. Epidemiology

MNG is endemic in regions with low iodine level in the soil, such as countries in the mountainous areas in South-East Asia, Latin America and Central Africa. The World Health Organization reported a worldwide iodine deficiency rate of 9. 8 – 56. 9% and total goiter prevalence of 4. 7 – 37. 3% by year 2003. [5] The Whickham study conducted in the 1970s found 15. 5% of participants had a palpable goiter with a female to male ratio of 4. 5 to 1. [6] In the iodine-deficient Danish population, the goiter prevalence is 9. 8 – 14. 6%. [7] And in the iodine sufficient areas of Framingham, Massachusetts and Connecticut, the goiter prevalence is 1 – 2%. [8-10] By ultrasound screening, the prevalence of nodular goiter worldwide ranges between 15 – 22. 6%. [11] Thyroid nodules are more commonly diagnosed in women, with incidence increasing with age and plateauing by the age of 60. Other risk factors for developing thyroid nodules and increased thyroid volume include number of childbirths, smoking and increased body mass index. [12-13]

3. Pathogenesis

The pathogenesis of MNG encompasses processes of diffuse follicular hyperplasia, focal nodular proliferation and eventual acquisition of functional automaticity. The development of MNG is a result of long-term exposure of the thyroid gland to proliferative stimuli, such as iodine deficiency, goitrogens and inborn error of thyroid hormone synthesis. All of the above results in insufficient thyroid hormone production and stimulate pituitary secretion of thyroid stimulating hormone (TSH).

TSH is a glycoprotein with stimulatory effect on the trophic and iodine metabolism pathway in the thyroid follicular cells. TSH binding to the cell membrane G protein-coupled receptor activates the cAMP and phospholipase C signalling pathways, which in turn upregulates the process of iodine uptake and organification, thyroglobulin synthesis, iodotyrosine coupling and iodothyronine (T3, T4) secretion, leading to a short-term response in thyroid hormone production. [14] In the long-term, TSH also stimulates proliferation of follicular cells to increase the functional mass of thyroid gland. Clinically, TSH stimulation results in enlargement of thyroid gland, increased radio-iodine uptake and increased T4 and T3 levels. (Figure 1)

Nodule formation is postulated to be the result of both an inherent and acquired heterogeneity in proliferative and functional upregulation of the follicular cells. The thyroid follicular cells are inherently heterogeneous with regard to thyroid hormone production and proliferation in response to TSH stimulation, such that under intermediate level of stimulation, a subpopulation of follicular cells outgrows other cells and expand into macroscopic nodules. [15] On the other hand, follicular cells acquiring activating somatic mutations in the cell proliferation pathways can expand clonally to form a nodule. About 60 – 70% of nodules form by the later mechanism and are monoclonal in origin. Somatic mutations leading to constitutive activation of TSH receptors are found in about 60% of autonomously functioning nodules. The remaining 40% of functioning nodules are TSH receptor mutation negative with poorly understood genetic mechanism behind.

An adenoma with reduced iodine uptake is scintigraphically detected as a "cold nodule". A defective iodine transport (membrane expression of sodium / iodine symporter protein) and iodine organification is implicated in the hypofunctionality. However, the molecular event accounting for the proliferative advantage is yet to be identified. [16] Unlike thyroid carcinomas, which also manifest as cold nodules in scintigraphy, *BRAF* and *ras* mutation are uncommon in benign cold adenoma. [17, 18] Recently, oestrogen was shown to stimulate growth of thyroid progenitor cells while simultaneously inhibiting the expression of sodium / iodine symporter mRNA, providing a possible explanation of growth / function dissociation in cold thyroid adenomas. [19]

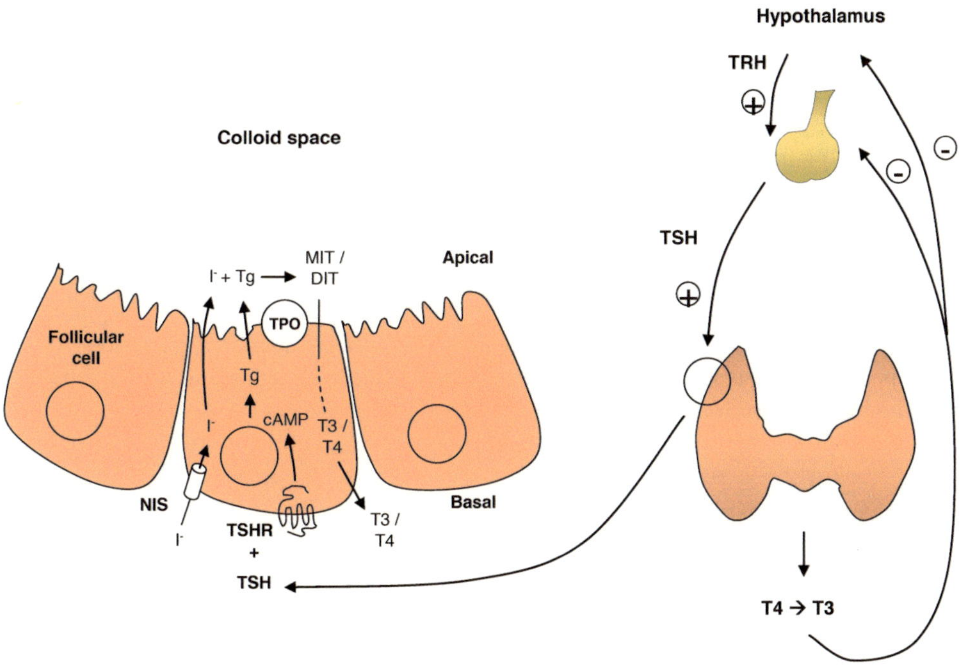

Figure 1. Regulation of thyroid hormone production

Although the majority of thyroid nodules are benign, about 5-10% of nodules may harbour a cancerous focus. In addition, it is known that about 6% of goiter patients eventually develop thyroid cancer, especially from MNG to thyroid cancer, suggesting a possible progression from benign thyroid lesions to malignant disease. [20] More recently, one group has identified a germline missense mutation (1016C>T) in TITF-1/NKX2. 1 encoding a mutant TTF-1 protein (A339V), which may contribute to predisposition for MNG patients to papillary thyroid carcinoma (PTC), further highlighting a causal link between these two diseases. [21] Ectopic expression of the A339V mutant protein in a normal rat thyroid PCCL3 cell line results in a significant up-regulation of cellular proliferation of these thyroid cells and promotes their TSH-independent growth, which was in part attributed to activated Stat3 survival signal in these cells.

4. Natural history

The natural history of MNG is nodular growth and acquisition of autonomy. Yet not all patients with nodular goiter will progress to develop compressive or thyrotoxic complications that indicates treatment intervention. The reported incidence rate of nodule growth is 39% of patients over a period of 5 years in the North America, 2 – 56% of patients over 2 – 5 years in European countries and 21% over 11 years in Japan. Nodule with cystic component is less likely to grow than solid nodules. Patient's age, gender or nodule size and function at presentation did not predict subsequent growth of nodules. Based on cross-sectional studies, the age-related increase in thyroid volume in patients with MNG is 4. 5% per year. [16, 22]

Functional autonomy develops in long-standing MNGs. Thyroid autonomy in euthyroid nodular goiters, as determined by presence of TSH suppression by thyrotropin releasing hormone (TRH) stimulation tests and failure of T3 suppression of radio-iodine uptake, was shown to precede development of biochemical and overt hyperthyroidism. Up to 40% of euthyroid goiters harbour areas of autonomy.

Transition to overt hyperthyroidism in euthyroid MNGs occurs at an incidence rate of 9 – 10% over a period of 7 – 12 years. Development of hyperthyroidism is more likely in patients with autonomously functioning nodules of larger than 3cm and an autonomous goiter volume of 16ml. Hyperthyroidism can be induced by exposing an autonomous gland to excessive iodine, such as the iodine-containing amiodarone. [23–25]

5. Clinical evaluation & investigation

Clinical evaluation of MNG aims at establishing diagnosis and clinical stage of disease, stratifying risk of occurrence of malignancy, identifying indications for thyroid ablation and addressing patient's concern.

Diagnosis of MNG is usually straight forward with the readily evaluable location of the thyroid gland. Clinically inconspicuous MNG are usually documented by imaging studies covering the neck and thoracic inlet performed for unrelated indications. MNGs with predominant retrosternal component are difficult to diagnose with patients undergoing prolonged investigations for symptoms of exertional or recumbent dyspnoea that mimic asthma, congestive heart failure or obstructive sleep apnoea. The tell-tail clue leading to thoracic inlet imaging and diagnosis of retrosternal goiter is frequently a flow-volume loop spirometry suggesting extra-thoracic airway obstruction or chest X-ray showing a mediastinal shadow causing tracheal deviation. Symptoms arising from airway irritation, compression and dragging by the goiter should be noted and addressed in patient counselling for treatment indications. Physical findings of nodule consistency and mobility, cervical lymphadenopathy, tracheal deviation, retromanubrial extension, thoracic outlet obstruction and thyrotoxicosis are determined. When thyrotoxicosis is suspected, the differential diagnosis of Grave's disease with nodules should be considered and the signs specific to Grave's disease, including ophthalmopathy and pre-tibial myxoedema be documented.

Serum thyroid stimulating hormone and free serum thyroxine levels are measured to determine the functioning status of the nodular goiter. A suppressed TSH level is commonly found in long-standing MNGs in which functional autonomy has developed. Hypothyroidism, on the other hand, may suggest Hashimoto thyroiditis and measurement of anti-thyroperoxidase antibody titre helps to confirm the diagnosis.

Thyroid scintigraphy using iodine-123 or technetium-99m is recommended for patients with suppressed serum TSH level to determine the relative iodine uptake of a nodule in contrast to its adjacent thyroid tissue. A hyperfunctioning nodule that can account for the thyrotoxicosis carries low risk of malignancy and further investigation is not required. An index nodule that is iso-or hypofunctional against the rest of thyroid gland has a reported malignancy risk of 3% to 15% and should be investigated with fine needle aspiration cytology (FNAC). [26-29]

Evaluating for risk of malignancy in MNG follows the same approach as in solitary thyroid nodules. Demographical risk factors include age of < 20 or > 60 years, male gender, history of head and neck irradiation, history of multiple endocrine neoplasia or family history of thyroid cancer. Suspicious symptoms include progressive enlargement, recent onset of voice change, airway irritation and compression. Objective physical findings of hard and fixed nodule, size > 4cm, cervical lymphadenopathy and vocal cord paralysis all points to features of local-regional invasion and prompts investigation for definitive diagnosis. If the rarer entity of medullary carcinoma is suspected from a positive family history or features of multiple endocrine neoplasia (type 2), spot serum calcitonin level should be measured as a screening test. A 33% risk of malignancy is reported in avid nodules detected by fluorodeoxyglucose positron emission tomography (^{18}FDG-PET), so such nodules should also undergo cytological evaluation. [30]

Use of ultrasound as routine clinical examination has compensated for the lack of sensitivity and precision of neck palpation alone in determining the number and size of nodules. Fifty percent of patients with single palpable thyroid nodule will demonstrate additional nodules when ultrasound exam is performed. More importantly, nodules with high risk features of malignancy, including irregular margin, lack of circumferential halo, heterogenous echogenecity, increased vascularity and presence of microcalcification, can be selected for cytological sampling.

FNAC is an accurate, safe, simple, and cost-effective investigation in the evaluation of nodular goiter. Diagnostic performance of FNAC is enhanced by ultrasound guidance in the identification of nodules with high risk features for aspiration. In complex cystic lesions, ultrasound guidance also allows positioning of needle to the solid component while avoiding acellular cystic area. Availability of pre-operative diagnostic information has increased diagnostic yield of thyroidectomies while reducing the number of surgeries performed for suspected malignancy by 35 – 75%. [31–33]

A review of diagnostic performance of FNAC reported a sensitivity of 65 – 98% and specificity of 72 – 100% for the detection of thyroid carcinoma. In general, the relative frequencies of FNAC findings in thyroid nodules are benign in 69%, suspicious 10%, malignant 4% and non-diagnostic in 17%. [34] In the "non-diagnostic" category, repeating FNA under ultrasound guidance will produce satisfactory specimen in 50% of the cases. The risk of malignancy in nodules with non-diagnostic cytology is 2 – 9%, and such lesions should be closely monitored or excised for histological evaluation. The category of "suspicious" cytology includes findings of follicular and Hurthle cell neoplasm. Differentiation between adenoma and carcinoma cannot be made because histological evidence of capsular or vascular invasion cannot be obtained from cytological examination. In patients referred for surgery for suspicious cytology, 20 – 30% are proven to have carcinoma on final pathology. [35-36] Molecular markers upregulated in thyroid carcinomas are being evaluated for their diagnostic value. Detection of protein markers (Galectin-3, HBME-1, cytokeratin-19, telomerase) by immunocytochemistry, gene mutations (BRAF, RAS, RET/PTC rearrangement, PAX8-PPARγ) by polymerase chain reaction (PCR), microRNAs by reverse transcriptase PCR, or multi-gene assays. [37] Yet a test with sufficient sensitivity that allows exclusion of malignancy in an indeterminate cytological category is still awaited. [38]

6. Treatment of MNG

MNG is benign disease with slow progression and at different stage of its natural history presents with different clinical problems. The clinical problem at earlier stage of disease before gross enlargement of the thyroid gland is usually a concerning dominant nodule, while later in the course patients tends to present with the mass effect of a voluminous goiter or hyperthyroidism. The indications of treatment include suspected or confirmed malignancy, thyrotoxicosis, goiters giving rise to compressive, irritative symptoms or cosmetic concern. Only the management of benign non-toxic MNG is discussed in the following text.

Asymptomatic non-toxic MNG with malignancy being ruled-out should be observed clinically or with ultrasound surveillance for nodule growth. TSH suppression by levothyroxine was shown to prevent increase in nodule size but nodule growth resumed after cessation of therapy. Long-term TSH suppression with levothyroxine is not recommended because of the increased risk of cardiac arrhythmia and osteoporosis associated with chronic subclinical hyperthyroidism. [39-40]

Evidence of significant mass effect of a nodular goiter, including symptoms of recumbent or exertional dyspnoea and signs of tracheal deviation and thoracic inlet obstruction, prompts amelioration by radio-iodine or surgery.

^{131}I radio-iodine is effective in reducing volume of euthyroid MNG with a response rate of 80%. Volume reductions at 1 to 3 years are up to 40 – 60% respectively, with half of volume reduction occurring within 3 months of treatment. The efficacy of radio-iodine is proportional to the absorbed radiation dose, which in turn depends on the goiter volume and functioning status. Therefore, in goiters with less than 20% radioactive iodine uptake, conventional ^{131}iodine therapy is not recommended as an unacceptably high dose of radioactivity would be required to achieve satisfactory goiter volume reduction. Pre-treatment with rhTSH before ^{131}iodine administration can stimulate radioactive iodine uptake and was shown by randomized controlled trials to increase goiter volume reduction by 35 – 56%. rhTSH-augmentation may therefore extend the application of ^{131}iodine therapy in euthyroid multinodular goiters by reducing the radioactive dose requirement, especially in goiters with low radioactive iodine intake. [41] Adverse effects of radio-iodine include radiation thyroiditis in 3%, transient thyrotoxicosis in 5% and later hypothyroidism in 22 – 58% in 5 – 8 years after therapy. For large goiters, radio-iodine is probably an inferior option due to incomplete volume reduction, requirement of higher radiation dose and, transient post-treatment increase in thyroid volume leading to risk of airway compression.

Surgery provides instantaneous relief of pressure effects and cosmetic concern of MNG. Subtotal thyroidectomy carries low risk of recurrent laryngeal nerve injury and hypoparathyroidism but results in a recurrence rate up to 40% in the long term. Total thyroidectomy can achieve a negligible recurrence rate [42] and carries low complication rate in specialized centers, with < 1% risk of permanent recurrent laryngeal nerve injury or hypoparathyroidism, even in the elderly population where massive goiters are more common. [43] Due to the loss of normal tissue plane and anatomical relationship between the thyroid tissue, recurrent laryngeal nerve and parathyroid glands, reoperating on a previously explored surgical field carries a 3-to 10-fold increase in risk of permanent recurrent laryngeal nerve damage or hypoparathyroidism, rendering sub-total thyroidectomy the less preferred option. [44] Total thyroidectomy has an added advantage in case of incidentally diagnosed thyroid carcinoma, which is diagnosed in about 10% of MNG specimens [45], that completion thyroidectomy is avoided. Other forms of thyroid resection, namely hemithyroidectomy or hemithyroidectomy with contralateral subtotal resection (Dunhill's operation) may have merits in the management of selected patient group, such as those with predominantly unilateral disease and without pre-operative suspicion of malignancy. Hemithyroidectomy has the advantage of preserving thyroid function in 65 – 88% of cases and avoiding life-long thyroxine replacement. [46-47] A summary of management of MNG is schematically presented in Figure 2.

TRH, thyrotropin releasing hormone; TSH, thyroid stimulating hormone; Tg, thyroglobulin; NIS, sodium-iodine symporter; TPO, thyroperoxidase; DIT, di-iodotyrosine; MIT, monoiodotyrosine.

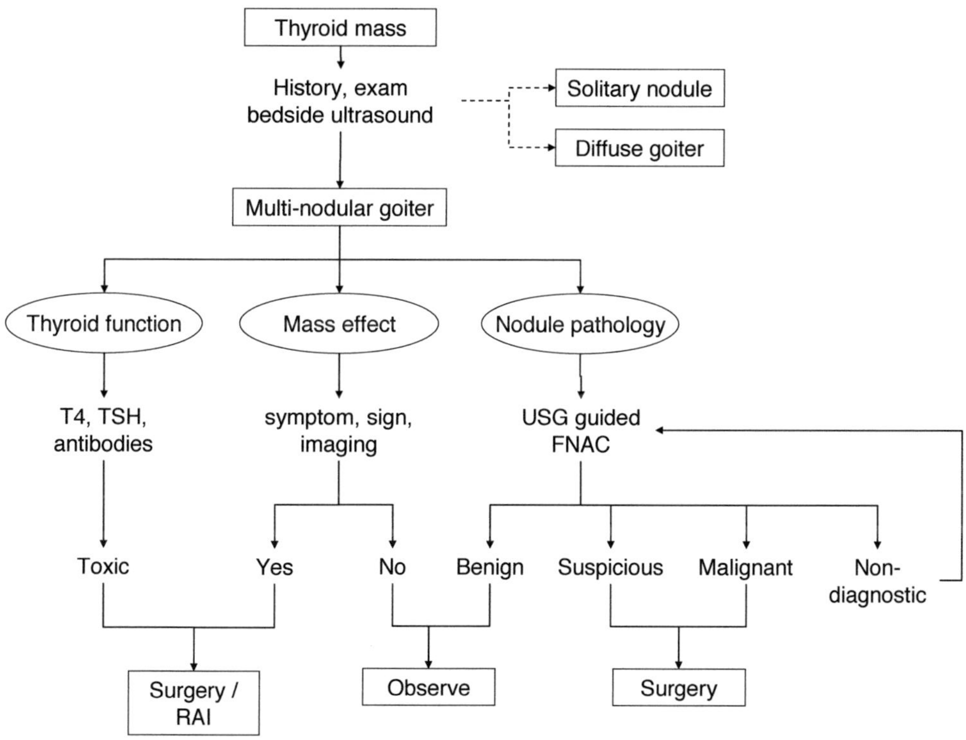

Figure 2. Management of a multinodular goiter (MNG)

Author details

Shi Lam and Brian Hung-Hin Lang*

*Address all correspondence to: blang@hku.hk

Department of Surgery, The University of Hong Kong, Hong Kong SAR, China

References

[1] Teng W, Shan Z, Teng X, Guan H. Effect of iodine intake on thyroid diseases in China. N Engl J Med. 2006 Jun 29;354(26):2783-93.

[2] Langer P. Discussion about the limit between normal thyroid and goiter: minireview. Endocrine regulations 1999

[3] Ramelli F, Studer H, Bruggisser D. Pathogenesis of thyroid nodules in multinodular goiter. Am J Pathol. 1982 Nov;109(2):215-23.

[4] De Smet MP. Pathological anatomy of endemic goitre. Monogr Ser World Health Organ. 1960;44:315-49.

[5] WHO, Iodine Status Worldwide, WHO Global Database on Iodine Deficiency, World Health Organization Department of Nutrition for Health and Development, Geneva, Switzerland, 2004.

[6] TunbridgeWM,Evered DC, Hall R, Appleton D, Brewis M, Clark F, Evans JG, Young E, Bird T, Smith PA The spectrum of thyroid disease in a community: the Whickham survey. Clin Endocrinol (Oxf) 1977; 7:481–493

[7] Knudsen N, Perrild H, Christiansen E, Rasmussen S, Dige-Petersen H, Jørgensen T. Thyroid structure and size and two-year follow-up of solitary cold thyroid nodules in an unselected population with borderline iodine deficiency. Eur J Endocrinol 2000; 142:224–230

[8] Vander JB, Gaston EA, Dawber TR. Significance of solitary nontoxic thyroid nodules. Preliminary report. N Engl J Med 1954; 251:970

[9] Baldwin DB, Rowett D. Incidence of thyroid disorders in Connecticut. JAMA 1978; 239:742–744

[10] Vander JB, Gaston EA, Dawber TR. The significance of nontoxic thyroid nodules. Final report of a 15-year study of the incidence of thyroid malignancy. Ann Intern Med 1968; 69:537–540

[11] Wang C, Crapo LM. The epidemiology of thyroid disease and implications for screening. Endocrinol Metab Clin North Am 1997; 26: 189–218

[12] Laurberg P, Jørgensen T, Perrild H, Ovesen L, Knudsen N, Pedersen IB, Rasmussen LB, Carlé A, Vejbjerg P. The Danish investigation on iodine intake and thyroid disease, DanThyr: status and perspectives. Eur J Endocrinol. 2006 Aug;155(2):219-28.

[13] Guth S, Theune U, Aberle J, Galach A, Bamberger CM. Very high prevalence of thyroid nodules detected by high frequency (13 MHz) ultrasound examination. Eur J Clin Invest. 2009 Aug;39(8):699-706.

[14] Szkudlinski MW, Fremont V, Ronin C, Weintraub BD. Thyroid-stimulating hormone and thyroid-stimulating hormone receptor structure-function relationships. Physiol Rev. 2002 Apr;82(2):473-502.

[15] Studer H, Peter HJ, Gerber H. Natural heterogeneity of thyroid cells: the basis for understanding thyroid function and nodular goiter growth. Endocr Rev. 1989 May; 10(2):125-35.

[16] Paschke R. Molecular pathogenesis of nodular goiter. Langenbecks Arch Surg. 2011 Dec;396(8):1127-36.

[17] Krohn K, Reske A, Ackermann F, Müller A, Paschke R. Ras mutations are rare in solitary cold and toxic thyroid nodules. Clin Endocrinol. 2001 Aug;55(2):241-8.

[18] Krohn K, Paschke R. BRAF mutations are not an alternative explanation for the molecular etiology of ras-mutation negative cold thyroid nodules. Thyroid. 2004 May; 14(5):359-61.

[19] Xu S, Chen G, Peng W, Renko K, Derwahl M. Oestrogen action on thyroid progenitor cells: relevant for the pathogenesis of thyroid nodules? J Endocrinol. 2013 Jun 1;218(1):125-33

[20] Arora N, Scognamiglio T, Zhu B, Fahey TJ 3rd. Do benign thyroid nodules have malignant potential? An evidence-based review. World J Surg. 2008 Jul;32(7):1237-46.

[21] Ngan ES, Lang BH, Liu T, Shum CK, So MT, Lau DK, Leon TY, Cherny SS, Tsai SY, Lo CY, Khoo US, Tam PK, Garcia-Barceló MM. A germline mutation (A339V) in thyroid transcription factor-1 (TITF-1/NKX2. 1) in patients with multinodular goiter and papillary thyroid carcinoma. J Natl Cancer Inst. 2009 Feb 4;101(3):162-75.

[22] Berghout A, Wiersinga WM, Smits NJ, Touber JL. Interrelationships between age, thyroid volume, thyroid nodularity, and thyroid function in patients with sporadic nontoxic goiter. Am J Med. 1990 Nov;89(5):602-8.

[23] Bähre M, Hilgers R, Lindemann C, Emrich D. Thyroid autonomy: sensitive detection in vivo and estimation of its functional relevance using quantified high-resolution scintigraphy. Acta Endocrinol (Copenh). 1988 Feb;117(2):145-53.

[24] Elte JW, Bussemaker JK, Haak A. The natural history of euthyroid multinodular goitre. Postgrad Med J. 1990 Mar;66(773):186-90.

[25] Wiener JD, de Vries AA. On the natural history of Plummer's disease. Clin Nucl Med. 1979 May;4(5):181-90.

[26] Campbell JP, Pillsbury HC 3rd. Management of the thyroid nodule. Head Neck. 1989;11:414-425.

[27] Gharib H, Goellner JR. Fine-needle aspiration biopsy of the thyroid: An appraisal. Ann Intern Med. 1993;118:282-289.

[28] La Rosa GL, Belfiore A, Giuffrida D, et al. Evaluation of the fine needle aspiration biopsy in the preoperative selection of cold thyroid nodules. Cancer. 1991;67:2137-2141.

[29] Slowinska-Klencka D, Klencki M, Sporny S, Lewinski. A. Fine-needle aspiration biopsy of the thyroid in an area of endemic goitre: Influence of restored sufficient iodine supplementation on the clinical significance of cytological results. Eur J Endocrinol. 2002;146:19-26.

[30] Are C, Hsu JF, Ghossein RA, Schoder H, Shah JP, Shaha AR. Histological aggressiveness of fluorodeoxyglucose positron-emission tomogram (FDG-PET)-detected incidental thyroid carcinomas. Ann Surg Oncol. 2007 Nov;14(11):3210-5.

[31] Werk Jr EE, Vernon BM, Gonzalez JJ, Ungaro PC, McCoy RC 1984 Cancer in thyroid nodules: a community hospital survey. Arch Intern Med 144:474–476

[32] Asp AA, Georgitis W, Waldron EJ, Sims JE, Kidd 2nd GS 1987 Fine needle aspiration of the thyroid: use in an average health care facility. Am J Med 83:489–493

[33] Hamburger JI 1987 Consistency of sequential needle biopsy findings for thyroid nodules: management implications. Arch Intern Med 147:97–99

[34] Gharib H, Goellner JR. Fine-needle aspiration biopsy of the thyroid: an appraisal. Ann Intern Med. 1993 Feb 15;118(4):282-9.

[35] Baloch ZW, Fleisher S, LiVolsi VA, Gupta PK 2002 Diagnosis of"follicular neoplasm": a gray zone in thyroid fine-needle aspiration cytology. Diagn Cytopathol 26:41–44.

[36] Sahin M,Gursoy A, Tutuncu NB, GuvenerDN2006 Prevalence and prediction of malignancy in cytologically indeterminate thyroid nodules. Clin Endocrinol (Oxf) 65:514–518.

[37] Hodak SP, Rosenthal DS; American Thyroid Association Clinical Affairs Committee. Information for clinicians: commercially available molecular diagnosis testing in the evaluation of thyroid nodule fine-needle aspiration specimens. Thyroid. 2013 Feb; 23(2):131-4.

[38] Kato MA, Fahey 3rd TJ 2009 Molecular markers in thyroid cancer diagnostics. Surg Clin North Am 89:1139–1155

[39] Papini E, Petrucci L, Guglielmi R, et al. Long-term changes in nodular goiter: a 5-year prospective randomized trial of levothyroxine suppressive therapy for benign cold thyroid nodules. J Clin Endocrinol Metab. 1998;83:780-783.

[40] Wemeau JL, Caron P, Schvartz C, et al. Effects of thyroid-stimulating hormone suppression with levothyroxine in reducing the volume of solitary thyroid nodules and improving extranodular nonpalpable changes: a randomized, double-blind, placebo-controlled trial by the French Thyroid Research Group. J Clin Endocrinol Metab. 2002;87:4928-4934.

[41] Fast S, Nielsen VE, Bonnema SJ, Hegedüs L. Time to reconsider nonsurgical therapy of benign non-toxic multinodular goitre: focus on recombinant human TSH augmented radioiodine therapy. Eur J Endocrinol. 2009 Apr;160(4):517-28.

[42] Snook KL, Stalberg PL, Sidhu SB, Sywak MS, Edhouse P, Delbridge L. Recurrence after total thyroidectomy for benign multinodular goiter. World J Surg. 2007 Mar;31(3): 593-8.

[43] Lang BH, Lo CY. Total thyroidectomy for multinodular goiter in the elderly. Am J Surg. 2005 Sep;190(3):418-23.

[44] Lima N, Knobel M, Cavaliere H, Sztejnsznajd C, Tomimori E, Medeiros-Neto G 1997 Levothyroxine suppressive therapy is partially effective in treating patients with benign, solid thyroid nodules and multinodular goiters. Thyroid 7:691–697.

[45] Gandolfi PP, Frisina A, Raffa M, Renda F, Rocchetti O, Ruggeri C, Tombolini A. The incidence of thyroid carcinoma in multinodular goiter: retrospective analysis. Acta Biomed. 2004 Aug;75(2):114-7.

[46] Piper HG, Bugis SP, Wilkins GE, Walker BA, Wiseman S, Baliski CR. Detecting and defining hypothyroidism after hemithyroidectomy. Am J Surg. 2005 May;189(5): 587-91.

[47] Rayes N, Steinmüller T, Schröder S, Klötzler A, Bertram H, Denecke T, Neuhaus P, Seehofer D. Bilateral subtotal thyroidectomy versus hemithyroidectomy plus subtotal resection (Dunhill procedure) for benign goiter: long-term results of a prospective, randomized study. World J Surg. 2013 Jan;37(1):84-90.

Section 3

Hyperthyroidism

Chapter 3

Imaging in Hyperthyroidism

Javier L. Pou Ucha

Additional information is available at the end of the chapter

http://dx.doi.org/10.5772/58324

1. Introduction

Abnormalities in the thyroid anatomy or physiology often arise when the clinician suspect hyperthyroidism or hypothyroidism detecting on physical examination a goiter or a thyroid nodule and confirms the suspicion by serum measurements of thyroxine (T4), or thyroid stimulating hormone (TSH).

Hyperthyroidism is the result of several diseases that may be located in the thyroid gland (primary), as well as in other locations (secondary), or be the product of an overeating of high-iodinated foods or being an undesirable effect of some drugs (amiodarone, antitussives). They will have different expressions in the clinical, laboratory and diagnostic imaging.

Primary hyperthyroidism is the most common condition where diseases like Graves Basedow disease, toxic multinodular goiter and toxic adenoma are the most common pathologies. Although rare, also the hyperthyroidism associated with thyroid carcinoma [1], extracervical ectopic thyroid tissue [2], mutation with activation of the TSH receptor [3], activating mutations of the stimulatory G protein in the McCune-Albright syndrome [4], Struma Ovarii [5] and medications such as the excess of iodine intake (Jod-Basedow phenomenon).

The secondary hyperthyroidism is characterized by an increased thyroid hormone caused by extrathyroid pathologies like the TSH high secreting pituitary adenoma [7], thyroid hormone resistance syndrome [8], human chorionic gonadotropin secreting tumor [9].

Within the thyrotoxicosis without hyperthyroidism will be the acute, subacute and silent thyroiditis and other causes such as medication with amiodarone, radiation, adenoma infarction or excessive thyroid hormone intake (factitious hyperthyroidism). These diseases will present a clinical picture similar to hyperthyroidism.

All these pathology will need to be studied using various imaging techniques (Figure 1).

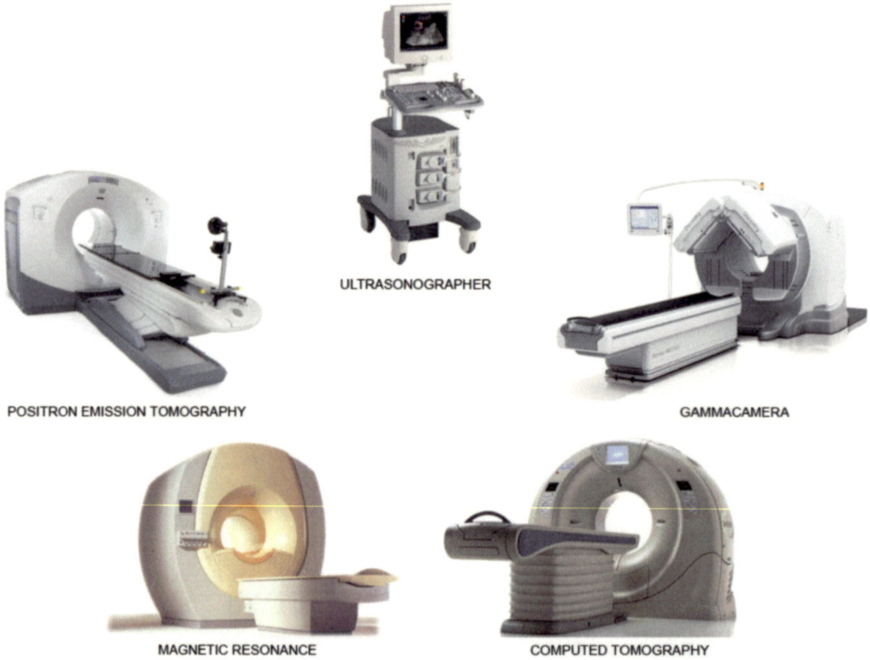

Figure 1. Medical imaging devices used in Radiology and Nuclear Medicine Departments.

Imaging studies will be in the first line for thyroid exploration techniques. There will be others that will serve to confirm or distinguish between thyroid pathologies as well as to locate pathology in extracorporeal way when it is secondary.

2. Introduction to imaging studies

Ultrasonography is a technique of first choice, based on the study of the thyroid gland by the emission and reception of ultrasound signal that according to its characteristic of reflection of sound wave in the different tissues studied will display them in different graduations of gray color on a scale that will go from white to black. Main advantages are their cost, non-invasive and that they not emit ionizing radiation. Within the disadvantages will be the need for experienced staff.

Then we will have a second imaging technique that will be of great importance in the study of hyperthyroidism, the scintigraphy, a non-invasive technique that through the use of radioactive material will be able to assess not only anatomy and glandular function, but exploring the whole body searching for extraglandular pathology. Of additional contribution will be the Radioactive Iodine Uptake (RAIU), is a test that evaluate the thyroid function,, it measures how much radioactive iodine is taken up by the thyroid gland in a certain time period, normally obtaining values in a few hours (4-6), 24 hours, and 48 hours.

And two imaging methods of high resolution, computed tomography (CT) and magnetic resonance imaging (MRI) techniques are used to assess cervical gland pathologies as well as extracervical level giving a greater resolution than other imaging studies. It is useful in the surgical planning and for their subsequent evaluation and monitoring. MRI will allow improved visualization of soft tissues and the identification of pathologies at thoracic as in abdominopelvic level.

When an intraglandular lesion is identified in thyroid, ultrasound technique will be useful for the intralesional correct approach and extraction of material by the Fine Needle Aspiration Biopsy (FNAB) for the cytopathology evaluation (Figure 2).

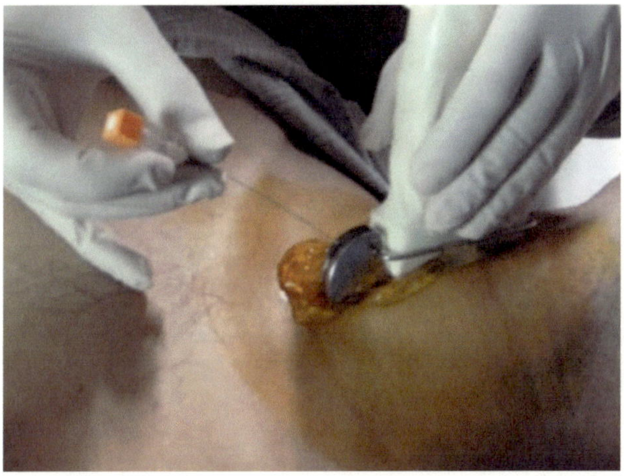

Figure 2. Fine needle aspiration biopsy guided by ultrasonography.

FNAB is the cornerstone in the solitary thyroid node assessment detected in the clinical exam as well as the evaluation of the dominant node in multinodular goiter disease.

In places where a nodule or a lymph node is difficult to be identified by fisical exam, or if there are multiple nodules, an echo-guided biopsy provides high precision for the nodule/ganglion sampling.

As we mentioned above the procedure requires skilled and experienced hands as well as an experienced cytopathologist. Even more, in experienced hands, 10% approximately of the biopsies are non diagnostics.

Thyroid nodules are discovered by palpation in a 3-7 percent of cases and by ultrasound in a 20-76% in the general population [10].

3. Ultrasonography

The ultrasound images tend to be reserved for those cases in which there are doubts about whether it is a nodule or palpable nodule is inside the thyroid. They are also used to distinguish between a suspicious nodule and a prominent lobe or thyroid hemiagenesis, to distinguish between a solitary nodule and a multinodular goiter, for the evaluation of a thyroid mass when cytology is not diagnostic.

Thyroid nodules are common. The most palpable nodules are benign (solid, cystic, mixed) being the minor, less than 10%, malignant [11]; however, the risk of malignancy in nodule rises in children, adolescents, and adults. The risk is substantially increased if the patient has been previously irradiated by head and neck pathology [12].

Multiple publications have documented that certain sonographic features by B-mode ultrasound and Doppler color, Figure 3, (hypoechogenicity, irregular margin, microcalcifications, intralesional vascular signals) are suggestive of malignancy [13-17].

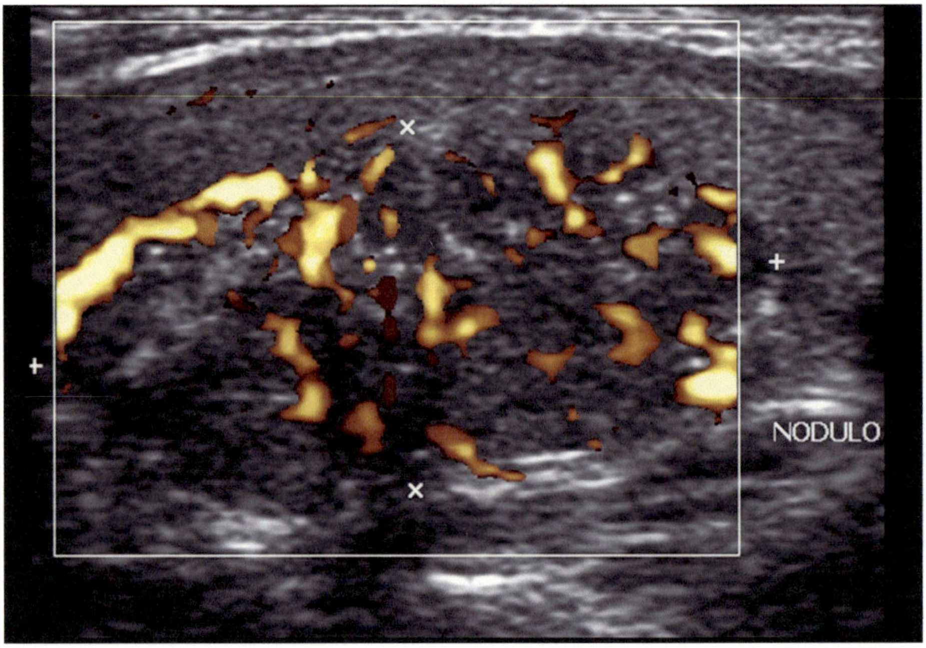

Figure 3. Colour Doppler of a thyroid nodule. In color is displayed the vascular distribution inside the nodule, showing periferic and central vascularization. The image shows multiple microcalcifications too, being in relation to papillary carcinoma. (Image courtesy by Dr. Alejandro Blando)

Ultrasound clearly defines the thyroid gland, it is more sensitive than scintigraphy in the detection of thyroid nodules and determines their intra/extra glandular location. Ultrasound is done when a clinician suspect the presence of a thyroid nodule or for the confirmation of the location inside or outside the gland.

Although radiation dose in scintigraphic studies and RAIU are extremely low and that there is no known health risk up to date, the ultrasonography avoid ionizing radiation and always it is used as initial imaging technique for the gland evaluation in children. Also, the ultrasonography is the initial imaging method for pregnancy assessment. In the presence of a nodule,

http://dx.doi.org/10.5772/58324

the ultrasonography will be helpful in determinate his composition (cystic, solid, miced). The ultrasound technique has an important limitation, being unable to differentiate between malignant and benigne nodule, only giving an estimation.

Ultrasonography also can be used for the degree of the nodule growth in patients under suppresing therapy. Their limitations are the necesity of experienced operator, high interoperator variability in the nodule identification and the uncertain signification of the thyroid micronodule in the moment of the detection in the adult population. The ultrasonography is so sensitive and the nodules so prevalent that may be difficult to be interpreted in some situations.

4. Doppler

Also the Doppler Ultrasonography is useful for the thyroid gland evaluation. It meassures the vascular flow in the inferior thyroid artery, being 6 ml/min in norml gland and increased more than 5-folds in hyperthyroidism. Doppler is very useful in Graves Disease for the global flow increase assessment (Figure 4), also the therapeutic response control showing a flow constant reduction and the posterior increase in case of recurrence.

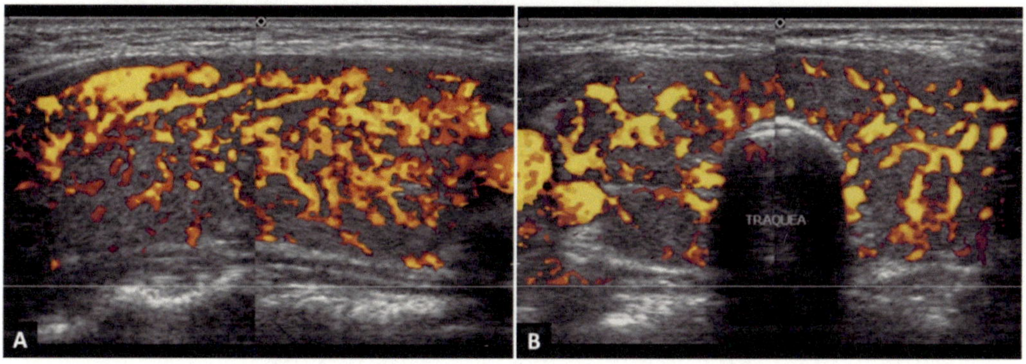

Figure 4. Color Doppler Ultrasound of the Thyroid Gland in longitudinal view (image A) as in transversal view (image B). High and diffuse hypervascular thyroid related to Graves Disease ("Thyroid Inferno Sign"). (Image courtesy by Dr. Alejandro Blando).

In the last years also it has also been evaluated the Doppler utility in the nodule feature determination between malignancy and benign as weel as inflamatory or malignant lymph nodes [18].

5. Elastography

Even more, recent studies shows that are ultrasopnography techniques that reduce the false negative probability using the Elastography Ultrasonographyic method, first described in thyroid lesions in 2005 by Lyshchik et al. [19] This method consist in the evaluation in real time (RTE) of a region of interest during the aplication of external force with the probe of the ultrasonography, the software meassure the tissue displacement wich is visualized in color scale depending on the nodular/extranodular consistency. It has been reported as a great tool that could optimize the thyroid nodule management because of his high sensitivity and specificity in the prediction of thyroid carcinoma (Figure 5). [20,21]

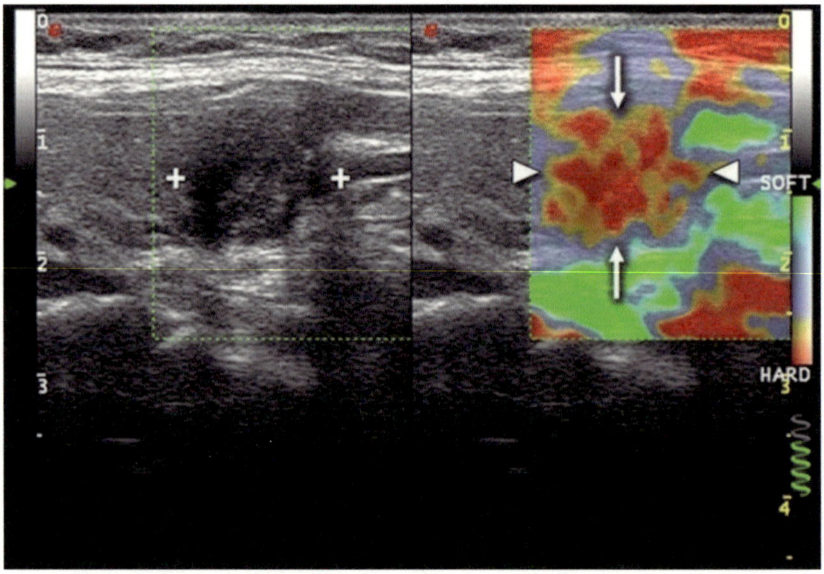

Figure 5. Dual Modality US Imaging. There is a small hypoecoic solid nodule related to papillary carcinoma (image at the left). Elastography method (image at the right) showing a nodular stiffness, hence the lack of nodular elasticity represented as red colour between arrows. (Image courtesy by Dr. Alejandro Blando)

6. Thyroid scintigraphy and radioactive iodine uptake

Thyroid assessment by radionuclides can contribute to the management of the patient under thyroid disease suspicious.

Thyroid scintigraphy helps to determinate the gland location, morfology and functional features (Figure 6).

Unlike ultrasonography, the scintigraphy assess the thyroid nodule and gland physiology.

Hot nodules (Figure 7) acumulates I-123 or Tc-99m in a major degree than normal thyroid, they are very uncommon to express malignancy and FNAB or surgery can be avoided.

Warm nodules acumulates radiotracers in the same intensity as normal thyroid tissue. They are low probably to be malignant, but doctors would try FNAB depending on the size, consistency and clinical presentation.

http://dx.doi.org/10.5772/58324

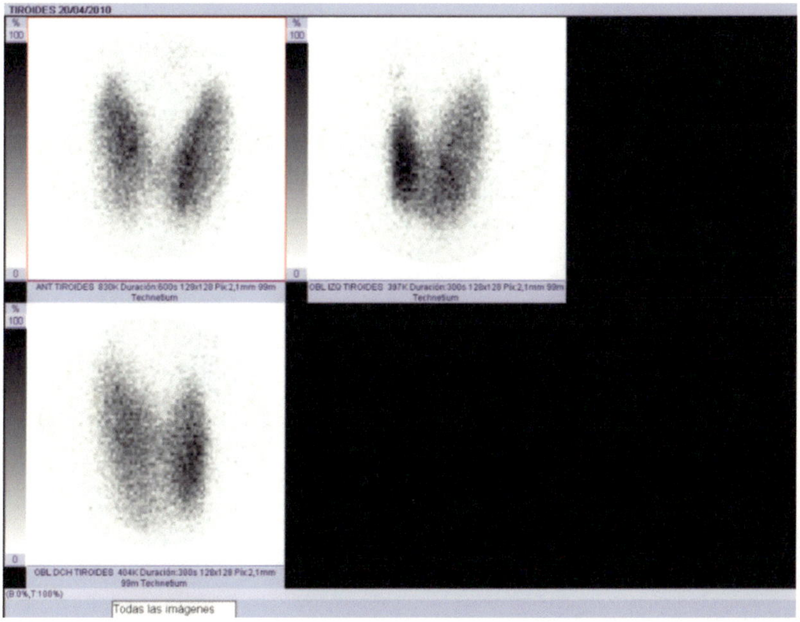

Figure 6. Thyroid Scintigraphy with Tc-99m-Pertecnetate. Anterior, Left Oblique and Right Oblique projections (top left, top right and botom right respectivelly) magnified with pin-hole collimator. Showing a normal thyroid gland with a normal radiotracer distribution.

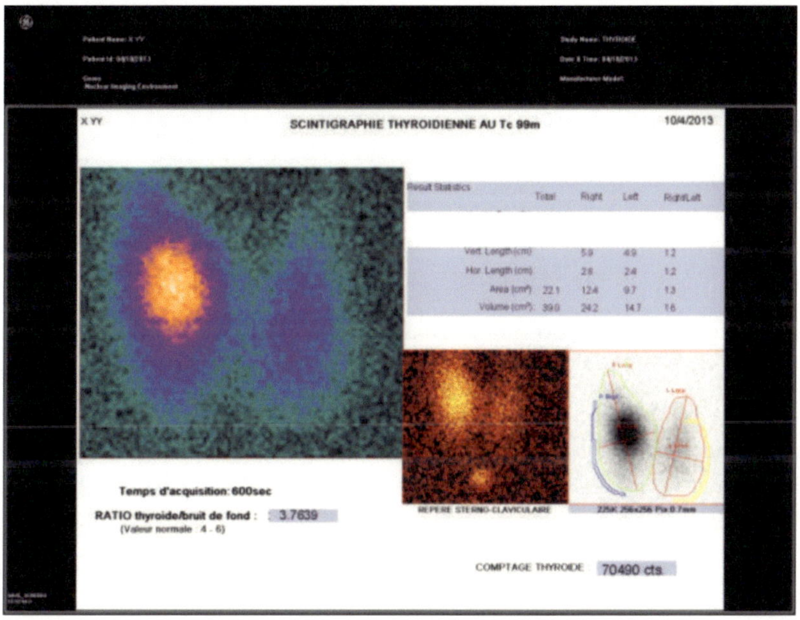

Figure 7. Thyroid Scintigraphy with Tc-99m-Pertecnetate in anterior projection. High focal uptake in right lobe related to Toxic Nodular Adenoma. (Image courtesy by Dr. Charles Bouirsot)

Cold nodules (Figure 8) lacks of radioisotope acumulation, they do not trap Tc-99m nor organify I-123 either. They have a 10-20 % of probability of malignancy [22], for this reason, the thyroid scintigraphy can be useful when a FNAB result is uncertain [23].

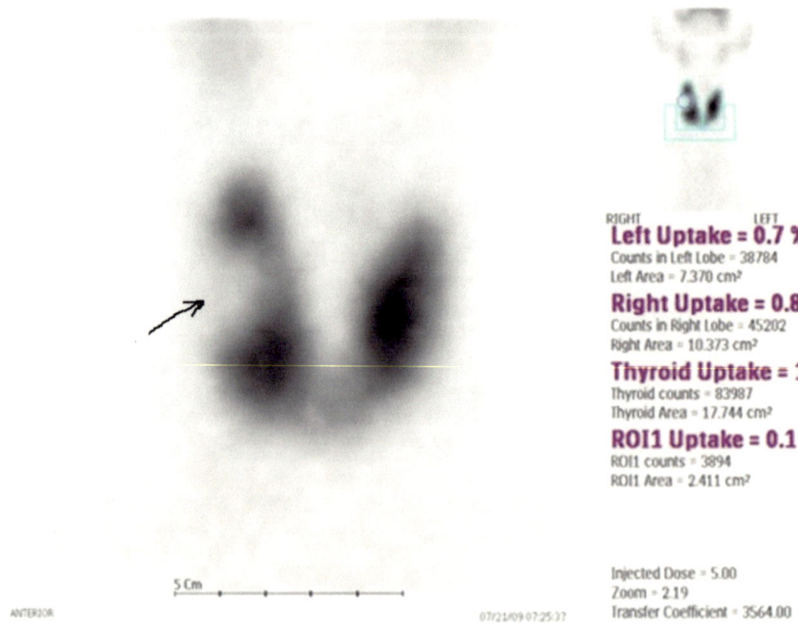

Figure 8. Thyroid Scintigraphy with Tc-99m-Pertecnetate in anterior projection. The image display a cold nodule (arrow) in the right lobe. (Image courtesy by Dr. Charles Bouirsot)

The presence of toxic multinodular goiter diminish the malignancy risk. The typical multinodular scintigraphic image shows areas of high and low uptake of radiotracer and always the two thyroid lobes affected (Figure 9). There are last articles that inform that multinodular goiter and solitary nodules have the same risk of malignancy.

Nevertheless, the presence of a dominant cold nodule it will be recomended a FNAB (Figure 10).

Radioactive Iodine Uptake complements the thyroid scan, and can meassure the percentage of glandular iodine uptake in order to find utility to the I-131 therapy (Figure 11). There are pathologies in which uptake will be negligible and not I-131 therapy will be needed such as subacute Thyroiditis, struma ovarii, or factitious hyperthyroidism.

The functional and structural information given by the Scintigraphy thyroid and thyroid uptake combined with physical exam and hormonal serology always allows a correct diagnosis and a logical therapeutic approach or next diagnostic procedures.

It is important to distinguish between hyperthyroidism associated with an increased iodine uptake (Graves, BMN, toxic adenoma disease) and a decreased uptake (Thyroiditis, factitious

http://dx.doi.org/10.5772/58324

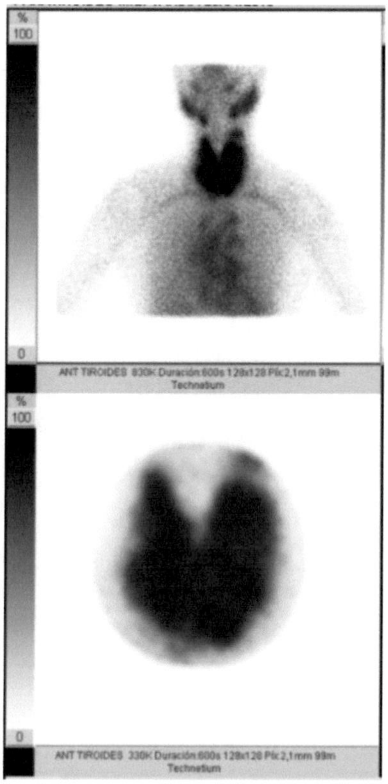

Figure 9. Thyroid Scitigraphy with Tc-99m-Pertecnetate, anterior projection images with different collimators (paralel hole and pin-hole, top and bottom respectivelly). The images displayed show a great hyperactivity with heterogeneous distribution in an enlarged thyroid gland (goiter) related to multinodular goiter.

hyperthyroidism, struma ovarii, functioning metastasis of thyroid carcinoma, extracervical ectopic thyroid tissue), because the treatment for these two categories of hyperthyroidism is going to be different.

The diagnosis of Graves disease can be based on clinical data and laboratory. A thyroid scintigraphy and a thyroid uptake curve can be usefull to confirm the Graves disease when it is a hyperthyroidism without signs of proptosis, pretibial myxedema and exophthalmos.

Thyroid scan shows a homogeneous uptake of radiotracer in both lobes. Sometimes the Graves disease can be confused with toxic Multinodular goiter, but both can be easily recognized by a thyroid scintigraphy. This differentiation is important because the therapeutic dose is much higher for toxic Nodular goiter.

Occasionally, a silent or subacute thyroiditis can be confused with Graves disease because in both situations the patient is hyperthyroid with abnormal analytic function. The patient with thyroiditis may have fever, pain and local inflammation, but it could be confused with an infection or inflammation of upper air tract. It could also happen that at the time of the elevated thyroid hormones in blood the clinic of thyroiditis had already disappeared.

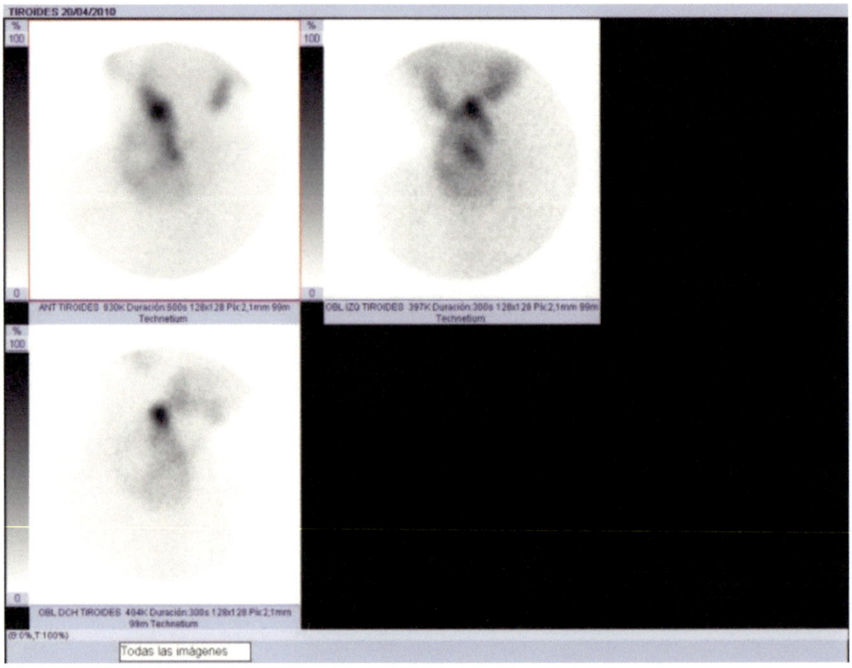

Figure 10. Thyroid Scintigraphy with Tc-99m-Pertecnetate. Anterior, Left Oblique and Right Oblique projections (top left, top right and botom right respectivelly) magnified with pin-hole collimator. Showing a right enlarged thyroid lobe (patient with hemithyroidectomy) with heterogenous distribution of the radiotracer. There is a hot nodule in the upper pole and a cold area at the right of the midlower part of the lobe.

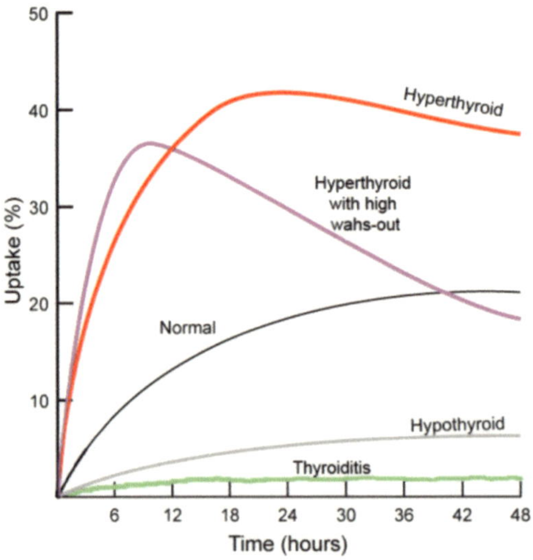

Figure 11. Radioactive Iodine Uptake Curve Plot. The image shows different uptake intensity (in percentage) depending on the thyroid disease represented in time (hours).

http://dx.doi.org/10.5772/58324

Because of glandular inflammation in acute or subacute Thyroiditis, this is not able to trap Tc-99m or organify I-123, consequently, the capture of 24 hours will be close to 0% (Figure 12).

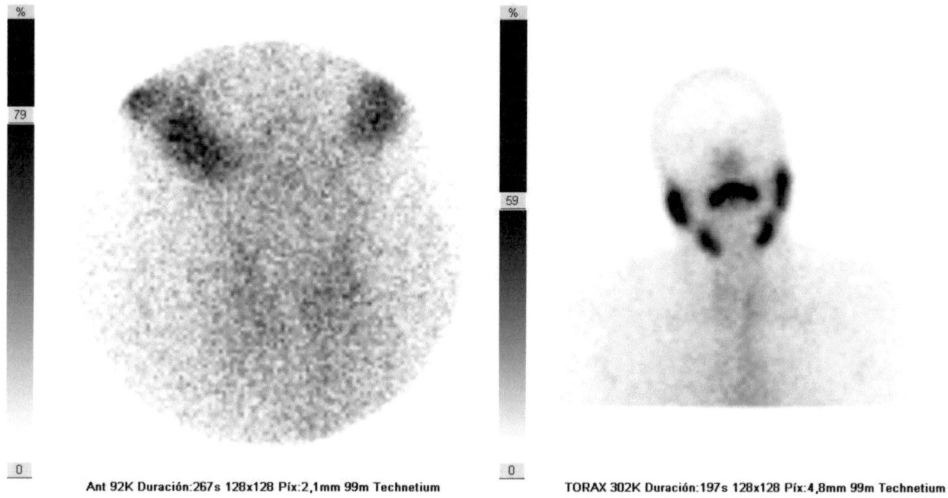

Figure 12. Thyroid Scintigraphy with Tc-99m-Pertecnetate in anterior projection with two different collimators (pin-hole and paralel hole, left and right respectivelly). The image displayed show no uptake of radiotracer by the thyroid gland.

The scintigraphy can be used to distinguish between the thyroiditis and Graves disease.

Another problem that can arise is that of a patient with hyperthyroidism in which we do not know if the pathology is toxic adenoma or toxic multinodular goiter. Thyroid scintigraphy is suitable technique for their differentiation. The importance of the difference between toxic adenoma, multinodular goiter and Graves disease is that the first two needs higher therapeutic dose.

Another situation is that the factitious hyperthyroidism where the scintigraphy will help showing absence of glandular uptake and a radioactive iodine uptake value of 24 hours close to 0%. The difference between thyroiditis and factitious hyperthyroidism will be through laboratory, where the values of TG and Ac anti thyroid (AAT) will be the key.

Extremely rare conditions where a hyperthyroidism due to struma ovarii will supress the thyroid gland activity uptake. 24-Hour uptake will be close to 0%. If this condition is suspected, the solution will be a whole body Tc-99m scintigraphy or MRI imaging of the pelvis. A case of struma ovarii is displayed in Figure 13.

There are also rare situations like functioning thyroid carcinoma metastases where they are going to be seen enhanced hot spots dispersed in multiple parts of the body (Figure 14).

When a mass in neck or retrosternal area is detected and the suspicion could be a goiter, Thyroid Scintigraphy will be of great use to confirm this suspicion. With the help of a cutaneous

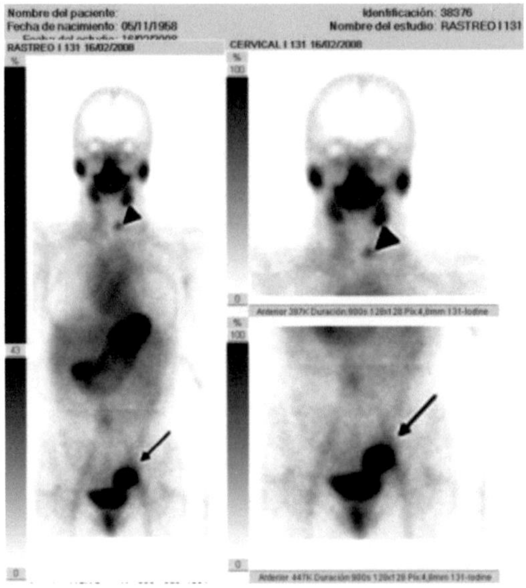

Figure 13. Thyroid Scintigraphy with I-131 in a patient under control for his thyroidectomy. There are displayed partially wholebody scan and craneocervical and pelvic statics views in anterior projection. There is a fical uptake at cervical level and a high activity mass lesion at the left hemipelvic region. This images is related to Struma Ovarii.

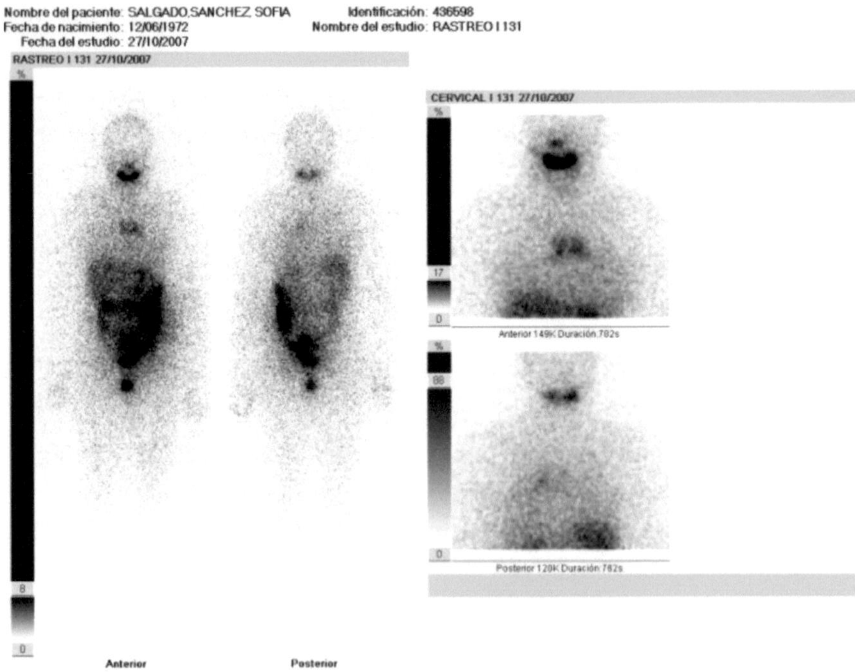

Figure 14. Thyroid Scintigraphy with I-131. Wholebody scanning in anterior and posterior views (at left) and cervico-mediastinal statics in anterior and posterior views (at right, top and bottom respectively).

radioactive labelling at the level of the suprasternal notch location cervicomediastinal thyroid or thyroid nodule in study can be defined with great precision.

A retrosternal goiter may be the manifestation of a multinodular goiter, which characteristically will presents with decreased radiotracer uptake of the area. There has been publicated a case of hyperthyroidism for multinodular ectopic goiter (Figure 15) where can be observed the great utility that will have the anatomical as well as functional images [2].

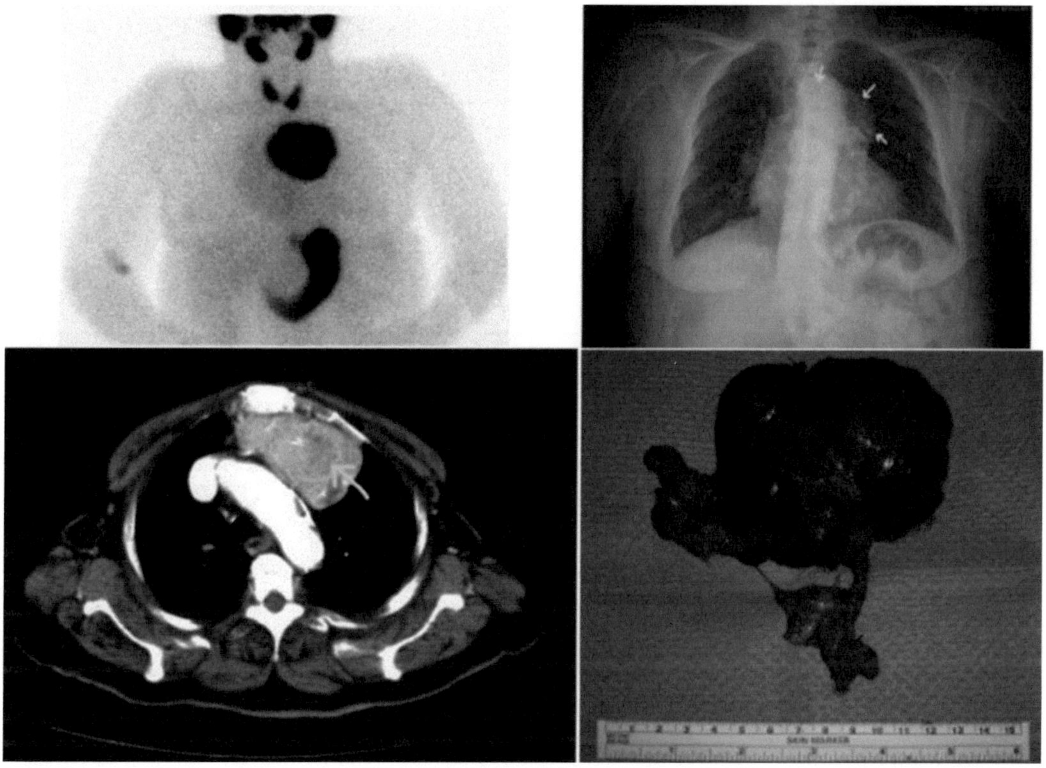

Figure 15. Thyroid Scintigrahpy with I-131 radiotracer, Chest Radiograph, Axial contrast enhanced CT scan at mediastinum level and a the ectopic goiter extracted by surgery (Top left, top right, bottom left, bottom right, respectivelly).

Thyroid scintigraphy can also differentiate between benign adenomatous nodule or a hot nodule. The scintigraphy is made after intravenous administration of thyroid hormone and can differentiate between a hot nodule if this decrease its level of uptake or will still be hot when we are in the presence of a autonomous node. It will be useful to measure the therapeutic approach, where is going to be useful to use thyroid hormone in order to decrease the size of the hot nodule not being useful to adenomatous autonomous nodules.

Scintigraphic characteristics between I-123/I-131 and Tc-99m	
I-123 / I-131	**Tc-99m**
• Half life: 13,22 Hs / 8 days	• Half life: 6,02 Hs
• Energy: 159 keV / 354 keV	• Energy: 140 keV
• Administration path: oral	• Administration path: intravenous
• Trasported actively to the intracelular space (Trapped)	• Transported actively to the intracelular space (Trapped)
• Bounded to thyrosine (Organified)	• NOT bounded to thyrosine (NOT organified)
• The scintigraphy will show tissue distribution of both functions (Trapped and Organified)	• The scintigraphy will show distribution of the function of Trap but no of organification.
• 3-4 hs pos oral administration imaging	• 10-30 minutes pos intravenous administration
• Thyroid nodule evaluation	• Thyroid nodule evaluation
• Nodular function assessment	• Nodular function assessment
• To determine retrosternal mass	• To determine retrosternal mass
• To confirm the presence of Graves Disease	• To confirm the presence of multi nodular goiter
• To confirm the presence of multi nodular goiter	• To confirm the presence of toxic adenoma
• To confirm the presence of toxic adenoma	• The Thyroid uptake is not standardized like I-123 y Tc-The measure of thyroid uptake has NO standard like I-123 y I-131, but can be evaluated in order to see the capacity of the glandular trap.
• It is useful in Radioactive Iodine Uptake study and to determine the I-131 dose for radiotherapy.	

7. Positron emission tomography

PET/CT study is a nuclear medicine imaging based on the gamma acquisition coming from the aniquilation of the posittron emited by a radiotracer administered intravenously, that in their majority of nuclear medicine centers is going to be F-18-FDG (fluorodeoxyglucose), useful for the measurement of the glucose metabolism in the wholebody, being higher in those very active and normal tissue (heart, brain, brown adipose tissue, Waldeyer ring), pathologic tissue (adenomas, multinodular goiter, Graves disease, autoinmune disease, cancer) and the radiotracer's collecting and excreting system (kidney, ureter, urinary bladder).

Primary hyperthyroidism will present a pathological increase in the activity of the thyroid gland, which can be presented as a homogeneous hyperactivity as is the typical case of Graves disease or can be a focal hyperactivity like toxic adenoma, which must be studied by FNAB since the focal hyperactivity may also been caused by malignant processes such as papillary or follicular carcinomas.

A recent publication relates the hyperthyroidism with an increase in the glucose metabolism by the brown adipose tissue. That means a problem in the assessment in the cervical soft tissue surrounding the thyroid gland because sometimes it is difficult to determine if the increased focal activity comes from a lymph node, metastasis or brown adipose tissue [24].

The PET study also is useful for assessing patients with hyperthyroidism and its mental behavior change. An article has been published in which there is a relationship between hyperthyroidism and alteration in brain glucose metabolism, showing a decrease in glucose activity at the level of the limbic system (uncus and inferior temporal gyrus), metabolic activation in the lower area of the parietal lobe and posterior cingulated level which was related to depression and anxiety, this last symptom was also associated with the increased metabolic activity at the level of the bilateral sensory associative cortex [25]

Multiple retrospective studies have reported that incidentalomas in thyroid gland with increased focal uptake of F-18 FDG has been found in 1.2 to 4.3% of healthy patients under study by PET/CT [26-29].

It was also suggested that a diffuse increase of the uptake into the thyroid gland was more in relation with benign lesion such as chronic thyroiditis or Graves disease [30].

We display in Figure 16 a normal thyroid gland with a normal F-18 FDG activity.

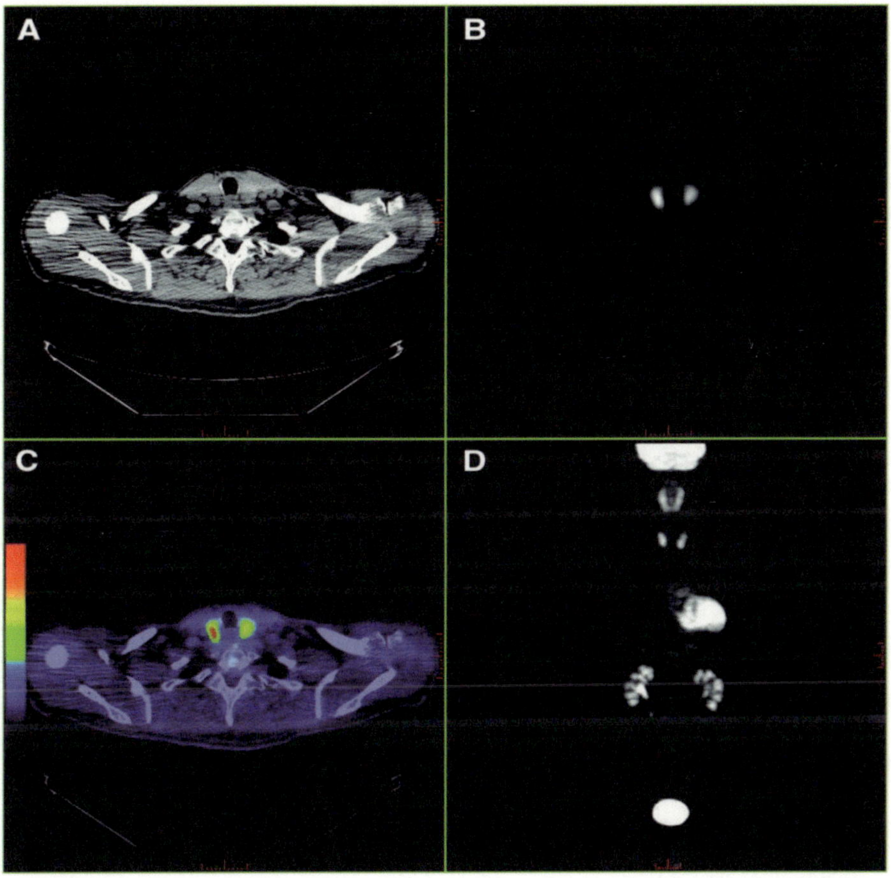

Figure 16. PET/CT scan at the thyroid gland level. Axial CT scan, emission image at thyroid level, axial PET/CT hybrid image and MIP emission image from mid-brain to bladder. The image displayed show an homogeneous activity in both thyroid lobes related to normal gland activity.

Although focal lesions with a high SUV (> 10) had a high probability of malignancy, the thyroid lesions with SUV < 10 have not demonstrated a high probability of benign lesion.

Inside those non-FDG radiotracers, the I-124 used for volumetric meassure for dosimetric planning in the treatment of hyperthyroidism with I-131, being their results better than those obtained by ultrasonography or conventional scintigraphy [31-33]. Although I-124 is not generally available and its use is limited to specialized centres.

Either, it has been done multiple studies with the radiotracer Ga-68 DOTATOC in an attempt to find differences between benign and malignant thyroid diseases, but no good conclusion were obtained. An increased DOTATOC uptake (target to background ratio >3.4) was found in hot nodules, disseminated thyroid autonomy, and in most cases (5 of 8) of active Hashimoto's disease. In Ga-68 DOTATOC PET, normal thyroid glands show a clearly detectable radiotracer uptake with a large variability and significantly higher target to background ratios in male patients. All patients with thyroid autonomy and most patients with active Hashimoto's disease have an increased thyroid DOTATOC uptake [34].

8. Computed tomography and magnetic resonance imaging

Both studies are useful for the anatomic description in high resolution of the thyroid gland, their nodes compositions, the adjacent structures characteristics when a thyroid goiter is present (trachea and esophagous principally), ophtalmopaties associated to Graves Disease, pituitary gland in secondary hyperparathyroidism, mediastinal structures in ectopic goiters and pelvic alteration when a struma ovarii exist.

They will be useful in the gland meassurement for the surgery planning or metabolic therapy with I-131.

In pos-therapy control period, both imaging studies are going to be useful for the follow-up of the cervical and extracervical region.

One of the most undesirable effects that might occur in a thyroid enhanced contrast CT is the induction of a thyrotoxicosis or thyroid storm [35-39].

9. Characteristic of imaging reports

9.1. Ultrasonography report

- Classification of a palpated nodule. eg solid, cystic, mixed
- Evaluate adjacent structures
- Determining the location of a palpable lump (within or outside of the thyroid)
- Identifying a cause for *Hyper*thyroidism

http://dx.doi.org/10.5772/58324

- Post surgical complications eg abscess, oedema
- Multi Nodular Goiter: Follow up nodules
- Guidance of injection, aspiration or biopsy
- Relationship of normal anatomy and pathology to each other

9.2. Scintigraphic report

- Configuration of the thyroid gland (homogeneity, nodules, size, location)
- Nodules activity (hot-warm-cold) respect to normal thyroid parenchima
- Extracervical pathologic activities
- Wholebody physiologic activities
- Thyroid Radioiodide Uptake Curve (RAIU)

9.3. Positron emission tomography report

- Metabolic feature of the thyroid gland (homogeneity, size, location)
- Nodular metabolic activity respect the normal thyroid parenchima
- Metabolic activity of Thyroid Goiter
- Semicuantification by SUV (Standard Uptake Value)
- Metabolic scanning of the whole body
- Metabolic activity of the pituitary gland, mediastinum and genitals (secondary hyperthyroidism)

9.4. Computed tomography report

- Configuration of thyroid gland (homogeneity, nodules, size, location)
- Nódules density (solid, cystic, mixed, calcium inside, abscess)
- Cervical and mediastinal lymphadenopathies
- Extracervical metastatic lesions (cranial, thorax, abdomen, pelvis, limbs)

9.5. Magnetic resonance imaging report

- Configuration of thyroid gland (homogeneity, nodules, size, location)
- Nódules density (solid, cystic, mixed, abscess)
- Cervical and mediastinal lymphadenopathies
- Extracervical metastatic lesions (cranial, thorax, abdomen, pelvis, limbs)

10. Metabolic radiotherapy

This therapy has a high success rate and carries a minimum risk. More than 80% of patients are successfully treated with a single dose. The disadvantages are minimal between them:

- Hypothyroidism (0-45 %)
- cervical compressive symptoms (2-4 days post administration of I-131)
- acute inflammation
- post-radiation thyroiditis (1-5%) (5-10 days post administration of I-131)
- exacerbation of thyrotoxicosis (7-10 days post administration of I-131)
- development of Graves (< 1%) disease
- acute sialitis

If there is no suspicion of malignancy, metabolic radiotherapy is indicated when the goiter causes local symptoms, such as dyspnoea or dysphagia. It is the therapy of choice, particularly in elderly patients, with diseases that increase the risk of surgical results or have a recurrence in post-surgery period (they have 10 times more likely to suffer damage to the laryngeal nerve).

The radiation dose to the thyroid following an administration of I-131 depends on:

- administered dose
- glandular size
- homogeneity in glandular distribution
- percentage of uptake at 24 hours
- Time of the I-131 inside the gland.

Patients with multi nodular goiter or toxic adenoma need one radioactive dose greater than grave's disease to achieve an euthyroid state.

10.1. Meassuring procedure

The pretherapy dosimetry should include the following tasks [40]:

- Target mass delineation by sonography or other suitable procedure.
- Quantification of the tracer activity with a dose calibrator.
- Measurement of the tracer activity with the test device, probe or gamma camera, with the activity located in the phantom or in free air with the relevant count rate correction.
- Verification that the observed count rate per activity matches the expected sensitivity value of the device.
- Administration of the tracer activity with accurate documentation

- If liquid 131I-NaI is administered, measurement of the residual activity and determination of the activity administered and the corresponding count rate.
- In-vivo measurements of the 131I uptake in the target tissue at the times stated in section Time lines.
- Calculation of the radioiodine activity needed for therapy according to section Data evaluation.

10.2. Potential sources of error

The evaluation of the therapeutic activity necessary to administer a specified target dose might be erroneous due to [40]:

- Errors in target volume determination
- Inappropriate attenuation correction (no or inadequate phantom)
- Contamination of the phantom
- Incorrect distance between the detector and the patient or phantom
- Deviation of the individual target tissue depth from the calibration depth
- Inappropriate centring of the probe over the phantom or the target tissue (target tissue partially outside the probe's FoV)
- Instability of the electronics of the measuring device, especially if quality control is inadequate
- Variation in background count rate (e.g. from radiation emitted by other patients) for the different uptake measurements
- Reduced or delayed absorption due to recent food intake
- Recent administration of another radionuclide
- Unfavourable choice of timing of the uptake measurements

11. Nanoparticles and future vision

According to Ramsden [41], increased vascularity in the thyroid can occur in hyperplastic goiter, Graves' disease and cancer, and may be associated with a vascular hum because of increased blood flow.

Interestingly, in experimental induction of goiter by low Iodine and thiouracil in rats, Wollman et al. [42] showed that the capillaries within the thyroid clearly enlarged within 3 days of treatment, and by 20 days, they surrounded the follicles with a continuous endothelial sheet. There was both fusion of capillaries and mitosis of endothelial cells.

Data suggest that, in human thyroid tumors, angiogenesis factors seem involved in neoplastic growth and aggressiveness.

The thyroid is an excellent model for the integrated control of angiogenesis, because of the vascularity of the thyroid gland, and its capacity to increase its blood flow in disease [43].

Biomolecular nanotechnology defined as "the threedimensional positional control of molecular structure to create materials and devices to molecular precision" recently has grown to the multifaceted industry providing new approaches to the old problems [44].

Nanodevices can receive the natural chemical messages transmitted from and between cells simply by eavesdropping on the natural molecular message traffic. Of course, mechanical (e.g., cytoskeletal) and electrical (e.g., ionic) cellular emanations may also be detectable by nanodevices [44].

Nanoparticles have emerged as agents for diagnosis and treatment with the distinction of being manipulated in their surface structure, thereby allowing a longer intravascular circulation period, physical and chemical manipulation of nergy, and being directed specifically to the target, achieving a target cell-specific uptake, allowing increased detection sensitivity through pathological signal amplification [45].

The application of nanoparticle-labelbased all-in-one dry-reagent immunoassay for thyroid stimulating hormone was reported by Huntinen et al. [46]. The magnetic properties of magnetic nanoparticles (MNPs) allow them to be imaged via magnetic resonance imaging (MRI) and targeted to a particular region by an externally applied MF (magnetic field). Once loaded with drug, MNPs can be targeted to a region of interest through an externally applied MF, and the drug released over a period of weeks. This helps to achieve optimal dosing by reducing the systemic toxicity of the drug, and decreases the likelihood of drug resistance that would result from insufficient drug present. Through MRI imaging, the biodistribution of MNPs and indirectly the drug concentration may be determined [47].

Mousa et al. [48] described methods of treating subjects having conditions related to angiogenesis including administering an effective amount of a polymeric nanoparticle form of thyroid hormone agonist, partial agonist or an antagonist to promote or inhibit angiogenesis in the organism.

Huang et al. [49] demonstrated an implementation of a time-resolved luminescence (TRL) assay for the sensitive and selective detection of thyroglobulin (Tg), a thyroid cancer marker, in homogeneous solution using water-soluble alpha-Dmannose-conjugated Au nanodots (Man-Au NDs). They employed those nanodots as a luminescence sensor for the detection of the thyroid-cancer marker thyroglobulin (Tg) in homogeneous solutions. Because luminescence quenching of the Man-Au NDs by Con A is inhibited by Tg selectivity, scientists obtained a highly sensitive and selective assay for Tg.

Many drugs can be delivered as NP and the opportunities for applying single and combined experimental medical therapy are almost inexhaustible.

http://dx.doi.org/10.5772/58324

12. Future works

The other idea is to investigate the effect of ionizing radiation and cancerogens on vascular structures observed in thyroid tissues. That research might elucidate the pathological changes similar to those which occur in nuclear atomic disaster survivors and provide knowledge for the implementation of drugs for radiation damage prevention and cancer treatment.

Could be interesting to develop more works into the endocrine imaging field in order to improve the differentiation between benign and malignant thyroid lesions.

Regarding the nanotechnology applied to the sphere of endocrine cancers and thyroid disease in particular, it is difficult to predict all the effects of NP to the alive human organism and that is why the major sources of experimental evidence are animal studies where tumors are produced unnaturally and NP are delivered during various stages of pathological process.

Acknowledgements

I would like to express my sincere appreciation to Ms Melina Masciotra for her great contribution to this chapter to english translation.

Author details

Javier L. Pou Ucha

Nuclear Medicine Department, Hospital Provincial de Rosario, Rosario, Argentina

Author is a permanent Member of the European Association of Nuclear Medicine

References

[1] Steffensen FH, Aunsholt NA. Hyperthyroidism associated with metastatic thyroid carcinoma. Clin Endocrinol (Oxf). 1994 Nov;41(5):685-7

[2] Pou Ucha J, Loira Bamio F, Campos Villarino LM, Serena Puig A, Nuño Vázquez-Garza J, Pena González E. Hyperthyroidism due to an ectopic intrathoracic thyroid. Rev Esp Med Nucl. 2009 Jan-Feb;28(1):15-7

[3] Sunthornthepvarakui T, Gottschalk ME, Hayashi Y, Refetoff S. Brief report: resistance to thyrotropin caused by mutations in the thyrotropin-receptor gene. N Engl J Med. 1995 Jan 19;332(3):155-60

[4] Mastorakos G, Mitsiades NS, Doufas AG, Koutras DA. Hyperthyroidism in McCune-Albright syndrome with a review of thyroid abnormalities sixty years after the first report. Thyroid. 1997 Jun;7(3):433-9

[5] Dunzendorfer T, deLas Morenas A, Kalir T, Levin RM. Struma ovarii and hyperthyroidism. Thyroid. 1999 May;9(5):499-502

[6] El-Shirbiny AM, Stavrou SS, Dnistrian A, Sonenberg M, Larson SM, Divgi CR. Jod-Basedow syndrome following oral iodine and radioiodinated-antibody administration. J Nucl Med. 1997 Nov;38(11):1816-7

[7] Hamilton CR Jr, Adams LC, Maloof F. Hyperthyroidism due to thyrotropin-producing pituitary chromophobe adenoma. N Engl J Med. 1970 Nov 12;283(20):1077-80

[8] McDermott MT, Ridgway EC. Thyroid hormone resistance syndromes. Am J Med. 1993 Apr;94(4):424-32

[9] Hershman JM. Human chorionic gonadotropin and the thyroid: hyperemesis gravidarum and trophoblastic tumors. Thyroid. 1999 Jul;9(7):653-7

[10] Hegedüs L. Clinical practice. The thyroid nodule. N Engl J Med 351:1764-1771

[11] Ezzat S, Sarti DA, Cain DR, Braunstein GD. Thyroid incidentalomas. Prevalence by palpation and ultrasonography. Arch Intern Med 154:1838-1840

[12] Favus MJ, Schneider AB, Stachura ME, Arnold JE, Ryo UY, Pinsky SM, Colman M, Arnold MJ, Frohman LA. Thyroid cancer occurring as a late consequence of head-and-neck irradiation. Evaluation of 1056 patients. N Engl J Med 1976; 294:1019-1025

[13] Solbiati L, Osti V, Cova L, Tonolini M. Ultrasound of thyroid, parathyroid glands and neck lymph nodes. Eur Radiol 11:2411-2424

[14] Kim EK, Park CS, Chung WY, Oh KK, Kim DI, Lee JT, Yoo HS. New sonographic criteria for recommending fine-needle aspiration biopsy of nonpalpable solid nodules of the thyroid. Am J Roentgenol 178:687-691

[15] Görges R, Eising EG, Fotescu D, Renzing-Köhler K, Frilling A, Schmid KW, Bockisch A, Dirsch O. Diagnostic value of high-resolution B-mode and power-mode sonography in the follow-up of thyroid cancer. Eur J Ultrasound. 2003 Feb;16(3):191-206

[16] Fukunari N, Nagahama M, Sugino K, Mimura T, Ito K, Ito K. Clinical evaluation of color Doppler imaging for the differential diagnosis of thyroid follicular lesions. World J Surg. 2004 Dec;28(12):1261-5

[17] Fukunari N. Thyroid ultrasonography B-mode and color-Doppler. Biomed Pharmacother. 2002;56 Suppl 1:55s-59s

[18] Belzarena C, Lago G, Lang R, et al. Propuesta 2000 para el tratamiento y seguimiento del carcinoma diferenciado de tiroides. Endocrinología y nutrición 2001; 48(3): 70-77

[19] Lyshchik A, Higashi T, Asato R, Tanaka S, Ito J, Mai JJ, Pellot-Barakat C, Insana MF, Brill AB, Saga T, Hiraoka M, Togashi K. Thyroid gland tumor diagnosis at US elastography. Radiology. 2005 Oct;237(1):202-11

[20] Rago T, Santini F, Scutari M, Pinchera A, Vitti P. Elastography: new developments in ultrasound for predicting malignancy in thyroid nodules. Clin Endocrinol Metab 92:2917-2922

[21] Unlütürk U, Erdoğan MF, Demir O, Güllü S, Başkal N. Ultrasound elastography is not superior to grayscale ultrasound in predicting malignancy in thyroid nodules. Thyroid 2012 Oct;22(10):1031-8

[22] Arturi F, Russo D, Schlumberger M, du Villard JA, Caillou B, Vigneri P, Wicker R, Chiefari E, Suarez HG, Filetti S. Iodide symporter gene expression in human thyroid tumors. Clin Endocrinol Metab 83:2493-96

[23] Pino Rivero V, Montero García C, Keituqwa Yáñez T, Rejas Ugena E, Blasco Huelva A. The use of scintigraphy and fine needle aspiration biopsy (FNAB) in thyroid surgery and review of literature. An Otorrinolaringol Ibero Am. 2003;30(2):161-9.

[24] Lahesmaa M, Orava J, Schalin-Jäntti C, Soinio M, Hannukainen JC, Noponen T, Kirjavainen A, Iida H, Kudomi N, Enerbäck S, Virtanen KA, Nuutila P. Hyperthyroidism increases brown fat metabolism in humans. J Clin Endocrinol Metab. 2013 Oct 23 [Epub ahead of print]

[25] Schreckenberger MF, Egle UT, Drecker S, Buchholz HG, Weber MM, Bartenstein P, Kahaly GJ. Positron emission tomography reveals correlations between brain metabolism and mood changes in hyperthyroidism. J Clin Endocrinol Metab. 2006 Dec; 91(12):4786-91

[26] Cohen MS, Arslan N, Dehdashti F, Doherty GM, Lairmore TC, Brunt LM, Moley JF. Risk of malignancy in thyroid incidentalomas identified by fluorodeoxyglucose-positron emission tomography. Surgery. 2001;130:941–946

[27] Kang KW, Kim SK, Kang HS, Lee ES, Sim JS, Lee IG, Jeong SY, Kim SW. Prevalence and risk of cancer of focal thyroid incidentaloma identified by 18F-fluorodeoxyglucose positron emission tomography for metastasis evaluation and cancer screening in healthy subjects. J Clin Endocrinol Metab. 2003;88:4100–4104

[28] Chen YK, Ding HJ, Chen KT, Chen YL, Liao AC, Shen YY, Su CT, Kao CH. Prevalence and risk of cancer of focal thyroid incidentaloma identified by 18F-fluorodeoxyglucose positron emission tomography for cancer screening in healthy subjects. Anticancer Res. 2005;25:1421–1426

[29] Yi JG, Marom EM, Munden RF, Truong MT, Macapinlac HA, Gladish GW, Sabloff BS, Podoloff DA. Focal uptake of fluorodeoxyglucose by the thyroid in patients undergoing initial disease staging with combined PET/CT for non-small cell lung cancer. Radiology. 2005;236:271–275

[30] Yasuda S, Shohtsu A, Ide M, Takagi S, Takahashi W, Suzuki Y, Horiuchi M. Chronic thyroiditis: diffuse uptake of FDG at PET. Radiology. 1998;207:775-778

[31] Eschmann SM, Reischl G, Bilger K, Kupferschläger J, Thelen MH, Dohmen BM, Besenfelder H, Bares R. Evaluation of dosimetry of radioiodine therapy in benign and malignant thyroid disorders by means of iodine-124 and PET. Eur J Nucl Med Mol Imaging. 2002 Jun;29(6):760-7

[32] Matheoud R, Canzi C, Reschini E, Zito F, Voltini F, Gerundini P. Tissue-specific dosimetry for radioiodine therapy of the autonomous thyroid nodule. Med Phys. 2003;30:791–8

[33] Canzi C, Zito F, Voltini F, Reschini E, Gerundini P. Verification of the agreement of two dosimetric methods with radioiodine therapy in hyperthyroid patients. Med Phys. 2006;33:2860–7

[34] Lincke T, Orschekowski G, Singer J, Sabri O, Paschke R. Increased gallium-68 DOTA-TOC uptake in normal thyroid glands. Horm Metab Res. 2011 Apr;43(4):282-6

[35] Blum M, Weinberg U, Shenkman L, Hollander CS. Hyperthyroidism after iodinated contrast medium. N Engl J Med. 1974 Jul 4;291(1):24-5

[36] Hehrmann R, Klein D, Mayer D, Ploner O. Risk of hyperthyroidism in examinations with contrast media. Aktuelle Radiol. 1996 Sep;6(5):243-8

[37] Alkhuja S, Pyram R, Odeyemi O. In the eye of the storm: iodinated contrast medium induced thyroid storm presenting as cardiopulmonary arrest. Heart Lung. 2013 Jul-Aug;42(4):267-9

[38] Rhee CM, Bhan I, Alexander EK, Brunelli SM. Association between iodinated contrast media exposure and incident hyperthyroidism and hypothyroidism. Arch Intern Med. 2012 Jan 23;172(2):153-9

[39] Grady D. Another reason to be cautious about imaging: comment on "association between iodinated contrast media exposure and incident hyperthyroidism and hypothyroidism". Arch Intern Med. 2012 Jan 23;172(2):161

[40] Eur J Nucl Med Mol Imaging. 2013 Jul;40(7):1126-34

[41] Rhee CM, Bhan I, Alexander EK, Brunelli SM. Association between iodinated contrast media exposure and incident hyperthyroidism and hypothyroidism. J Endocrinol. 2000 Sep;166(3):475-80

[42] Wollman SH, Herveg JP, Zeligs JD, Ericson LE. Blood capillary enlargement during the development of thyroid hyperplasia in the rat. Endocrinology. 1978 Dec;103(6): 2306-14

[43] Ramsden JD. Angiogenesis in the thyroid gland. J Endocrinol. 2000 Sep;166(3):475-80

[44] Freitas, R.A., Nanomedicine. 1999, Austin, TX: Landes Bioscience

[45] Pou Ucha, Javier L. (2013). Nanoparticles in bioimaging. In Arun Kumar, et al (Ed.), Nanomedicine in Drug Delivery. Boca Ratón, FL: Taylor & Francis Group; 2013 (pp. 187-212).

[46] Huhtinen P, Pelkkikangas AM, Jaakohuhta S, Lövgren T, Härmä H. Quantitative, rapid europium(III) nanoparticle-label-based all-in-one dry-reagent immunoassay for thyroid-stimulating hormone. Clin Chem. 2004 Oct;50(10):1935-6

[47] Varadan, Vijay K., Linfeng Chen, and Jining Xie, "Magnetic nanomaterails, nanotubes, and nanomedicine", Chapter 9, "Nanomedicine-Design of particles, sensors, motors, implants, robots, and devices", Artech House, 2009

[48] Mousa SA, Davis PJ, Hercbergs A (2009). Nanoparticle and polymer formulations for thyroid hormone analogs, antagonists and formulations and uses thereof.United States Patent and Trademark Office Pre-Grant Publication

[49] Huang CC, Hung YL, Shiang YC, Lin TY, Lin YS, Chen CT, Chang HT. Photoassisted synthesis of luminescent mannose-Au nanodots for the detection of thyroglobulin in serum. Chem Asian J. 2010 Feb 1;5(2):334-41

Chapter 4

Complications of Hyperthyroidism

Irmak Sayin, Sibel Ertek and Mustafa Cesur

Additional information is available at the end of the chapter

http://dx.doi.org/10.5772/58196

1. Introduction

Some clinical views which appear during hyperthyroidism can be called complications of hyperthyroidism. These clinical events are as follows.

1. Thyrotoxic heart disease
2. Progressive infiltrative ophtalmopathy in hyperthyroidism
3. Hyperthyroidism and bone
4. Thyroid chrisis
5. Thyrotoxic periodic paralysis
6. Thyrotoxicosis related psychosis and convulsion
7. Thyrotoxicosis related diabetes mellitus

2. Thyrotoxic heart disease

2.1. Effects of hyperthyroidism on heart-from pathophysiology to clinical complications

Cardiovascular signs and complications are generally the first alarming signs of hyperthyroidism for any physician. Effects of thyroid hormones on the heart and cardiovascular system could be direct or indirect. Palpitations and exercise intolerance are the most frequent signs [1, 2]. Although effects of iodization and world-wide use of radiocontrast agents may change the incidence, overt hyperthyroidism is common and affects 2-5% of the population [3,4]. In hyperthyroid patients mortality is increased 20% and the major causes of death are cardiac problems [5]. Atrial fibrillation is the most common and fearful arrythmic complication of hyperthyroidism which occurs in an estimated 10-25% of all overtly hyperthyroid patients [6]. Susceptibility to arrhythmic effects of thyroid hormones may have a genetic basis and recently the studies on molecular details of cardiac actions of thyroid hormones revealed some important knowledge [7]. Meanwhile, the cause of hyperthyroidism may also change the cardiovascular risk; patients with toxic multinoduler goitre have higher cardiovascular risk than patients with Graves' disease, probably because of older age, and patients with Graves disease may have autoimmune complications, such as valvular involvement, cardiomyopathy and pulmonary arterial hypertension [8]. Effects of thyroid hormones on the heart may be grouped as molecular or cellular mechanisms and hemodynamic effects. On the other hand, thyroid hormones have 2 types of effects on every tissue; genomic effects which occur more slowly, and non-genomic effects. Severity of hyperthyroidism may also cause differences in clinical presentation of the patient, overt hyperthyroidism and subclinical hyperthyroidism bring differing degrees of risks to patients.

2.2. Molecular and cellular mechanisms of thyroid hormone effects on heart

Both T3 and T4 are lipophylic and they pass through the cellular membranes and the conversion of T4 to T3 occurs in many cells. Triiodothyronin (T3) is the active thyroid hormone and it has genetic and cellular effects on cardiac muscle and blood vessels. It acts on THRs (thyroid hormone receptors) in the nucleus, creating dimers of 9-cis-retinoic acid receptor (RXR) (9): the formed complexes recognize some specific DNA consensus sequences, the thyroid response elements (TRE), located in the enhanced region of the genes initiate the transcription [9].

In myocytes, thyroid hormones act on many TREs, such as alpha myosin heavy chain fusion (MHC-α), sarcoplasmic reticulum calcium-activated ATPase (SERCA), the cellular membrane Na-K pump (Na-K ATPase), β1 adrenergic receptor, cardiac troponin I, atrial natriuretic peptide (ANP) [10-12] and some genes are also suppressed such as β-myosin heavy chain fusion (MHC-β), adenylic cyclase (IV and V) and the Na-Ca antiporter [13].

Thyroid hormone upregulates α, but downregulates β-chain in myocytes [14]. The final effect of thyroid hormones in animal studies is an increased rate of V1 isoform of MHC (MHCα/α) synthesis that is characteristically faster in myocardial fibre shortening [13,15]. A similar effect has been also observed in preliminary human studies [16,17].

Thyroid hormones also have effects on SERCA, which is responsible for the rate of calcium uptake during diastole, by actions on calcium activated ATPase and its inhibitory cofactor phospholamban [18,19]. Thyroid hormones enhance myocardial relaxation by upregulating expression of SERCA, and downregulating expression of phospholamban. The greater reduction in cytoplasmic calcium concentration at the end of the diastole increases the magnitude of systolic transient of calcium and augments its ability for activation of actin-myosin subunits. As a confirmation, phospholamban deficient mice showed no increase in heart rate after thyroid hormone treatment [20].

On the plasma membranes, T3 exerts direct extragenic actions on the functions other ion channels such as Na/K ATPase, Na/Ca++exchanger, and some voltage gated K channels (Kv

1.5, Kv 4.2, Kv 4.3) affecting myocardial and vascular functions [21,22] coordinating electrochemical and mechanical responses of myocardium [23,24]. It prolongs the activation of Na channels in myocardial cells [25] and induces intracellular Na uptake and secondary activation of the Na-Ca antiporter, which can partly explain the positive inotropic effect. T3 exerts direct effect on L-type calcium channels resulting in abbreviation of action potential duration and possibly L-type calcium channel mRNA expression [26,27].

The strong inotropic activity of thyroid hormones is probably due to an increased number of β-adrenergic receptors [28]. Circulating cathecholamine levels are in fact the same, but G protein and β-receptors increase [29]. The sensitivity of cardiovascular system to adrenergic stimulation does not change by thyroid hormones [30,31]. The changes in the heart rate result from both an increase in sympathetic tone and decrease in parasympathetic tone [32,33].

These genomic effects fail to explain the fast actions of thyroid hormones on the cardiovascular system. Non-genomic effects promote rapid changes, such as increased cardiac output [34-36]. The hemodynamic consequences of hyperthyroidism and nongenomic changes on plasma membranes occur acutely and contribute to these rapid changes. Studies indicate that thyroid hormone activates acute phosphorylation of phospholamban, and that also partly explains the homology between thyroid hormone and adrenergic system on the heart [32].

In an experimental study on rats, thyroid hormones upregulate connexin-40, a gap junction protein of myocardium important for the transport of electrical activity, and this may be one of the pathogenetic mechanisms of atrial fibrillation in hyperthyroidism [37]. In another animal study the authors suggested that the connexin-43 phosphorylation was downregulated by T3 in diabetic rats and decrease adaptation of heart to hyperglycemia and this may render the heart prone to ventricular arrythmias [38]. In fact thyroid hormone receptor alpha 1 is predominantly expressed in cardiac myocardium and may have an important role in cardiac myoblast differentiation by ERK kinase dependent process, but its clinical relevance is not known [39]. Also ERK (extracellular signal-regulated kinase) pathway may have a role in negative cardiac remodelling and decreased cardiac contractile function in hyperthyroidism, by inhibition of the Raf-1/ERK pathway by T3 [40,41].

Meanwhile, the thyroid hormone may have direct (without autonomous nervous system) effects on the sinoatrial node [42,43] and oxidative stress in animal studies [44]. The heart rate increases due to increased sinoatrial activity, a lower threshold for atrial activity, and a shortened atrial repolarisation [45,46]. Together with hemodynamic changes, i.e. the volume preload increases due to activation of the renin-angiotensin system [47], contractility increases due to increased metabolic demand and the direct effect of the thyroid hormone on heart muscle [48] and systemic vascular resistance decreases because of triiodotyronine-induced peripheral vasodilatation [49]. The result is a dramatic increase in cardiac output [50].

Local type 2 iodothyronine deiodinase up-regulation may also be involved in cardiac remodelling via activation of thyroid hormone signalling pathways involving Akt and p38 MAPK (mitogen-activated protein kinase) in thyrotoxic-dilated cardiomyopathy [51]. Animal studies show the effects of thyroid hormones on soluble fractions of 5′-nucleosidase activity, via protein kinase C-related pathway [52]. Preclinical studies blocking Akt by angiotensin-II type

2 receptor blocker showed that this blockage might prevent thyroxine-mediated cardiac hypertrophy [53]. Meanwhile, hypertrophied myocytes may be susceptible to apoptotic stimulation by angiotensin II in hyperthyroidism [54].

Studies on rats show that mitochondrial ultrastructure was damaged in T3 treated hyperthyroid rat heart, leading to energy depletion and cardiac dysfunction [55]. Another study on hamsters revealed that long term hyperthyroidism cause increased left ventricular interstitial fibrosis, significant cardiac hypertrophy and deleterious cardiac remodeling characterized by myocyte lengthening, chamber dilatation, decreased relative wall thickness, increased wall stress, and impaired global cardiac function whereas cardiomyocyte functions may be enhanced [56]. Some animal studies Show beneficial effects of angiotensin receptor blockers on myocytes as improved left ventricular longitudinal strain, heart rate and reduced cardiomyocyte width, affecting structural remodelling beyond the anti-tachycardic effect of beta-blockers [57].

2.3. Hemodynamic effects of thyroid hormones

Hemodynamic effects of thyroid hormones are generally nongenomic and faster, by direct effects on the heart and blood vessels. In the peripheral vascular system, the rapid use of oxygen, increased production of metabolic end products and relaxation of arterial smooth muscle fibres by thyroid hormone cause peripheral vasodilatation [21]. This fall in peripheral vascular resistance (PVR) plays the central role in all hemodynamic changes caused by thyroid hormones [58]. Decreased PVR causes an increase in heart rate and selective increase in blood flow of some organs (skin, skeletal muscles, heart), and a fall in diastolic pressure with consequent widening of pulse pressure. Vasodilatation without an increase in renal blood flow causes reduction in renal perfusion and activation of the renin-angiotensin system which causes sodium retention and increased blood volume [59]. In addition, thyroid hormones regulate erythropoietin secretion and increased red cell mass may also contribute to blood volume increase [60]. Improved diastolic relaxation and increased blood volume increased left ventricular end-diastolic volume (LVEDV). Reduced PVR and increased LVEDV means increased preload and decreased afterload, thus the stroke volume increases. Increased stroke volume and increased heart rate leads to a doubling or tripling of cardiac output which cannot be solely explained by the increased metabolic rate of the body [61].

The importance of the contribution of decreased systemic vascular resistance to the increase in systemic blood flow in patients with hyperthyroidism is evidenced by studies in which the administration of arterial vasoconstrictors, atropine and phenylephrine, decreased peripheral blood flow and cardiac output by 34% in patients with hyperthyroidism but not in normal subjects [62,63].

2.4. Clinical aspects of hyperthyroidism and subclinical hyperthyroidism on heart

Increased rate and strength of the heart contractility, together with an exaggerated response of heart rate to exercise is present in hyperthyroid patients who describe this as palpitations. Diurnal heart rate variations are generally preserved. The most common ECG abnormality is sinusal tachycardia and shortened PR interval, and frequently intra-atrial conduction is prolonged, which is seen as increase in P wave duration. Intraventricular conduction delay in the form of right bundle branch block is present in around 15% of patients, and atrioventricular block may also occur due to unknown reasons. The most common rhythm disturbance in hyperthyroid patients is sinus tachycardia [32]. Its clinical impact however is overshadowed by that of patients with atrial fibrillation. The prevalence of atrial fibrillation (AF) and less common forms of supraventricular tachycardia in this disease ranges between 2 to 20 percent [64,65]. AF is generally accompanied by rapid ventricular response. It is more common in men and its significance increases by age, after 40 years [65]. As in the case of angina or heart failure, the development of AF should not be attributed only to hyperthyroidism, and the underlying organic heart diseases should be investigated.

Atrial fibrillation usually reverses to a sinus rhythm by achievement of a euthyroid state, if the patient is younger and the duration of hyperthyroidism is not long. The beta-adrenergic blockade may be effective in controlling the ventricular rate. Increased plasma clearance of beta-blockers may necessitate higher doses [66]. Among them propranolol has the advantage of blocking the conversion of T4 to T3 in peripheral tissues, however other cardioselective beta-blockers have a longer half-life and can be equally effective on the heart. In cardiac arrhythmias intravascular infusion of calcium blockers should be avoided due to the risk of a further fall in PVR [67]. It is still controversial whether the patients with AF should have anticoagulant therapy to prevent systemic embolization. It is advised to evaluate each patient on a case-by-case basis, and determine the risk of bleeding over embolization [68,69]. In younger patients with hyperthyroidism and AF, who do not have other heart disease, hypertension, or independent risk factors for embolization, the risk of anticoagulant therapy may suppress its benefits. But it would be appropriate to administer anticoagulant agents to older patients with known or suspected heart diseases, or AF with longer duration. When oral anticoagulants will be used, it should be considered that hyperthyroid patients will need smaller doses than euthyroid ones, due to faster elimination of vitamin-K dependent clotting factors [70].

In the patients with AF the maintenance of sinus rhythm is not possible until the euthyroid state is restored, so electrical cardioversion is not recommended without confirming the euthyroid status.

Many hyperthyroid patients experience exercise intolerance and exertional dyspnea, in part because of weakness in the skeletal and respiratory muscle [71] and also due to inability to increase heart rate or lower vascular resistance further, as normally occurs in exercise [72]. The tem "high output heart failure" has not been used in recent decades, because it is clear that the heart is still able to increase cardiac output at rest and with exercise. In the setting of low vascular resistance and decreased preload, the cardiac functional reserve is compromised and cannot rise further to accommodate the demands of submaximal or maximal exercise [73]. About 6% of thyrotoxic patients develop heart failure and less than 1% develop dilated cardiomyopathy with impaired left ventricular systolic dysfunction, due to the tachycardia-mediated mechanism leading to an increased level of cytosolic calcium during diastole, with reduced contractility of the ventricle and diastolic dysfunction, often with tricuspid regurgitation [74]. In the recent study of Yue et al, diastolic dysfunction was more prominent in thyrotoxic patients older than 40 years of age, whereas in younger ones marked reduction in peripheral vascular resistance and increased cardiac output were prominent [75].

Hyperthyroidism may complicate or cause pre-existing cardiac disease because of increased myocardial oxygen demand, increased contractility and heart rate, and may cause silent coronary artery disease, anginas or compensated heart failure and even endothelial dysfunction [76]. Treatment of heart failure with tachycardia should include a beta-blocker, by considering its contraindications in each patient. Furosemide may help to reverse the volume overload, but digoxin is less beneficial when compared with euthyroid heart failure patients because there may be relative resistance to its action, due to greater blood volume (distribution) and the need to block more Na-K-ATPase in myocardium [70].

Subclinical hyperthyroidism is a state characterised by low serum thyrotropin levels and normal serum thyroid hormone concentrations. Over recent decades this state has also been found to be associated with some abnormalities in cardiac function. Enhanced systolic function and impaired diastolic function due to slowed myocardial relaxation may cause increased left ventricular mass in these subjects, together with increased heart rate and arrhythmias by similar mechanisms as overt hyperthyroidism [77,78]. In people over 60 years of age subclinical hyperthyroidism was associated with a tripled risk of atrial fibrillation during a 10-year follow-up period [79]. In a recent cross-sectional study with 29 patients, subclinical hyperthyroidism was found to be related with impaired functional response to exercise with low oxygen consumption and exercise threshold, together with slower heart rate recovery [80].

Besides antithyroid treatment strategies, beta-blocker therapy reduces heart rate and improves left ventricular mass, but positive inotropic response persists. This subclinical hyperthyroidism is associated with increased cardiovascular mortality [81]. In the study of Heeringa et al with 1,426 patients, it was shown that even the high-normal thyroid function may increase the risk of AF [82]. Besides increased AF and thromboembolic events, increased left ventricular mass and left ventricular function may be the reason. Thus, it is advised to measure serum thyrotropin in all elderly patients with systolic hypertension, a widened blood pressure, recent-onset angina, atrial fibrillation and any exacerbation of ischemic heart disease and treat it [72,83].

3. Progressive infiltrative ophtalmopathy in hyperthyroidism

3.1. Hyperthyroidism and eye disease

Thyroid eye disease (TED), also called thyroid-associated ophthalmopathy (TAO) and Graves' ophthalmopathy (GO), affects 25–50% of patients with Graves' disease [84]. Regardless of whether hyperthyroidism occurs first, the signs and symptoms of GO become manifest in 85% of patients within 18 months [85]. The clinical features are usually mild. Most common symptoms are; ocular irritation with redness and tearing,, sensitivity to light, double vision, blurring of vision, and feeling a pressure sensation behind the eyes. On physical examination, extraocular muscle dysfunction, proptosis, periorbital and eyelid edema, conjunctival chemos, lid lag and retraction (or stare), or exposure keratitis may be detected [86]. Most patients experience only the minor congestive signs of TAO (chemosis, injection, lid edema), with improvement in several months without treatment. Approximately 28% of TAO cases are severe and symptomatic for several years. Symptoms and signs include, restricted motility leading to diplopia, exposure keratopathy, optic neuropathy and loss of vision [87,88].

TAO can be divided into two clinical stages; congestive and fibrotic. In the congestive or inflammatory stage, auto-immunity leads to inflammatory cellular infiltration of the muscles and transformation of fibroblasts into adipose tissue. The fibrotic stage is characterized by fibrosis which causes proptosis and strabismus [89,90].

3.2. Pathophysiology

In TAO, the most important pathological changes are enlarged extraocular muscles and increased orbital fat. These changes result from a complex interplay among orbital fibroblasts, immune cells, cytokines, auto-antibodies, genetics, and environmental factors [84].

Interactions between orbital fibroblasts, immune cells, cytokines and autoantibodies

Patients with TAO, orbital tissue is infiltrated by inflammatory cells (T helper type 1 (Th1) and T helper type 2 (Th2) lymphocytes, B lymphocytes, mast cells, and macrophages) [91,92]. These cells release cytokines which participate in tissue reactivity and remodeling. Normally, the antigens to which lymphocytes respond are foreign, and several tolerance mechanisms act to prevent the development of reactivity to self-antigens or autoimmunity, but these tolerance mechanisms sometimes fail and autoimmunity develops [93,94]. Fibroblasts are a highly interactive cell type, described as "sentinel cells" [95]. They, respond to immune stimulation and actively participate in the inflammatory pathway [96,97]. In patients with TAO, orbital fibroblasts synthesize excess glycosaminoglycans (GAGs), including hyaluronan. These can differentiate into adipocytes, leading to the accumulation of fat [98]. Orbital fibroblasts do not express the IL-1 receptor antagonist at levels found in other fibroblasts, but also display lymphocyte costimulatory molecules such as CD40. These differentations result in excessively high levels of Cox-2 and PGE_2 in response to proinflammatory cytokines [99,100]. T lymphocytes in the orbital tissue interact with fibroblasts. This interaction results with activation and proliferation of fibroblasts, synthesis of extracellular macromolecules, and differentiation to adipocytes [101]. A summary of this model for the pathogenesis of TED is depicted in Figure 1 [102].

Autoantigen expression by orbital fibroblasts results in T lymphocyte accumulation to the orbit [103]. The autoantigen may be a TSH receptor (TSH-R) or an insulin-like growth factor-1 receptor (IGF-1R) [103,104]. T lymphocytes in the orbital tissue induce fibroblast proliferation and hyaluronan synthesis. This result in orbital tissue remodeling [101]. Stimulation of orbital fibroblasts by T lymphocytes results in production of chemokines (e.g. IL-16, RANTES) and cytokines (e.g. IL-6). These molecules initiate migration of T and B lymphocytes to the orbital tissue and increase fibroblast presentation of autoantigens [97,101,105). Costimulatory molecules, adhesion molecules, and cytokines like IFNγ, IL-1β, and TNFα play an important role in the interaction between T lymphocytes and fibroblasts. One of the communication pathways of T lymphocytes and orbital fibroblasts is the CD40-CD40 ligand pathway [97,100,101]. In TAO orbital fibroblasts express high levels of CD40 [97,106]. Activation by CD40L induces hyaluronan synthesis, IL-6 and IL-8, Cox-2 and PGE2 [97,101,107].

T lymphocyte-mediated activated fibroblasts release factors which promote and activate the proliferation of T lymphocytes. In this way fibroblasts perpetuate inflammation [101,108]. Antonelli et al. found that orbital fibroblasts from TAO patients may modulate the activity of T lymphocytes through the production of CXCL10. Serum CXCL10 levels were higher in active TAO patients than in those with inactive disease. CXCL10 release enhances the migration of T lymphocytes into the orbital tissue. These lymphocytes secrete IFNγ and TNFα. There is a positive feedback between CXCL10 and IFNγ – TNFα. Peroxisome proliferator-activated receptor-gamma (PPAR-γ) activation has an inhibitory role in this process [108]. Feldon et al. found that activated human T lymphocytes drive the differentiation of human fibroblasts to adipocytes. They showed that human T cells, when activated, strongly express Cox-2 and produce PGs, possibly 15d-PGJ_2, that are PPAR-γ ligands and human T cells also produce PGD_2. These findings showed that PGD_2 converts to the PGJ series of PGs with the final product being 15d-PGJ_2, a notable potent PPAR-γ ligand [109-111]. Feldon et al. also showed that human orbital fibroblasts express PPAR-γ and that 15d-PGJ_2, PGD_2, and 15d-PGD_2 strongly induce adipogenesis [109]. Natural and synthetic activators of PPAR-γ stimulate lipid accumulation and the expression and secretion of adiponectin [112,113]. PPAR-γ levels are higher in orbital tissue from patients with active TAO [108,114].

Chen et al. showed higher mRNA levels of a macrophage chemoattractant called C-C motif chemokine ligand-2 (CCL2)/monocyte chemoattractant protein-1 (MCP-1) and dense infiltration with macrophages in the orbital fat compared with normal controls [115].

3.3. Smoking

There is a strong and consistent association between smoking and TAO [116]. But the exact mechanism by which smoking affects TAO is not known. Formation of superoxide radicals and tissue hypoxia could be responsible. Cigarette smoke either contains or can generate a variety of oxidants and free radicals [117]. Orbital fibroblasts can be induced by tissue hypoxia (5% CO_2 and 95% N_2) and superoxide radicals, thus they proliferate and synthesize GAGs [118,119]. Mack et al. cultured orbital fibroblasts, obtained from patients undergoing orbital decompression for severe GO. They showed that, inreased human leukocyte antigen (HLA-DR) expression of orbital fibroblasts occurred in response to nicotine and tar only in the presence of interferon-γ. These findings suggest that there is an interaction between smoking and orbital immune responses [120]. Many studies demonstrated a dose-response relationship between the numbers of cigarettes smoked per day and TAO [121]. Smokers suffer more severe TAO than non-smokers. Smoking increases the progression of TAO after radioiodine therapy for hyperthyroidism [116]. Eckstein et al. demonstrated that smoking influences the course of TAO during treatment in a dose dependent manner. The response to treatment is delayed and considerably poorer in smokers [122]. Pfeilschifter et al. showed that former smokers had a significantly lower risk for the occurrence of proptosis and diplopia than active smokers with a comparable lifetime cigarette consump

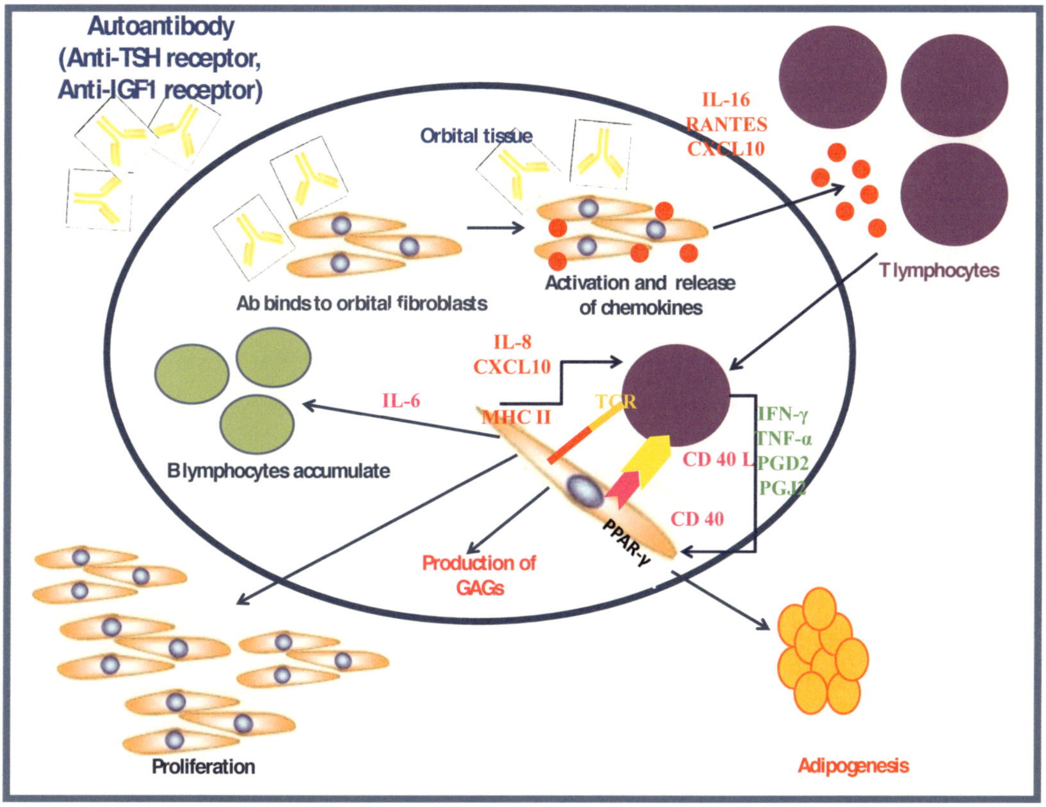

(Data adapted from reference 102)

Figure 1. Pathophysiology of thyroid eye disease

3.4. Genetics

For the development of TAO the presence of autoimmune thyroid disease appears to be necessary, but not sufficient [124]. The interaction between genetic and environmental factors plays a major role for the development of TAO in a patient with autoimmune thyroid disease. TAO and autoimmune thyroid disease share a common etiology; regardless of which occurs first, the other develops within 18 months in 80% of affected patients [125]. Polymorphic variations in individual somatic genes or groups of genes known to be involved in thyroid autoimmunity might also predispose to TAO.

Thymic stromal lymphopoietin (tslp) gene promoter polymorphisms

The role of TSLP in Th17 cell differentiation implicates TSLP in the pathogenesis of TAO. Tsai et al. genotyped 470 patients with TAO at 3 single nucleotide polymorphisms (SNPs) in TSLP and determined the serum concentrations of TSLP in 432 patients and 272 controls. They showed that TSLP polymorphisms are associated with TAO and that expression levels of TSLP are higher in patients than in control subjects. In addition, they concluded that TSLP mediates the differentiation of CD4+T cells into Th17 cells. According to this study the *TSLP* gene may be a relevant candidate gene for susceptibility to TAO. *TSLP* genotypes may be used as genetic markers for the diagnosis and prognosis of TAO [126].

Toll-like receptor gene polymorphisms

Toll-like receptors (TLRs) are a family of pattern-recognition receptors, which play a role in eliciting innate/adaptive immune responses and developing chronic inflammation. Liao et al evaluated 6 TLR-4 and 2 TLR-9 gene polymorphisms in 471 GD patients (200 patients with TAO and 271 patients without TAO) from a Taiwan Chinese population. There was no statistically significant difference in the genotypic and allelic frequencies of TLR-4 and TLR-9 gene polymorphisms between the GD patients with and without TAO. In the sex-stratified analyses they showed that the association between TLR-9 gene polymorphism and the TAO phenotype was more pronounced in the male patients. Their data suggest that TLR-9 gene polymorphisms are significantly associated with increased susceptibility of ophthalmopathy in male GD patients [127].

Polymorphisms of B7 molecules (CD80 and CD86)

Liao et al. evaluated genotypes of CD80 and CD86 polymorphism in GD patients. They found that the frequency of C allele at position rs_9831894 of the CD86 gene is different in patients with GD (with and without TAO). They showed that the G-A haplotype has a protective effect in the development of TAO among patients with GD. Their data suggest that the polymorphisms of the CD86 gene may be used as genetic markers for making the diagnosis and prognosis of TAO [128].

Interleukin-1beta (IL1β) polymorphisms

Recent studies have demonstrated that IL1β plays a role in the development of TAO by inducing adipogenesis and accumulation of GAGs and prostaglandin E2 (PGE2) [129,130]. Liu et al. found that the SNPs rs3917368 and rs1143643 in the 3′ UTR and intron regions of *IL1β* and patients with the genotypes containing both rs3917368 A/A and rs1143643 A/A may bear a higher risk of developing TAO. Thus we can speculate that *IL1β* polymorphisms can be related with the development of TAO in GD [131].

Cytotoxic T lymphocyte antigen-4

Vaidya et al. firstly reported an association between *CTLA-4A/G* polymorphism at codon 17 and TAO [132], but this data was not confirmed by Allahabadia et al. in a larger cohort of patients [133]. Daroszewski et al. evaluated the relation between soluable CTLA-4 level and clinical manifestation of TAO and CTLA-4 gene polymorphisms. They found higher levels of Serum sCTLA-4 in the TAO group than in controls. The level of sCTLA-4 was higher in severe TAO patients than in non-severe cases. They showed for the first time that the presence of the *CTLA-4* gene polymorphisms Jo31 and CT60 were related with elevated sCTLA-4 levels [134]. These data suggest that the polymorphisms of the *CTLA-4* gene may be used as a genetic marker for making the diagnosis and prognosis of TAO. The role of sCTLA-4 and its full-length cell-bound analogue in autoimmunity remains uncertain.

PPAR-γ gene polymorphism

The PPAR-γ transcription factor is involved in both adipogenesis and inflammation which have been implicated in the pathogenesis of TAO. Alevizaki et al. found no difference in the distribution of the Pro(12)Ala PPAR-γ gene polymorphism between GD patients with and without TAO. But they showed that PPAR-γ polymorphism carriers had lower TSH-Rab levels and lower clinical activity scores (CAS). According to this study patients with TAO who have this polymorphism are associated with less-severe and less-active disease [135].

IL-23R polymorphisms

Huber et al. demonstrated that two IL-23R polymorphisms (rs10889677 and rs2201841) were associated with TAO. According to this study we can speculate that these variants may induce TAO by changing the expression and/or function of IL-23R, by promoting a pro-inflammatory signaling cascade [136].

Protein tyrosine phosphatase-22

Lymphoid protein tyrosine phosphatase (LYP, aka PTPN-22) represents another negative regulator of T cell activation. Syed et al. found an association between certain single nucleotide polymorphisms (SNPs) in the protein tyrosine phosphatase (PTP) called PTPN12 and increased risk of mild/moderate ophthalmopathy [137]. But this data should be confirmed in larger studies.

Nuclear factor (NF)-[kappa]B1

Kurylowicz et al. showed a correlation between a polymorphism in the NF-[kappa]B1 gene promoter (-94ins/del adenine, thymine, thymine, guanine) and the development of TAO [138].

Human leukocyte antigen (HLA)

HLA class I-II genes are related for the development of TAO [139]. Akaishi et al. found TAO patients with major extraocular muscle involvement have had a higher frequency of the HLA-DRB1*16 allele, but patients with minor extraocular muscle involvement have had a higher frequency of the HLA-DRB1*03 allele [140]. In another study an association between HLA-A11,-B5,-DW12 and-DR14 and TAO has been found [141,142].

3.5. Cytokines

Autoimmune thyroid disease involves the activation of multiple cytokine networks. Serum IL-6 levels were greater in the patients with TAO than in those without eye disease [143] and both Th1-and Th2-derived cytokines were elevated in TAO patients compared with control samples [144]. Chen et al. found that the exaggerated capacity of orbital fibroblasts to express high levels of both IL-6 and its receptor in an anatomic site-selective manner could represent an important basis for immune responses in TAO [145]. Higher serum levels of IL-17 were obtained in TAO patients than in controls. Serum IL-17 concentration had significant correlation with CAS [146]. Significantly higher PAI-1 [147] and IgE levels [148] were found in TAO patients than in the control groups.

3.6. Imaging procedures in TAO

Ultrasound (US)

US is of primary importance in orbital pathology because of its safety, non-invasiveness, short time of investigation, low cost, lack of radiation and application without need to prepare the patient. In endocrine orbitopathy; the A scan demonstrates echographical widening of the peripheral orbital space and a widening of the muscle echo, while the B scan shows a high internal echo of the connective tissue septa, increased reflection of the muscle belly and distension of the retrobulbar optic nerve sheaths, enlargement of lacrimal gland and dilatation of the superior ophthalmic vein [149]. Although it has many advantages, US cannot effectively display the muscles at the apex of the orbit. US is not as effective as other diagnostic procedures in delineating the relationship of orbital pathology to contiguous structures, nor is it reliable in imaging lesions of either the posterior orbit or those involving the bone walls [150].

Computed tomography (CT)

According to differential X-ray absorption CT can differentiate normal and abnormal structures of different tissue density. In CT orbital fat images as a black, low-density area, while in contrast to this extraocular muscles and the optic nerve image as higher-density areas [151]. The primary areas of orbital involvement are extraocular muscles, and CT findings correlate with clinical impressions of the severity of extraocular muscle enlargement [152]. Muscle involvement on CT of TAO is usually limited to the non-tendonous portion of the muscle. Due to compression of the optic nerve by enlarged extraocular muscles near the orbital apex, optic nerve dysfunction can be seen in TAO [153]. Other findings that may be noted on CT are lachrymal gland enlargement, a dilated superior opthalmic vein, muscle belly enlargement and increase in orbital fat volume [154,55]. CT imaging is a non-invasive, simple, fast, and cost effective imaging procedure. Furthermore, having high sensitivity and correlation with clinical findings, CT imaging should be considered first during diagnostic evaluation of TAO.

Magnetic resonance imaging (MRI)

Pulse sequences that examine T2 in MRI can estimate the water content of tissues. In TAO lymphocytes infiltrate the orbital tissue that causes fibroblast stimulation. Fibroblasts produce large amounts of GAGs. By binding large amounts of water, GAGs cause edema. Increased water content of thickened extra-ocular muscles cause elevated T2 [156]. In TAO there are two different phases with disease activity. Medical treatment can be effective in the active stage. Therefore, for predicting the outcome of medical management the evaluation of disease activity is important. Yokoyama et al. investigated whether MRI could assess the disease activity in TAO. They found that MRI is not only a useful tool for detection of extraocular muscle enlargement, but also for assessment of disease activity in TAO [157]. In conclusion, MRI is useful to assess TAO. But cost and availability are current limitations of this modality. Therefore, MRI should be used for the management of TAO in specialized patients and clinics.

Octreoscan (OCT)

It is thought that radionuclide accumulation is probably due to binding to somatostatin receptors on lymphocytes, myoblasts, fibroblasts and endothelial cells. Another explanation is local blood pooling due to venous stasis by the orbital inflammation [158,159]. Krassas et al. found that OCT positivity is higher in Graves' patients with than in those without ophthalmopathy, and higher in patients with active TAO than in those with inactive TAO [160]. Postema et al. demonstrated that OCT positivity correlates with activity of the TAO such as high CAS [161]. Thus, a positive orbital OCT means clinically active TAO, in which immunosuppressive treatment might be of therapeutic benefit [162]. However, limitations such as cost, non-negligible radiation burden, non-specific examination for TAO, and finally, lack of evaluation of eye muscle swelling restrict the widespread use of this technique [163]. Orbital OCT is mainly indicated to select patients with TAO who will benefit from immunosuppression [162].

3.7. Other diagnostic techniques

Kuo et al. were first described in a positron emission tomography (PET/CT) study in a patient with TAO. The detection of inflammation by 18F-fluorodeoxyglucose (FDG) uptake was sensitive and objectively demonstrable by this semi-quantitative imaging method [164]. García-Rojas et al. carried out the first prospective study. FDG uptake of extra-ocular muscles was statistically different between patients with and without TAO. In cases with TAO where clinical doubt exists, PET/CT provides valuable and useful information for the diagnosis, characterization, and therapeutic decision [165]. Further research is required to define the role of FDG-PET/CT in the management of TAO.

Another tool to measure orbital inflammation is the uptake of radioactively labeled substances, such as ^{67}Gallium (Ga) citrate [166] and ^{99m}Technetium (Tc)-labeled agents [167,168]. In medical literature there are few studies about these nuclear imaging techniques.

3.8. Clinical classification systems

The treatment for TAO varies according to the level of disease activity. Thus, methods have been proposed to determine whether TAO is active (33). There are two main scoring systems [169,170]:

1. NOSPECS (No signs or symptoms; Only signs; Soft tissue involvement with symptoms and signs; Proptosis; Eye muscle involvement; Corneal involvement; Sight loss)

2. CAS (Clinical Activity Score) systems.

Neither NOSPECS nor CAS are both specific and completely reliable, but CAS is a simple office-based tool. The modified NOSPECS criteria include lid retraction, soft tissue inflammation, proptosis, size difference, extra-ocular muscle involvement, corneal defects, and optic nerve compression [169]. CAS demonstrates the presence or absence of seven symptoms or signs that indicate inflammation (Table-1) [171].

The score ranges from 0 to 7, with 0 to 2 characteristics indicating inactive TAO and 3 to 7 characteristics indicating active TAO. The CAS has a high predictive value for the outcome of immunosuppressive treatment in TAO. The main determinant of therapeutic outcome is disease activity, not disease duration [172]. In addition, the severity of disease should be assessed (Table-2). Dysthyroid optic neuropathy, corneal breakdown or both indicate that the TAO is sight-threatening and requires immediate treatment [116].

• Spontaneous retrobulbar pain
• Pain with eye movement
• Redness of the eyelids
• Redness of the conjunctiva
• Swelling of the eyelids
• Swelling of the caruncle
• Conjunctival edema (chemosis)

Table 1. Components of the Clinical Activity Score

• Lid aperture	• Exophthalmos
• Swelling of the eyelids	• Subjective diplopia score
• Redness of the eyelids	• Eye muscle involvement
• Redness of the conjunctivae	• Corneal involvement
• Conjunctival edema	• Optic nerve involvement
• Inflammation of the caruncle or plica	

Table 2. Assesment of Disease Severity

3.9. Management

Smoking and TAO

Patients should be encouraged to quit smoking. In an observational study smoking cessation has been associated with a decreased risk of the development of exophthalmos and diplopia in patients with Graves' disease [171].

Management of hyperthyroidism in patients with TAO

Uncontrolled thyroid functions (both hyper-and hypothyroidism) are related to severe TAO. Patients with hyperthyroidism can be treated with anti-thyroid drugs (ATDs), radioactive iodine (RAI) therapy and surgical therapy. Some different studies have shown improvement in TAO [173] by indirect beneficial effects [174] and a gradual decrease in TSH-receptor antibody (TRAb) levels during ATDs treatment [175]. There are confliciting reports in medical literature about RAI therapy and severe TAO [176,177]. But this association cannot be excluded. This risk can be eliminated by therapy with oral glucocorticoids (GCs) after RAI therapy and avoiding post-treatment hypothyroidism [116]. Thyroidectomy is an effective treatment choice for the definitive cure of hyperthyroidism. Wilhelm et al. showed that near-total/total thyroidectomy is safe and superior to subtotal thyroidectomy for management of hyperthyroidism in Graves' disease [178]. According to the European Group on Graves' Orbitopathy (EUGOGO) Consensus Statement; ATD therapy and thyroidectomy do not affect the course of TAO. No particular ATD or regimen, nor any type of thyroidectomy (subtotal or total) has been demonstrated to have any advantages in terms of outcome of TAO in hyperthyroidism [116].

3.10. Pharmacologic treatments

TAO represents a complex therapeutic problem. Currently available pharmacologic treatment options result in a partial or absent response of the ophthalmopathy. Up to date available treatments for TAO are as follows:

Glucocorticoids

Glucocorticoids (GCs) are effective treatment options in TAO because of their antiinflammatory and immunosuppressive actions (96). Moreover they decrease GAGs synthesis and secretion by orbital fibroblasts [180].

GCs can be administrated by oral, local (retrobulbar or subconjunctival) and intravenous routes. Oral GCs are generally used in high doses (prednisone, 60–100 mg/day or equivalent doses of other steroids) and for long-time periods (several months). It has been demonstrated that high-dose oral GCs are effective on soft tissue changes and optic neuropathy. But when its dose is tapered down and/or withdrawn, recurrence of active eye disease is a frequent problem [181]. In slightly more than 60% of cases (range: 40–100%) favorable effects of high-dose oral GCs are reported. GCs have also been used intravenously. In most studies effects have been observed on inflammatory signs and optic nerve involvement. But the effects on extra-ocular muscle involvement, and especially proptosis, have not been constantly impressive [90].

In most studies patients treated with intravenous GCs have had more favorable results compared with patients treated with oral GCs [18,183]. But in almost all studies treatment with intravenous GCs have been associated with, in the interpulse periods, or followed by (often prolonged) treatment with oral GCs. Moreover there have been biases in patient selections (different degrees of disease activity and duration). Bartalena et al. compared the efficacy and safety of three doses of intravenous (IV) methylprednisolone (2.25, 4.98, or 7.47 g in 12 weekly infusions) in patients with moderate to severe and active TAO. They demonstrated that the use of a cumulative dose of 7.47 g of methylprednisolone provides short-term advantage over lower doses. This benefit was transient and associated with slightly greater toxicity. According to this study we can speculate that an intermediate-dose regimen be used in most cases and the high-dose regimen be reserved to the most severe cases of TAO [184]. Systemic glucocorticoid therapy relates with some side effects and complications. Therefore, local (retrobulbar or subconjunctival) glucocorticoid therapy has been raised. But in most studies local glucocorticoid therapy had been less effective than systemic administration. As a result, local glucocorticoid therapy can be a treatment option in patients with active ophthalmopathy and with major contraindications to the systemic administration [181].

GCs are generally used for severe and active TAO [90]. Furthermore, patients with sight-threatening dysthyroid optic neuropathy should be treated with high-dose intravenous or oral glucocorticoid agents [116]. Additionally, there are some case reports in medical literature, who had severe complicatons related with high-dose glucocorticoid pulse therapy [185].

Somatostatin (SST) analogues

SST receptors (SSTR) are expressed in many tissues, including activated lymphocytes. OCT was proposed as a method to evaluate orbital inflammation in TAO. The use of the SST analog, octreotide, was first reported in TAO patients by Chang et al [186]. Uysal et al. evaluated the effect of octreotide treatment in nine patients with TAO. Seven of the patients showed improvement in CAS. Proptosis improved either slightly or significantly in seven patients. None of the patients has showed deterioration in the eye according to their findings [187]. A major disadvantage of octreotide is its short half-life, which requires multiple injections. To overcome this limitation, new long-acting SST analogs (lanreotide / octreotide-LAR) have been developed. Stan et al. carried out a randomized, double-blind, placebo-controlled trial of octreotide-LAR for treatment of TAO. In octreotide-LAR-treated patients, the CAS improved with a greater degree than in the placebo group. They noted improvement in eyelid fissure width, which suggest that octreotide LAR treatment may be effective in TAO patients with significant lid retraction [188]. In another study Krassas et al. aimed to investigate the orbital Indium-111-pentetreotide activity after treatment with octreotide and lanreotide in patients with TAO. All patients treated with SST analogs had a negative follow-up OCT, whereas controls had a positive OCT. Both NOSPECS score and CAS had improved in the treatment group, but there have been no changes in control subjects [189]. Most common side effects of SST analog therapy in TAO patients were mild gastrointestinal symptoms occurring during the first week of treatment. Because of minimal side effects and proven efficacy, SST analogs could be a treatment option in selected patients. But we need further large, multi-center, prospective and randomized clinical trials and a comparable series of patients with other established treatment options, to achieve more accurate outcomes. In addition, the high cost of this treatment must also be taken into account.

Intravenous immunoglobulins (IVIG)

Antonelli et al. was published as the first non-randomized study on the use of IVIGs for TAO. They treated 7 patients with high-dose IVIGs alone (400 mg/kg/day for 5 consecutive days; the cycle was repeated five times at 3-week intervals) and 7 patients with IVIGs associated with orbital radiotherapy. The results were compared with a historical group of patients previously treated with high-dose GCs and orbital radiotherapy. They found that IVIGs, either alone or combined with orbital radiotherapy, had improved the ocular conditions. This result did not differ from those obtained in the historical group [190]. In a randomized trial by Kahaly et al. 19 patients with active TAO were treated with a 20-week course of oral prednisolone (P, starting dose 100 mg/day), and 21 received 1g immunoglobulin/kg body weight for 2 consecutive days every 3 weeks. The immunoglobulin course was repeated six times. The degree of clinical improvement between two groups was not significant. There was a marked reduction of thyroid antibody titres in the immunoglobulin group. Side effects were more frequent and severe during P than during immunoglobulin therapy [191]. But another study by Seppel et al. failed to show any beneficial effects of IVIGs in TAO [192]. In summary, treatment studies with IVIGs include small numbers of patients and all of them are not randomized. In addition to this, treatment is quite expensive and is related with disease transmission using plasma-derived products. More prospective, randomized and controlled trials, which includes large series of patients are required to obtain more accurate results.

Immunosuppressive drugs

a. Cyclosporine A (CyA): The first report by Weetman et al. showed that CyA had positive effects on ocular-muscle function, visual acuity, exophthalmos and orbital muscle swelling [193]. Prummel et al. compared two groups of 18 patients each of which were treated with either cyclosporine or prednisone. At the end of the study, treatment response was observed in 11 patients treated with prednisone, but only in 4 patients treated with cyclosporine [194]. Weissel et al. treated 8 patients with TAO, all of whom had compressive optic nerve disease (CON), by a combined treatment with CyA and cortisone. CON disappeared completely in all patients [195]. In summary, the use of CyA has been reported in several studies. Given the side effects of CyA, some of which can be severe, it should not be considered as a first-line treatment in TAO. The use of CyA might be maintained in patients who are resistant to GCs alone, and in whom the persistent activity of the disease warrants a continuing medical intervention. According to the recent European Thyroid Association survey CyA or azathioprine were indicated as suitable therapeutic options by only 6% and 2% of respondents respectively [196].

b. Methotrexate (MTX): MTX is not a novel drug, but it has not systematically been evaluated in TAO management. Smith et al. carried out the unique study on the use of MTX for non-infectious orbital inflammatory disorders like TAO. They included 14 patients, and three of them had TAO. All three patients with TAO had an improvement in their ocular conditions after MTX treatment [196] According to the recent European Thyroid Association survey MTX was indicated as a therapeutic option by only 1% of respondents [197]. MTX has many dose-dependent and reversible side effects and should not be used as a first-line treatment. In patients with GC dependency, it can be used at low doses with the aim of reducing the dose of GCs. However, to clarify the effectiveness of MTX in TAO management we need more controlled and randomized prospective studies.

Antioxidants

Bouzas et al. carried out a prospective, nonrandomized, comparative study on the effects of the antioxidant agents allopurinol and nicotinamide in TAO patients. Ocular conditions significantly improved in antioxidant-treated patients, more than placebo-treated patients [198]. Yoon et al. investigated the inhibitory effect of quercetin on inflammation in cultured whole orbital tissue. Quercetin had a significant suppression of tissue IL-6,IL-8, IL-1β and TNFα mRNA expression in cultured orbital tissues from three TAO samples relative to untreated control tissue [199]. Marcocci et al. demonstrated that selenium administration (100 μg twice daily) significantly improved quality of life, reduced ocular involvement, and slowed progression of the disease in patients with mild TAO [200].

There is limited data about treatment TAO with antioxidants. We need larger, prospective and randomized trials to clarify the role of antioxidant agents in the treatment of TAO.

Cytokine antagonists

Chang et al. aimed to determine the effects of pentoxifylline (Ptx); a cytokine antagonist, on fibroblasts derived from patients with Graves' ophthalmopathy. Ptx treatment caused a dose-dependent inhibition of serum-driven fibroblast proliferation and glycosaminoglycan synthesis [201]. Balazs et al. showed that Ptx has had beneficial effects on inflammatory symptoms of TAO and associated laboratory parameters [202]. In another study Ptx has improved the quality of life (QOL) of patients in the inactive phase of TAO [203]. According to these studies Ptx may be an effective and promising drug in the treatment of TAO.

TNF-α antagonists

Paridaens et al. assessed the effect of etanercept on clinical signs in TAO. After treatment the mean CAS and ophthalmopathy index (OI) had decreased significantly. No adverse effects were noted [204]. İnfliximab administration resulted with a significant reduction of inflammation and improvement of visual function without noticeable short-term side effects in two patients with active TAO [205,206]. But randomized prospective clinical trials are needed to obtain whether TNF-α antagonists are effective in reducing the inflammatory symptoms of TAO, and can be administered safely for a long-term period without serious side effects.

Rituximab (RTX)

A patient with TAO, who was unresponsive to steroids, was treated with RTX. The CAS declined from 5 to 2 in 3 months and the patient had peripheral B-cell depletion [207]. When the effect of RTX therapy was compared with IV GCs, RTX had positively affected the clinical course of TAO, independently of either thyroid function or circulating antithyroid antibodies, including TSH receptor antibody [208]. Silkiss et al. demonstrated a statistically significant decrease in CAS from the baseline value. B-cell depletion had been observed and was well tolerated, and there were no adverse effects from the RTX infusions [206]. There is currently insufficient evidence to support the use of RTX in patients with TAO. We need large randomised conrolled trials (RCTs) for investigating the efficacy and safety of RTX versus placebo or corticosteroids in patients with active TAO to make adequate judgement of this novel therapy for this condition

Rapamycin

A case of TAO, with dysthyroid optic neuropathy, who was refractory to steroids and orbital decompression surgery reported. Symptoms, visual acuity, color plate testing, and visual fields of the patient had been improved; despite the prednisone tapering [210]. On the basis the pathogenesis of TAO, rapamycin can be considered as a therapeutic option. But we need more RCTs to assess the efficacy and safety of this drug.

Colchicine

A randomized clinical study showed that colchicine had a beneficial effect on the inflammatory phase of TAO. Therefore, it was equally effective when compared to the classic treatment with corticosteroids, but safer and better tolerated [211]. Due to the lack of controlled trials, it is not clear that these effects were related to the natural history of the ophthalmopathy or to the effects of the drug.

Thalidomide

Thalidomide plays a role in inhibiting adipogenesis of orbital fibroblasts in TAO [212]. Han et al. demonstrated the immunoregulatory effect of thalidomide on peripheral blood mononuclear cells in patients with TAO [213].

Peroxisome proliferator-activated receptor (PPAR) agonists / antagonists

Orbital fibroblasts from patients with TAO have treated with rosiglitazone, and the results suggested that TSHR expression in TAO orbital preadipocyte fibroblasts is linked to adipogenesis [214]. Several case reports of TAO exacerbation following the initiation of PPAR agonists have been reported in the literature [215,216]. These findings suggest that novel drugs which antagonize the PPAR signalling system can also be considered as a treatment option in TAO. The effects of PPAR-γ activation on CXCL10, CXCL9 and CXCL11 secretion in orbital fibroblasts and preadipocytes were evaluated. The inhibitory role of PPAR-γ activation in the process demonstrated [217,218].These studies suggest that PPAR agonists can also be considered as a treatment option in TAO. There are conflicting reports in the medical literature, regarding the use of PPAR agonists and antagonists in the treatment of TAO.

3.11. Radiotherapy

Radiotherapy (RT) is a treatment option in TAO because of its non-specific anti-inflammatory and specific immunosuppressive effects (lymphocytes infiltrating the orbital space are highly radiosensitive) [219]. Moreover RT reduces GAG production by orbital fibroblasts [220]. RT has especially benefical effects on soft tissue changes and optic neuropathy. Unfortunately, in longstanding TAO, the benefical effects for reduction in proptosis and the improvement in ocular motility are not satisfactory [90]. A systematic review and meta-analysis of eight randomized controlled trials showed that, in patients with moderate to severe TAO, RT 20 Gy is a valid therapeutic option which improves lots of ocular symptoms. According to medical literature the dose of 20 Gy can be considered the optimal dose for orbital RT of TAO. The cumulative dose is usually fractionated in 10 daily doses over a 2-week period to reduce the cataractogenic effect [221]. Higher cumulative doses of RT does not improve the effectiveness of treatment [222]. Combined use of GCs and orbital RT was found to be more effective than using either one alone (140). Orbital RT is usually well tolerated. It may be associated with a transient exacerbation of inflammatory eye signs and symptoms, but this is unlikely to occur if GCs are concomitantly administered. Cataract is a possible complication of irradiation to the lens. Radiation retinopathy is an extremely rare complication of RT. Systemic microvascular disease due to diabetes mellitus (DM) or to previous chemotherapy may increase the risk for radiation retinopathy [221].

A major concern about orbital RT is carcinogenecity. In a small cohort of patients treated with RT for TAO, there was no significant evidence of radiation-induced cancer death [224]. Wakelkamp et al. evaluated the frequency of long-term complications of orbital RT for TAO (radiation-induced tumors, cataract, and retinopathy) in comparison with GCs. Mortality has obtained similarly in the irradiated and nonirradiated patients [225]. Haenssle et al. reported pigmented basal cell carcinomas 15 years after orbital RT therapy for TAO [226]. The long-term treatment results seem to be satisfactory. But long-term follow up studies with greater numbers of patients are necessary to examine the risks and benefits more precisely. Orbital radiotherapy, when properly performed, appears to be a safe procedure with limited side effects.

3.12. Plasmapheresis

In the first report by Dandona et al., a patient with Graves's disease with acute progressive exophthalmos was treated with plasmapheresis. Their results has suggested that plasmapheresis could be a useful treatment option in acute and rapidly progressive ophthalmopathy [227]. Glinoer et al. observed significant clinical improvement immediately after plasmapheresis. The most significant effects were on soft tissue involvement, proptosis, intraocular pressure, and visual acuity [228]. In contrast to these, unfavorable effects of plasmapheresis have been reported [229,230]. Trials involving plasmapheresis provided conflicting results. We need RCTs to assess the efficacy and safety of plasmapharesis.

3.13. Total thyroid ablation

According to "shared" antigen(s) theory hypothesis; autoreactive T-lymphocytes which can recognize and interact with one or more antigens shared by the thyroid and the orbital tissue, trigger the event [231]. If this hypothesis is correct, in patients with appropriate genetic background and exposed to relevant environmental risk factors, the presence of thyroid tissue could be related with the development and progression of the ophthalmopathy [232,233]. A progressive decrease and disappearance of circulating auto-antibodies in initially antibody-positive thyroid cancer patients was demonstrated. This observation supports the theory that total thyroid ablation reduces thyroid autoimmunity [234]. Spinelli et al. reported major efficacy in the ophthalmopathy by total thyroidectomy(TT) [235]. De Bellis et al. evaluated the effect of TT alone or followed by post-surgical ^{131}Iodine with respect to methimazole treatment on the activity and severity of TAO. Patients in TT and ^{131}Iodine showed an early significant decrease and a further progressive reduction of the activity and severity of TAO during the follow-up, without statistically significant differences. These studies suggest that TT alone could be an appropriate alternative to improve TAO with a reduction of the cost/benefit ratio [236]. In conclusion, Total Thyroid Ablation (TTA) could be a possible treatment strategy for TAO. Its advantages are; better outcomes in the short term and a shorter period for the improvement of TAO. Because of its costs and risks TTA can not be recommended as a first-line treatment option in TAO.

3.14. Surgical therapy

Orbital decompression

The goal of orbital decompression is to provide increased space for the increased orbital tissue, by removing the bony or fatty components of the orbit. In this way it is effective on proptosis and on the other ocular manifestations. This treatment could not act on the pathogenesis of the diesease. Several techniques have been used to remove portions of one to four walls of the orbit. The decision for which surgical techniques could be used, depends on the experience of the orbit surgeon and the clinical situation of the patient [237].

The studies in the medical literature could not make any meaningful comparisons between the surgical techniques. In the previous studies because of the risks of surgery, orbital decompression has been used in patients with marked proptosis and optic nerve compression, especially if no beneficial effect was obtained with other treatments. But in recent years the indications of orbital decompression has expanded. Garrity et al. reviewed the records of 428 consecutive eye surgery patients at the Mayo Clinic. These were; optic neuropathy, severe orbital inflammation, proptosis, and glucocorticoid side effects [238]. According to the EUGOGO consensus statement on TAO; orbital decompression for exophthalmos (rehabilitative surgery) could be delayed for at least 6 months, until the orbitopathy has been inactive for a period, because surgery yields the best results when TAO is inactive. But in patients with TAO who are intolerant or non-responsive to GCs, orbital decompression can be considered in the active phase. In conclusion, orbital decompression seems to be an effective and safe treatment for patients with TAO [116].

3.15. Medical and surgical recommendations

Bartalena et al. within the EUGOGO consensus statement on TAO, published the set of medical and surgical recommendations shown in Figure 2.

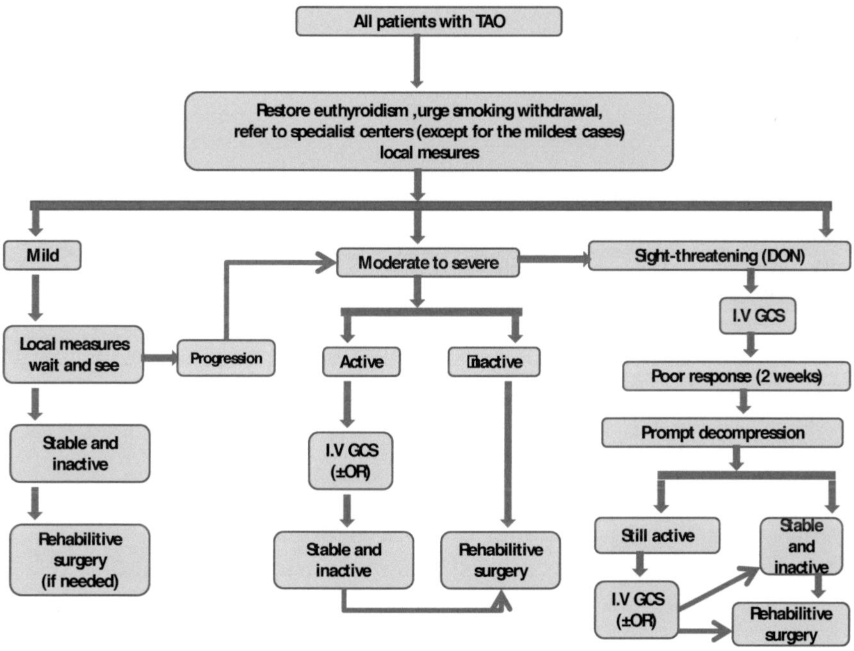

Commentary: Rehabilitative surgery includes orbital decompression, squint surgery, lid lengthening, and blepharoplasty/browplasty. I.V.GCs: intravenous glucocorticoids; OR: orbital radiotherapy; DON: dysthyroid optic neuropathy.

Figure 2. Management of Thyroid-Associated Oophthalmopathy (TAO)

4. Hyperthyroidism and bone

In 1891 Von Recklinghausen firstly described reduced bone mass in untreated hyperthyroidism. Thyroid hormones (3,3',5-triiodothyronine [T3] and 3,3',5,5'-tetra iodothyronine [T4]) act on normal bone growth, development and turnover in both children and adults [239,240]. Hyperthyroidism increases bone turnover, acting mainly on bone resorption, but also on osteoblast activity [241,242] [Figure-3]. As a result, hyperthyroidism is an important etiology of secondary osteoporosis [243].

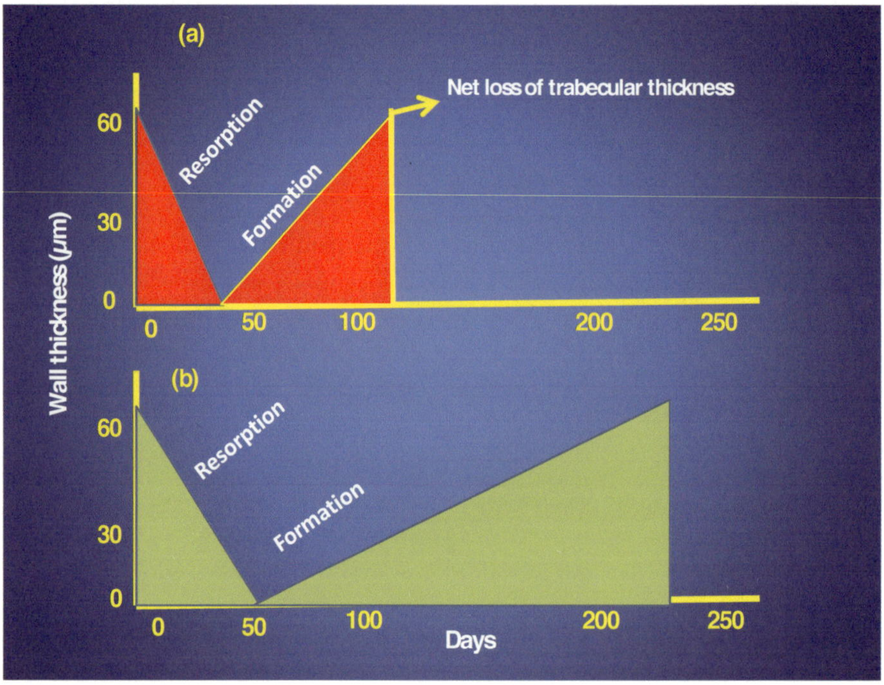

(Data adapted from reference 252).

Figure 3. Trabecular Bone Remoelling Cycle in (a) Hyperthyroid and (b) Normal Subjects

4.1. Mechanism

Direct stimulation of thyroid hormones on bone resorption in organ cultures have been demonstrated [244]. This action may be mediated by a nuclear T3 receptor [245,246]. Thyroid hormones may also affect bone calcium metabolism by a direct action on osteoclasts [247].

Besides the hormones of calcium metabolism, locally produced factors are important in maintaining normal bone metabolism. Serum interleukin-6 (IL-6) concentration increases in hyperthyroid patients and stimulates osteoclast production. Therefore, IL-6 may be an effector of the action of PTH on bone [248]. Thyroid hormones may influence the IGF-I/IGFBP system in vivo in hyperthyroidism. The anabolic effects of increased levels of IGF-I may be limited in hyperthyroidism due to the increases of inhibitory IGFBPs that can counteract the anabolic effects and contribute to the observed net bone loss [249]. T3 activates fibroblast growth factor receptor-1 (FGFR1) in bone and this can be related with the pathogenesis of skeletal disorders resulting from thyroid disease [250].

4.2. Changes in hyperthyroidism

Histological changes in hyperthyroidism

Thyroid hormones increase the activation of new remodeling cycles. These effects include predominantly increased osteoclastic activity. Although; excess osteoblastic activity, osteoid deposition (osteomalacia) and rarefaction (osteoporosis) were also described. These changes were observed both in trabecular and cortical bone ([51]. In 1978 Mosekilde & Melsen demonstrated a unique histomorphometric pattern; with evidence of both increased osteoblast and osteoclast activity in hyperthyroidism. These changes have given rise to a net loss of bone volume and were evident in both cortical and trabecular bone. But cortical bone has been rather more influenced (Figure-4) [252]. An *in-vitro* organ culture of fetal rat bone, demonstrated a direct stimulation of bone resorption by prolonged treatment with T4 or T3 [244].

Biochemical changes in hyperthyroidism

a. Calcium homeostasis in hyperthyroidism

The majority of patients with hyperthyroidism have normal or near normal total serum calcium levels. However, ionized serum calcium levels are elevated in most of the patients. Changes in serum calcium levels correlate with serum T3 levels [253,254]. Generally hypercalcemia in hyperthyroidism tends to be mild or asymptomatic. Severe (>15 mg/dl) and symptomatic hypercalcemia is rare [255]. Hypercalcemia usually resolves after attainment of euthyroid state by all therapeutic modalities, i.e. subtotal thyroid resection, antithyroid drugs and radioiodine therapy. Symptomatic hypercalcemia can be treated by rehydration, use of corticosteroids, calcitonin and phosphate therapy. Reduced renal tubular and intestinal calcium reabsorption leads to increased urinary and fecal calcium [241]. The hyperadrenergic state of hyperthyroidism contributes hypercalcemia [256]. These changes correlate positively with thyroid hormone levels and cortical osteoclastic activity. Hypercalcemia in hyperthyroidism is unrelated to the parathyroid hormone (PTH) levels [253,254].

b. Phosphorous homeostasis in hyperthyroidism

Most of the patients have increased serum phosphorous levels. But some studies have shown normal or low levels of serum phosphorous. Increased bone and tissue catabolisms which lead to excess input of phosphorous to the plasma, lower clearance and increased renal tubular reabsorption of phosphorous may lead to hyperphosphatemia in hyperthyroidism. These changes are related to suppressed PTH levels and direct effects of thyroid hormones. Antithyroid treatment normalizes serum phosphorous concentration [253].

c. Parathyroid hormone secretion in hyperthyroidism

The reduction of serum PTH levels has been reported for the first time by Bouillon and DeMoor [257]. This observation confirmed by other clinical trials. Increased serum calcium levels inhibit

PTH secretion, so there is an inverse relationship between serum PTH and calcium levels. Additionally, serum parathyroid hormone-related peptide (PTH-rP) levels increase in hyperthyroidism. In hyperthyroid patients, a significant elevation in PTH-rP levels was obtained when compared with healthy controls. After treatment, levels of PTH-rP declined. PTH-rP could be a factor in the pathogenesis of hypercalcemia in hyperthyroid patients [258].

d. Vitamin D in hyperthyroidism

Serum concentrations of 25-hydroxyvitamin D_3 (25(OH)D_3)and 1,25-dihydroxyvitamin D_3 (1,25(OH)$_2D_3$) in hyperthyroidism have been evaluated in many clinical trials. In most studies, serum 25(OH)D_3 levels were normal [255,259]. However, few studies in medical literature obtained lower serum 25(OH)D_3 levels in patients with hyperthyroidism than control subjects [260,261]. Karsenty et al. found a higher metabolic clearance rate of 1,25(OH)$_2D_3$ in hyperthyroid patients than in control subjects [262]. These changes in serum concentrations of 25(OH)D_3 and 1,25(OH)$_2D_3$ are probably unrelated with the direct effects of thyroid hormones on bone metabolism. It is postulated that lower levels of serum 25(OH)D_3 and 1,25(OH)$_2D_3$, can be related with reduced intestinal absorption [261]. Biochemical changes in hyperthyroidism are shown in Figure-2.

4.3. Evaluation of bone turnover in hyperthyroid patients and serum markers

Alkaline phosphatase (ALP)

Patients with hyperthyroidism have elevated levels of serum [263]. Total, liver, and bone ALP activities obtained significantly higher in hyperthyroid patients. Bone ALP level are more markedly elevated than liver ALP. Intestinal ALP does not differ significantly between hyperthyroid and normal subjects. These changes correlate positively with thyroid hormone levels. After a euthyroid state is achieved, serum ALP level remains elevated for a prolonged time. This means increased bone turnover continues even after restoration of hyperthyroidism [264].

Other serum markers

Serum pyridinoline (PYD) and deoxypyridinoline (DPD) [265,266]., osteocalcin [267]., carboxy-terminal propeptide of type 1 procollagen (P1CP) and carboxy-terminal telopeptide of type 1 collagen (1CTP) [268]., serum bone Gla protein (BGP) [269]. and serum osteoprotegerin (OPG) [270]. levels were obtained significantly higher in hyperthyroid patients than in control subjects. These laboratory parameters can be considered as reliable non-invasive markers of bone turnover in hyperthyroid patients. All markers were correlated with serum thyroid function tests and were normalized after a eutyhyroid state was achieved.

4.4. Clinical implications

Hyperthyroidism causes reduction in bone mineral density (BMD) assessed by the measurement of lumbar vertebrae and femur by dual energy X-ray absorptiometry (DEXA) [271]. Hyperthyroidism affects bone mineralization especially during the early post-menopausal period and the effect is mainly at the cortical bone [272]. However, hyperthyroidism could be associated with bone loss and may be a risk factor for the development of osteoporosis in pre-menopausal women [273]. It has been well established that hyperthyroidism leads to reduced BMD in female patients, but there is lack of acceptable data in male patients. Majima et al. evaluated BMD and bone metabolism in male patients with hyperthyroidism. The study demonstrated a high prevalence of cortical bone loss in male patients with hyperthyroidism, especially in elderly patients [274].

Also, endogenous subclinical hyperthyroidism can be a risk factor for osteoporosis. In several cross-sectional studies, BMD was decreased at multiple sites in pre-and post-menopausal women with endogenous subclinical hyperthyroidism [275-277]. This finding, however, was not confirmed in other cross-sectional observations in endogenous conditions [278]. Földes et al. demonstrated that numbers of pre-menopausal patients with endogenous sub-clinical hyperthyroidism BMD of the lumbar spine, femoral neck and the midshaft of the radius were not significantly decreased. But in post-menopausal women with long-lasting endogenous sub-clinical hyperthyroidism mean densitometric values were slightly, but significantly, lower [279]. Whether endogenous sub-clinical hyperthyroidism significantly affects bone metabolism and increases the risk of fractures remains controversial.

Prolonged hyperthyroidism due to L-thyroxine(L-T4) treatment has been associated with reduced bone mass and thus with the potential risk of premature development of osteoporosis. The effects of L-T4 treatment have been evaluated in many clinical trials. In several studies, bone mineral density was decreased at multiple sites in pre-and post-menopausal women treated with L-T4 [280,281]. In a study by Giannini et al. post-menopausal thyroidectomized patients showed significantly lower bone mass than pre-menopausal patients. A negative correlation between time since menopause and bone mass were obtained in post-menopausal L-T4 treated patients [282]. There is lack of acceptable data about the effects of L-T4 treatment on bone metabolism in male patients. A mild deleterious effect of thyroid hormone excess in the axial bone mass from male subjects obtained. Male patients with chronic TSH suppression by L-T4 or history of hyperthyroidism should be assessed by BMD [283]. However, several recent studies have failed to show such a harmful effect of L-T4 treatment on BMD [284-286].

It should be noted that other risk factors may affect BMD in hyperthyroid patients. These include a relative deficiency of insulin-like growth factor type I, dehydroepiandrosterone sulfate [287], vitamin D receptor (VDR) polymorphisms [288] and estrogen [289]. The question as to whether prolonged hyperthyroidism due to L-T4 treatment increases the risk of fractures also remains controversial.

4.5. Diagnosis

BMD measuring by DEXA scan is one of the best techniques to obtain the extent of bone changes in hyperthyroidism. DEXA scan offers monitoring for response to therapy and with little radiation it gives very reliable measurements [290]. Quantitative ultrasound (QUS) might give information about bone mass and also on bone elasticity and structure. Advantages are the lower expense, portability, and lack of radiation exposure [291]. Acotto et al. reported significantly lower QUS parameters in hyperthyroid patients in comparison with controls

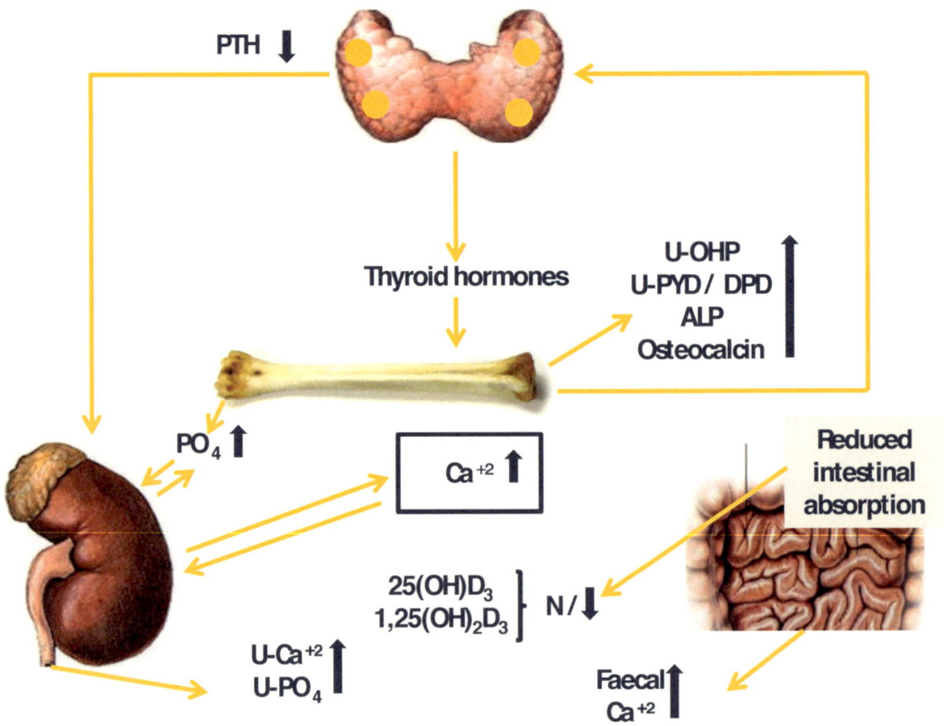

Abbreviations are as follows: calcium (Ca), alkaline phosphatase (ALP), 25 hydroxy vitamin D_3 (25 OH D), 1,25 dihydroxy vitamin D_3 (1,25 $(OH)_2D_3$), 24,25 dihydroxy vitamin D3 (S-24,25 (OH)2D), parathyroid hormone (PTH), phosphate (PO4), urinary calcium (U-Ca), urinary hydroxyproline (U-OHP), urinary phosphate (U-PO_4), urinary pyridinium and deoxypyrodinoline (U-PYD/DPD). (Data adapted from reference 292).

Figure 4. Biochemical Changes in Hyperthyroidism.

[292]. For practical use, the development of quality standards and criteria for diagnosing osteoporosis are necessary.

Prevention and treatment of reduced bone density

Patients with a history of hyperthyroidism and who are treated with L-T4 replacement/ supressive therapy should be considered at higher risk of reducing BMD and developing clinically significant osteoporosis. These patients should be encouraged to modify other risk factors for osteoporosis such as smoking, drinking excessive alcohol, low Ca^{+2} intake and lack of exercise [293]. In these patients adequate daily calcium intake should be provided. Kung et al. found that 1,000 mg. daily calcium supplementation prevents bone loss in post-menopausal women taking suppressive doses of L-T4 compared with a placebo [294]. Estrogen replacement therapy prevents a decrease of BMD in postmenopausal women with previous hyperthyroidism and subsequent L-T4 therapy [295,296]. These potentially beneficial effects of estrogen replacement on BMD in postmenopausal women with a history of thyroid disease suggests that estrogen administration should be encouraged in this group.

Titration of suppressive therapy to maintain serum TSH concentration between a slightly low (*e.g.* between 0.1-0.5 mU/l) range may prevent bone loss [297]. Guo et al demonstrated a reduction of L-T4 dose in post-menopausal women with suppressed serum TSH levels related with deceleration of bone turn over (serum osteocalcin and urinary excretion of bone collagen-derived pyridinium cross-links decreased) and increased BMD (lumbar/femoral) [298]. Careful titration of L-T4 dosage to maintain biochemical euthyroidism is the most important way to prevent the adverse effect of T4 on bone.

The major question is whether the decrease in BMD caused by hyperthyroidism can be reversible. Many clinical trials have obtained that there is some reversibilty of bone mass after treatment of hyperthyroidism [293,299-301]. Another question is whether antiresorptive treatment is effective on hyperthyroidism related osteoporosis. Two clinical trials evaluated the increase of BMD in osteoporotic/osteopenic hyperthyroid patients treated with only anti-thyroid drugs versus patients treated with anti-thyroid drugs and alendronate. The combination of anti-thyroid drugs and alendronate was found to be more efficacious than anti-thyroid therapy alone [302,303]. Majima et al. evaluated the efficacy of risedronate for the treatment of osteoporosis/osteopenia in patients with Graves' disease. The percentage increases in BMD at the lumbar spine and distal radius were significantly greater in patients treated with an anti-thyroid drug and risedronate than treated with an anti-thyroid drug only [304]. These findings conclude that bisphosphonates can be considered as a treatment option in decreased bone mass cases associated with hyperthyroidism. Kung et al. demonstrated intranasal calcitonin with calcium supplements was not more effective than calcium supplements alone in preventing bone loss induced by thyroxine suppressive therapy in post-menopausal women [305]. Jódar et al. designed a prospective study to evaluate the effects of antiresorptive therapy with nasal salmon calcitonin (CT) in hyperthyroid patients receiving standard medical treatment. They showed that treatment with nasal CT has no additional beneficial effect compared with the attainment of the euthyroid state [306]. But in another study by Akçay et al. the addition of intranasal calcitonin to the anti-thyroid drugs was found to be effective in preventing the degradation of bone [307]. More prospective, randomized and controlled trials, which include large series of patients, are required to obtain more accurate results about antiresorptive treatment in hyperthyroidism.

5. Thyroid storm

Thyroid storm (TS) [thyrotoxic crisis] is an uncommon, life-threatening condition reflecting the augmentation of the manifestations of thyrotoxicosis. Mortality rates are high (10-20%) and occur in less than 10% of patients hospitalized for thyrotoxicosis. TS occurs nine to ten times more commonly in women than in men, and the most common aetiology is Graves' hyperthyroidism. However, any aetiology of thyrotoxicosis can cause TS. This situation can be precipitated by a number of factors shown in Table-3 [308-312].

The pathophysiology of thyroid storm is not fully understood. The current theory is that; increased numbers of catecholaminergic receptors being exposed to increased catecholamine levels in states of stress. Decreased binding to thyroxine-binding globulin (TBG), markedly increase in free thyroid hormone levels may also play an important role [313].

• **Severe infections (pulmonary)**	• Direct trauma or surgical manipulation of the thyroid gland
• **Diabetic ketoacidosis (DKA)**	• Biological agents such as interleukin-2 and α-interferon
• **Surgery**	• Discontinuation of anti-thyroid medications or poor patient adherence to the treatment
• **Trauma**	• Cerebrovascular disease
• **Pulmonary thrombo-embolism**	• Myocardial infarction (MI)
• **Salicylates ***	• Exogenous thyroid hormone intake
• **Administration of large quantities of exogenous iodine ****	• Pregnancy
• **Radioactive iodine therapy**	• Unknown factors

*They increase the concentration of circulating free thyroid hormones to critical levels

**Such as iodinated contrast agents or amiodarone

Table 3. Precipitating Factors for Thyroid Storm

Clinical presentation of thyroid storm

Symptoms of thyroid storm are similar to those of hyperthyroidism, but they are more sudden, severe and extreme. The main findings are high fever (38-41° C) accompanied by excessive sweating and flushing. Other common symptoms include; altered mental status (confusion, agitation, overt psychosis, and in extreme cases, even coma), cardiovascular complications [tachycardia, cardiac arrhythmias (including atrial fibrillation), high systolic bood pressure, low diastolic bood pressure and congestive heart failure], diffuse muscle weakness, tremor or fasciculations and neuropsychiatric syndromes. Gastrointestinal involvement presents with nausea, vomiting, diarrhoea and abdominal pain. Liver dysfunction (cardiac failure with hepatic congestion or hypoperfusion, direct effect of the excess thyroid hormones) could be present with jaundice [309,314]. Elderly patients often present with apathy, stupor, cardiac failure, coma and minimal signs of thyrotoxicosis so-called apathetic thyroid storm [313].

The scoring system suggested by Burch and Wartofsky (Table 4) illustrates the typical features of thyroid storm [315]. The clinical symptomatology is sometimes difficult to distinguish from other medical emergencies [308]. Differential diagnosis of TS is shown in Table-5.

5.1. Diagnosis

Diagnosis depends on primarily clinical findings. There are no specific laboratory tests available. Serum thyroid hormone levels (i.e. free T3 [FT3] and free T4 [FT4]) are elevated with suppressed TSH levels (with the rare exceptions being states of thyroid hormone resistance or TSH secreting pituitary adenomas). An immediate search should begin for precipitating factors. Pregnancy should be excluded urgently in any woman of childbearing age with urinary or plasma assessment of human chorionic gonadotropin (HCG) levels. Routine

http://dx.doi.org/10.5772/58196

Clinical feature	Scoring points
1. Thermoregulatory dysfunction	
Temperature °F (°C)	
99-99.9 (37.2-37.7)	5
100-100.9 (37.8-38.2)	10
101-101.9 (38.3-38.8)	15
102-102.9 (38.9-39.4)	20
103-103.9 (39.5-39.9)	25
≥104 (40)	30
2. Cardiovascular dysfunction	
• *Tachycardia (beats per minute)*	
<99	0
99-109	5
110-119	10
120-129	15
130-139	20
≥140	25
• *Congestive heart failure*	
Absent	0
Mild (Pedal oedema)	5
Moderate (Bibasal rales or crackles)	10
Severe (Pulmonary oedema)	15
• *Atrial fibrillation*	
Absent	0
Present	10
3. Central nervous system dysfunction	
Absent	0
Mild (Agitation)	10
Moderate (Delirium, psychosis, extreme lethargy)	20
Severe (Seizures, coma)	30
4. Gastrointestinal-hepatic dysfunction	
Absent	0
Moderate (Diarrhoea, nausea/vomiting, abdominal pain)	10
Severe (Jaundice)	20
5. Previous episode of thyroid storm	
Absent	0
Present	10
TOTAL	
>45	Highly likely thyroid storm
25-44	Suggestive of impending storm
<25	Unlikely to represent storm

Table 4. Diagnostic Criteria for Thyroid Storm

biochemical tests, urinalysis, urine sediment, complete blood count, chest X-ray and related cultures should be made, to exclude infectious diseases. Electrocardiography (ECG) and cardiac enzymes should be procured, to exclude arrhythmia and myocardial infarction (MI) [313]. Leukocytosis, increased transaminase-bilirubin levels, hypoglycemia and lactic acidosis can be seen in laboratory evaluation [316,317].

Neurolept malignant syndrome	Hypertensive encephalopathy
Malignant hyperthermia	Alcohol withdrawal
Phaeochromocytoma	Benzodiazepine / barbiturate withdrawal
Hypoglycemia	Opioid withdrawal
Hypoxia	Heat stroke
Sepsis	Encephalitis / meningitis

Table 5. Differential Diagnosis of Thyroid Storm

5.2. Management

The patient should be managed in an intensive care unit. ABCDEs (i.e. airway; breathing; circulation; disability, i.e. conscious level; and examination) should be provided as soon as possible. Precipitant factors such as infection, trauma, MI, DKA, and other underlying processes should be managed as per standard care [313].

General supportive care

First of all haemodynamic stability should be provided. Supportive care includes cooling measures, intravenous (IV) fluid-electrolyte replacement and nutritional support. In order to control profound pyrexia cooling blankets and acetaminophen can be used. Salicylates should be avoided (increase the concentration of circulating free thyroid hormones). Tachyarrhythmias, which cause haemodynamic instability should be managed with cardioversion by defibrillation. Otherwise, tachyarrhythmias can be managed with appropriate anti-arrhythmic therapy. Diuretics, ACE inhibitors and digitalis can be used carefully for heart failure. Based on arterial blood gas (ABG) analysis and other assessments; ventilatory support, either with non-invasive positive pressure ventilation (NIPPV) or intubated ventilation, could be performed. In patients with severe agitation, medical intervention could be difficult. Sedatives such as haloperidol or a benzodiazepine can be used in this situation. Phenobarbital increases peripheral metabolism and inactivation of FT3-FT4. Chlorpromazine has the additional benefit of reducing body temperature through effects on central thermoregulation. However, these agents should be monitored for respiratory side effects. Nutritional support is important. This includes vitamin (e.g. thiamine) and glucose replacement (as liver glycogen stores are depleted during a thyroid storm) [313].

Thyroid-specific therapy

Thyriod-specific therapy includes; decreasing thyroid hormone synthesis, prevention of thyroid hormone release and decreasing peripheral action of circulating thyroid hormones [318]. In the treatment of thyroid storm, the five B's should be kept in mind. This includes 'Bs':

Block synthesis (i.e. antithyroid drugs); Block release (i.e. iodine); Block T4 into T3 conversion (i.e. highdose propylthiouracil [PTU], propranolol, corticosteroid and, rarely, amiodarone); Betablocker; and Block enterohepatic circulation (i.e. cholestyramine) [313].

Anti-thyroid drugs include PTU or carbimazole (or methimazole). PTU was preferred because of its more rapid onset of action, short half-life and inhibition of peripheral deiodinase enzyme-mediated conversion of T4 into T3. PTU could be administered orally or via a nasogastric (NG) tube, if the patient is not suitable for oral administration, both PTU and methimazole can be given as a rectal suppository or enema. PTU is administered with a loading dose of 600mg followed by a dose of 200-250 mg every 4-6 hours. Carbimazole (or methimazole) is administered at a dose of 20-30mg every 4-6 hours [318]. The major concern about PTU is hepatoxicity. In the thyroid storm management, there are not any comparative trials showing superiority of PTU over either carbimazole or methimazole. It's now recommended that using either carbimazole or methimazole in thyroid storm (unless there is a contra-indication such as pregnancy), and achieving T4 into T3 conversion inhibition just with beta-blockers and corticosteroids [319].

Iodine should be administered at least 1 hour after PTU or carbimazole (or methimazole) administration. In this way undesired tyrosine residue iodination and enrichment of thyroid hormone stores could be prevented. Iodine could be administered in various formulations (Table-6) [313].

In order to block the adrenergic effects of thyroid hormones betablockers should be administered immediately. A non-cardiac specific betablocker; propranolol can be used for this purpose. Propranolol has the advantages of being suitable for IV administration and of inhibition of peripheral T4-T3 conversion at high doses. Decompensated cardiac function, triggered with tachycardia, can be treated with beta-blockers. However, beta-blockers should be used with caution in patients with a history of heart failure. Cardioselective beta-blockers such as metoprolol or atenolol could be used in patients with asthma and chronic obstructive pulmonary disease, which are contra-indications for non-cardiac specific betablockers. If unfavorable cardiac effects are expected, a short-acting beta-blocker; esmolol, can be used as an alternative drug. Diltiazem, a calcium-channel blocker, can be used when there is absolute contra-indication for beta-blockers (Table-6) [313].

Thyroid hormones accelerate cortisol metabolism and may trigger an adrenal crisis. Thyroid crisis give rise to low plasma levels of ACTH and cortisol. Therefore, against a possible adrenal insufficiency, exogenous corticosteroid therapy should be administered [320]. Furthermore, corticosteroids inhibit peripheral conversion of T4 into T3 and have been shown to improve outcomes in patients with thyroid storm [318]. Hydrocortisone or an equivalent corticosteroid can be used for this purpose (Table-6). Then, the treatment should be withdrawn gradually, based on the required duration of steroid therapy.

Other possible treatment options are lithium carbonate, potassium perchlorate and cholestyramine. Lithium inhibits thyroid hormone release from the gland and reduces iodination of tyrosine residues. Lithium carbonate can be an alternative treatment option when there is a contraindication or previous toxicity history to thionamide therapy. The major concern about lithium carbonate is it's toxicity. Potassium perchlorat inhibits iodide transport into the thyrocyte [313]. Erdogan et al. demonstrated that the combination of thionamides, corticosteroids and potassium perchlorat for a short period could be effective in the treatment of amiodarone-induced thyrotoxicosis [321]. The most important side effects of potassium perchlorat are aplastic anaemia and nephritic syndrome. To inhibit the enterohepatic circulation of thyroid hormones, a T4 and T3 binding resin, cholestyramine can be used [322].

Emerging treatments

In spite of all treatment approaches, clinical improvement could not be obtained. In this situation, different treatment approaches can be tried in order to remove thyroid hormones from the circulation.

Plasmapheresis should be considered as a treatment option, especially when patients have failed or cannot tolerate conventional therapy. Plasmapheresis leads to amelioration of symptoms and a significant decline in thyroid hormone levels, providing a window to treat definitively with thyroidectomy [323,324]. In each session only small amounts of thyroid hormones can be removed from the circulation, therefore plasmapharesis can be repeated. Koball et al. reported a case of thyrotoxic crisis treated with plasmapheresis and single pass albumin dialysis. Thyroxine can be bound by albumin and removed by extracorporeal single-pass albumin dialysis (SPAD). The patient underwent two sessions of plasmapheresis without clinical response. After four SPAD treatments clinical status of the patient improved. According to this report SPAD represents a safe and efficient alternative to plasmapheresis [325].

Charcoal haemoperfusion has also been demonstrated to be effective in thyrotoxic states [326].

6. Thyrotoxic hypokalaemic periodic paralysis

Hyperthyroidism can be related with muscular disorders such as acute and chronic thyrotoxic myopathies, exophthalmic ophthalmoplegia, myasthenia gravis, and periodic paralysis [327]. The association between thyrotoxicosis and periodic paralysis was first described by Rosenfeld in 1902. Thyrotoxic hypokalaemic periodic paralysis (THPP) is a rare condition which occurs in 2% of patients with thyrotoxicosis. THPP is generally sporadic, but autosomal recessive or autosomal dominant cases have been reported and may be associated with certain HLA haplotypes [HLA-Bw46 / B5 / DRw8 / CW7] [328-330]. THPP has been reported in many ethnic groups such as Asian populations and Caucasians [331]. THPP appears almost exclusively (85%) in young men between the ages of 20-39 [327].

Many aetiological factors that can lead to hyperthyroidism may be associated with THPP. It has been reported that the most important aetiologic factor is Graves' disease according to large case series [332,333]. Other possible aetiological factors are subacute thyroiditis, silent thyroiditis [334], autonomously functioning thyroid nodules [335], thyrotropin-secreting pituitary adenomas [336,337], ingestion of excessive thyroxine [338], thyroxine-containing herbal and dietary supplements [339], iodine induced thyrotoxicosis with inadvertent use of iodine or with drugs containing iodine such as iodinate contrast agents or amiodarone

Medication	Dose	Notes
Inhibition of hormone synthesis		
Propylthiouracil (PTU)	600mg loading dose, followed by 200-250mg PO q4-6h	Additional inhibition of peripheraldeiodination However, recent warning from FDA regarding severe liver toxicity with PTU makes either carbimazole or methimazole first-choice thionamide
Carbimazole (or methimazole)	20-30mg PO q4-6h	
Inhibition of hormone release		
Potassium Iodide	5 drops PO q6-8h	Administer at least 1 hour after thionamide
Lugol's Solution	5-10 drops PO q6-8h	Administer at least 1 hour after thionamide
Iapanoic Acid	1000mg IV q8h for 24 h, followed by 500mg bd	Administer at least 1 hour after thionamide, infrequently available
Inhibition of peripheral effects of excess thyroid hormone		
Propranolol	1-2 mg/min IV q15min up to max 10mg 40-80mg PO q4-6h	IV dose initially if haemodynamically unstable
Esmolol	50 mg/kg/min IV -may increase by 50 mg/kg/min q4min as required to a max of 300 mg/kg/min.	Short acting
Metoprolol	100mg PO q6h	Cardioselective; use if known airways disease
Diltiazem	60-90mg PO q6-8h	Use if beta-blockers contraindicated IV formulation available
Supplementary management		
Hydrocortisone	100mg IV q6h	
Dexamethasone	2mg IV q6h	Care if significant hepatic dysfunction
Acetaminophen	1 g PO q6h	
Additional therapies		
Lithium Carbonate	Carbonate 300mg PO q8h	Monitor for toxicity
Potassium perchlorate	1 g PO od	Associated with aplastic anaemia
Cholestyramine	4 g PO q6-12h	and nephritic syndrome

PO, oral; IV, intravenous; q4-6h, every 4_6 hours; q6h, every 6 hours; q8h, every 8 hours; q4min, every 4 minutes; q15min, every 15 minutes;od, once daily; bd, twice daily.

(Data adapted from reference 313)

Table 6. Medical Management of Thyroid Storm

[340,341], interferon-alpha-induced thyrotoxicosis [342] and radioactive iodine therapy induced radiation thyroiditis [343]. Many precipitating factors can trigger THPP attacks (Table-7) [344-346].

Carbohydrate-rich meal	Cold
Strenuous exercise	Alcohol
Awakening in the middle of sleep	Glucocorticoids
Emotional stres	Injection of medicine
Radioactive iodine treatment	Upper respiratory tract infection
Menses	Trauma
Epinephrine	Insulin

Table 7. Precipitating factors

The pathophysiology of THPP is not certain. However, it can be explained by some mechanisms (Figure-5). A quick shift of potassium from the extracellular compartment to the intracellular compartment causes hypokalemia. This especially occurs in the muscles. Excess thyroid hormone and insulin levels, increased sensitivity of beta-receptors to catecholamines in thyrotoxicosis causes an increase in sodium/potassium-adenosine triphosphatase (Na/K-ATPase) pump activity [347,348]. This mechanism explains insulin and epinephrine induced paralytic attacks. Factors related with an increased insulin and epinephrine levels, such as carbohydrate rich meals, emotional stress, cold, trauma and infection trigger THPP. During exercise K releases from the skeletal muscles, but in the resting process K again returns to the intracellular compartment. Because of this transport of the potassium, periodic and paralytic attacks usually occur during resting time [349].

6.1. Clinical features

THPP attacks mostly occur in the late night or early morning and last from a few hours up to several days. Prodromal symptoms such as aches, cramps and stiffness can be seen [334]. The typical motor involvement in THPP begins from the lower limbs and ascends to the upper limbs. The muscles affected may be asymmetrical. The severity of attacks range from mild weakness to flaccid paralysis. Clinical improvement starts from the most recently affected muscles. Sensory function is not affected and deterioration of mental functions has never been seen [327]. Paralysis of respiratory, bulbar, and ocular muscles has been rarely reported in severe attacks of THPP. Respiratory muscle involvement can be fatal [350]. Deep tendon reflexes are markedly diminished or absent. Patients completely recover between the attacks [348].

6.2. Laboratory features

The cardinal laboratory finding in THPP is hypokalaemia. But normokalaemic TPP have been reported in some cases [351,352]. Severe hypokalaemia may trigger life-threatening arrhythmias and the severity of paralysis correlates with the degree of hypokalemia but not with the

http://dx.doi.org/10.5772/58196

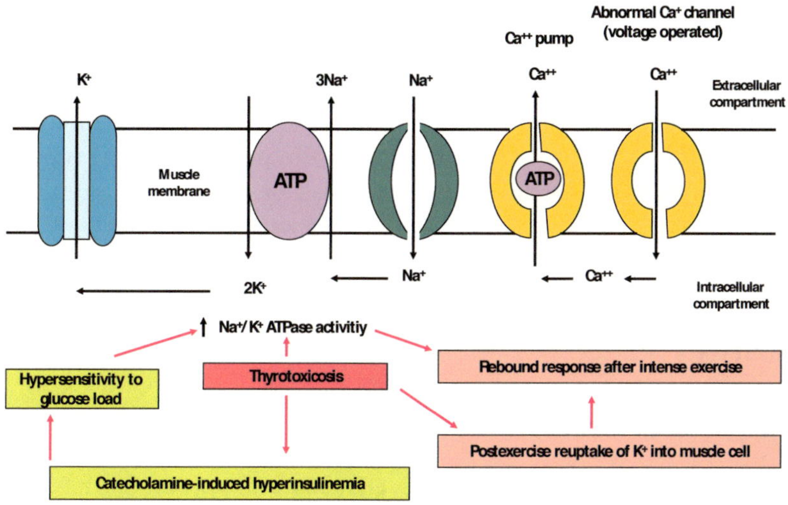

Figure 5. Pathophysiology of THPP

thyroid hormone level. Therefore the degree of hypokalaemia is important [353,354]. Hypophosphataemia and hypomagnesaemia could be obtained in THPP [332]. Hypokalemia can cause vasoconstriction in muscle arterioles and may lead to ischemic changes in sarcolemma. Thus hypokalaemia causes rhabdomyolysis [355]. Besides hypokalaemia, hypophosphataemia [356] and hyperthyroidism alone may cause rhabdomyolysis [357]. As a result of rhabdomyolysis, serum creatine phosphokinase (CPK) level increases [332,358]. ECG changes in THPP vary from nondiagnostic to those showing typical features of hypokalaemia and serious ventricular arrhythmias. Other possible ECG changes include rapid heart rate, high QRS voltage, and first-degree atrioventricular block [359,360].

6.3. Management

In cases of acute attacks of THPP immediate restoration and close monitoring of serum potassium is important. Potassium replacement can be done in two ways; oral or intravenous. Intravenous potassium has significant superiority to the oral route in the improvement of the clinical findings and it is the major choice if the patient shows signs of cardiac dysrhythmia, respiratory distress or is unable to take oral medications. Potassium replacement should not exceed 90 mEq/24h because of the possibility of rebound hyperkalemia [327,344,361]. A non-selective beta-blocker, propranolol, increases serum potassium and phosphate concentrations and ameliorates paralysis [362].

THPP does not disappear completely unless patients become euthyroid. Thus, the management of hyperthyroidism is the mainstay of therapy. Permanent treatment is so important and could be done by antithyroid drugs, radioiodine therapy or surgery [348]. Although glucocorticoids (GCs) have been used to treat hyperthyroidism, they have detrimental effects on insulin sensitivity. Thus GCs can mimic this physiologic process and induce attacks. Physicians should be aware of the risk of triggering THPP when using high-dose GCs in the thyrotoxic phase [363]. To prevent recurrence of attacks, precipitating factors should be avoided.

The use of propranolol is important during early treatment with anti-thyroid drugs or after radioactive iodine when the euthyroid status is not yet achieved. Propranolol also reduces the frequency and severity of attacks. If the patient's serum potassium level is between normal ranges, prophylactic potassium supplementation is not effective to prevent the attacks. Acetazolamide may worsen the attacks in THPP and should be avoided [364,365].

7. Thyrotoxicosis related psychosis and convulsion

7.1. Hyperthyroidism and central nervous system

The brain, particularly the limbic system (amygdala and hippocampus), has a large number of Tri-iodothyronine (T3) receptors. These receptors affect a variety of functions such as emotion, behavior, and long term memory [366]. Excess thyroid hormones affect neurotransmitters such as serotonin, dopamine, or second messengers. This could be a possible explanation for the relation between neuropsychiatric symptoms and hyperthyroidism [367]. Evidence suggests that the modulation of the beta-adrenergic receptor response to catecholamines in the central nervous system by thyroid hormones in thyrotoxic patients, may contribute to psychotic behavior [368].

As a result, people with thyroid dysfunction could be presented with a wide variety of neuropsychiatric symptoms such as anxiety, irritability, unstable mood, fatigue, insomnia, dementia, confusion state, depression, thyrotoxic crisis, seizures, pyramidal signs, chorea, attention deficit-hyperactivity disorder, sleepwalking (somnambulism)and Hashimoto's encephalopathy. "Apathetic thyrotoxicosis" is an unusual presentation of hyperthyroidism, characterised by depression, psychomotor slowing and apathy and occurring mostly in the elderly [369-371].

7.2. Psychosis

More than 150 years ago, von Basedow first described a psychotic illness, probably mania, in a patient with exophthalmic goitre [372]. More recent case reports have emphasised depressive [373], manic [374], paranoid [375] and schizophreniform features [372]. But psychotic reactions as the presenting feature of thyrotoxicosis is extremely rare, it was reported in 1% of cases and most patients who develop psychosis have been previously diagnosed with mania and/or delirium [376]. The occurrence of psychosis depends on the severity and duration of thyroid disease and the underlying predisposition of the individual to psychiatric instability [377].

Most of the cases caused by thyrotoxicosis or hyperthyroidism have been described in patients with Graves' disease or toxic multinodular goiter. Therefore, transient thyroiditis or factitious thyrotoxicosis can be related with neuropsychiatric symptoms, including organic psychosis [378]. Only one case each of postpartum thyroiditis [379] and subacute thyroiditis [377] have been reported related with psychosis. The relations between thyroid autoimmunity and anxiety disorders have been reported [380].

But it should be noted that psychiatric disorders can trigger hyperthyroxinemia [381]. Differential diagnosis between the two conditions is important. In such cases the TSH level is usually in the upper "normal" range and free thyroxine elevation is modest and transient and is usually seen within 1 week. This entity has not been established clearly, but may be considered a form of non-thyroidal illness [382].

7.3. Management

Treatment of hyperthyroidism by standard anti-thyroid drugs (propylthiouracil, methimazole, carbimazole) results with improvement in mental and cognitive symptoms. Psychiatric improvements parallel with improvements in endocrine symptoms. Trzepacz et a.l also showed that a similar improvement both in psychiatric and endocrine symptoms by two weeks of propranolol treatment could be obtained [383,384].

Because of their slow onset of action and potential toxicity, psychotropic drugs (lithium, benzodiazepines, antidepressants and antipsychotics) are not recommended as the primary treatment option for neuropsychiatric symptoms caused by hyperthyroidism. Dopamine receptor blockade with an antipsychotic such as haloperidol can be used in patients with severe neuropsychiatric symptoms. If there is an exhibited psychiatric disease before hyperthyroidism, β-adrenoceptor antagonists may not be effective and neuropsychiatric symptoms may remain after euthyroidism has been achieved, in which case psychotropic drug treatment should be given. Selective serotonin reuptake inhibitors, lithium and benzodiazepines can be used for the treatment of neuropsychiatric symptoms [366].

If therapy fails with the above-mentioned options, more radical approaches such as radioactive iodine ablation and thyroidectomy should be considered [377,385].

7.4. Convulsion

Seizures in hyperthyroidism have rarely been reported in medical literature. Most of the cases were related with Graves' hyperthyroidism [386-388]. Other aetiologic factors were massive levothyroxine ingestion [389], L-thyroxine treatment for hypothyroidism [390,391], subclinical hyperthyroidism [392] and Hashimoto's encephalopathy (HE) [393,394]. The pathophysiology of HE is not clear but increased antithyroid antibodies in all affected patients supports an autoimmune etiology. Generally, patients in medical literaure were euthyroid or hypothyroid. But Sakurai et al reported a case of HE associated with Basedow's disease presented with hyperthyroidism. Another possible aetiologic factor for seizures in hyperthyroidism may be superior sagittal sinus (SSS) thrombosis. Hyperthyroidism may cause hypercoagulabilty, venous stasis and could be related with thrombosis. All cases of seizures in SSS thrombosis in medical literature were known cases of hyperthyroidism [395-397].

The certain incidence of seizures in hyperthyroidism is still unknown. Song et al. recently informed a 0.2% prevelance in a retrospective study [398]. Seizures were seen more frequent in women than in men, but no differences in the pattern of clinical seizures or electroencephalography (EEG) were demonstrated between the two gender [399]. Most of the reports are for generations of childhood and young adults.

Hyperthroidism can exacerbate seizures and paroxysmal EEG abnormalities in patients with a diagnosis of epilepsy [390,400] or focal/generalized seizures only during thyrotoxicosis in patients without established epilepsy [401]. The mechanisms of seizure induction by thyroid hormones are not clear, but there are some possible explanations. Thyroid hormones may influence the activity of sodium potassium adenosine–triphosphatase, leading to severely altered concentrations of sodium in cerebral cells. In this way thyroid hormones trigger seizures by lowering the seizure threshold [402-405].

To confirm the diagnosis patients should be evaluated for the other causes of seizures. Any epileptic focus or organic lesion should not be obtained with EEG, CT or MRI. Hypoglycemia, hypoxemia, serum electrolyte imbalance, acid-base imbalance or possible central nervous system infections should be excluded [406]. Hyperthyroidism should be confirmed by low serum thyroid-stimulating hormone (TSH) and high concentrations of T4, T3, or both. EEG can be used as another diagnostic tool. Severity of hyperthyroidism correlates with EEG parameters [399]. Generally EEG abnormalities regress after a euthyroid state achieved. Thus EEG can be used to assess response to treatment [406]. The reversibility of EEG findings demontrates that seizures in hyperthyroidism are functional, not organic [407]. But EEG may not be positive in all cases of hyperthyroidism with seizures, and also positive EEGs in all cases of hyperthyroidism may not manifest clinical seizures [399].

7.5. Management

Treatment of hyperthyroidism with standard medical approaches (propylthiouracil, lugols iodine, propanolol and dexamethasone with additional vitamin B complex) have been shown to be effective in patients with seizures. Anti-epileptic drugs may have been useful when standard medical approaches were not adequate to control seizures. Thus, various anti-epileptic drugs (carbamazepine, phenytoin, sodium valproate, diazepam, or clonazepam) were used to treat seizures in the acute phase [399,408]. HE responds to glucocorticoids, immunosuppressive therapy and plasmapheresis which supports the autoimmune etiology. Seizure exacerbations usually remit when patients become euthyroid with treatment [409,410].

8. Thyrotoxicosis related diabetes mellitus

Glucose metabolism disorders can be seen in thyroid disorders, especially in hyperthyroidism. Hyperthyroid patients have a higher risk of developing diabetes mellitus. The pathogenesis is complex and there is lack of data about prevalence and severity in the literature [411].

8.1. Epidemiology

In young individuals with an autoimmune thyroid disease (as Graves' disease) it is common to develop type 1 diabetes. It is due to the alteration of the immune system which leads to a pathological reaction against self-antigens. In fact other autoimmune diseases like celiac disease can also occur. Thyroid auto-immunity is common in type 1 diabetic patients, with up to 27% of them having detectable titers of anti-thyroid peroxidase antibodies [412]. A prevalence study by Greco et al. confirmed the frequent association between Graves' disease and type 1 diabetes. Graves' disease often preceded diagnosis of type 1 diabetes, particularly in female subjects with a high age at diabetes onset [413].

In older patients, hyperthyroidism can be associated with type 2 diabetes. The pathogenetic mechanism can be explained by insulin resistance and metabolic derangement [414]. A study showed that patients on treatment for hyperthyroid Graves' disease were almost twice as likely to develop type 2 diabetes than the general population, although they were less likely to be overweight and were less likely to have family history. This suggests an association between Graves' disease and type 2 diabetes [415].

8.2. Genetic predisposition

Studies have been performed for HLA-DR3, HLA-DR4 CTLA-4, and PTPN22. These studies suggest that abnormalities in antigen presentation and T cell activation might play a significant role in the shared genetic etiology of type 1 diabetes and auto-immune thyroid disease [416].

8.3. Hyperthyroidism and glucose homeostasis

The effect of hyperthyroidism on glucose homeostasis is complex [417]. Hyperthyroidism stimulates increased metabolism in many tissues, leading to an increased demand for glucose [418]. Altough having insulin resistance, as long as pancreatic beta cell functions remain normal, overt diabetes does not develop in a hyperthyroidism.

Gastric emptying and intestinal absorption

It has been suggested that rapid gastric emptying and increased rates of intestinal absorption of glucose could be responsible for altered glucose tolerance in hyperthyroidism [419]. In contrast to this, recent studies found that gastric emptying has been decreased [420,421] or unchanged [422,423] in hyperthyroidism.

Liver

Hyperthyroidism can cause insulin resistance with direct and indirect effects on the liver. The direct effect is to increase basal hepatic glucose output by promoting gluconeogenesis and glycogenolysis [424]. A sympathetic pathway from the hypothalamic paraventricular nucleus to the liver has been proposed as a central pathway for modulation of hepatic glucose metabolism by thyroid hormone, which forms the indirect effect [425].

Peripheral tissues

Glucose uptake in peripheral tissues especially in the skeletal muscle have been found to be increased in hyperthyroisdism [426-429]. This increased uptake is mainly related with an increase in insulin-stimulated glucose oxidation rates [430-433]. Furthermore, reduced glycogenogenesis and insulin-stimulated nonoxidative glucose elimination results with intracellular glucose being redirected towards glycolysis and lactate formation [428,429,434]. The release of lactate from peripheral tissues back to the liver contributes to the Cori cycle where more hepatic glucose is being produced [434-436]. In the adipose tissue, lipolysis increases in the fasting state. This results with an increased production of glycerol and nonesterified fatty acids (NEFA). Increased glycerol generated by lipolysis and increased amino acids generated by proteolysis are used for gluconeogenesis. NEFA stimulate gluconeogenesis and provide substrate to other tissues such as muscle, for oxidation [437].

Cytokines

There is an interaction between thyroid hormones and adipose tissue derived cytokines. Effects of thyroid hormones on production rates and plasma levels of these cytokines could be used to explain mechanisms of insulin resistance in hyperthyroidism. Adipose tissue derived cytokines are adiponectin, leptin, interleukin-6, tumor necrosis factor-α, resistin and visfatin. There are conflicting reports about the role of these cytokines to insulin resistance in hyperthyroidism [418].

Insulin and glucagon secretion

Decreased [438-442], normal, or even increased [437,443] levels of plasma insulin have been reported in hyperthyroidism. There are conflicting reports about insulin secretion in hyperthyroidism. But it is more consistent that insulin degradation increases. Hyperthyroidism augments renal clearance of insulin [428,444,445]. Another important pathologic change induced by long-term hyperthyroidism has been shown to be irreversible pancreatic damage [446-448]. Secretion and metabolic clearance rates of glucagon have been found increased in hyperthyroidism [449]. Increased levels of growth hormone and catecholamines that accompany hyperthyroidism may further contribute to insulin resistance. Interorgan communication in hyperthyroidism are shown in Figure-6 [418].

8.4. Subclinical hyperthyroidism and glucose homeostasis

Subclinical hyperthyroidism could be endogenous and exogenous. Both of them have also been associated with insulin resistance in some studies [450,451]. But there are conflicting reports in the literaure about insulin resistance in exogenous subclinical hyperthyroidism. Yavuz et al. have reported reduced insulin sentivity in these patients [452,453]. In contrast to this Heemstra et al. have reported that insulin sensitivty was not altered [454]. According to its cronicity and higher T3 levels endogenous subclinical hyperthyroidism may have a larger impact on glucose homeostasis when compared to exogenous subclinical hyperthyroidism [451].

8.5. Impact of hyperthyroidism on diabetes

In some young women with Type 1 diabetes, glucose control may fluctuate following childbirth due to post-partum thyroiditis, when a state of hyperthyroidism is followed by hypothyroidism. Routine screening of TSH is recommended in such patients 6-8 weeks following delivery [455]. Thyrotoxicosis and diabetic ketoacidosis can occur simultaneously. In this

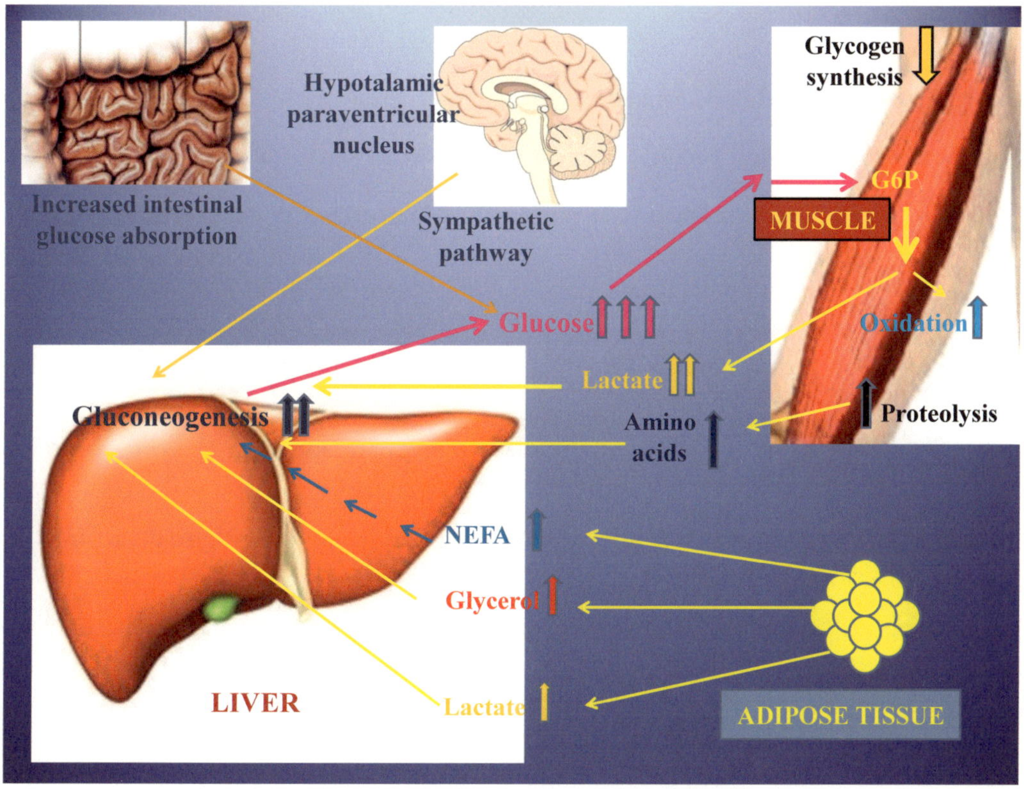

(Data adapred from reference 418)

Figure 6. Interorgan Communications in Hyperthyroidism

instance the combination could be fulminant and potentially life threatening. The first goal of treatment is to maintain electrolyte balance to avoid cardiac arrest [456].

As far as hyperthyroidism affects glucose homeostasis and causes insulin resistance, the patients need more insulin administration for glycemic control. Moon et al. reported a case of hyperglycemic hyperosmolar state (HHS) associated with Graves' hyperthyroidism. HHS rarely associates with Graves' hyperthyroidism but this unusual relation should be considered [457].

9. Conclusion

In conclusion all types of thyrotoxicosis may induce severe systemic complications which may affect morbidity, even mortality of the disease. Prompt and effective treatment of the complications and proggresing to euthyroidism is important for the management.

Author details

Irmak Sayin[1], Sibel Ertek[2] and Mustafa Cesur[2]

1 Ufuk University, Medical Faculty, Department of Internal Medicine, Turkey

2 Ufuk University, Medical Faculty, Department of Endocrinology and Metabolic Disease, Turkey

References

[1] Ghandour A, Reust C. Hyperthyroidism: a stepwise approach to treatment. J Fam Pract 2011;60(7) 388-395.

[2] Palitzsch KD. Prevention and multimodal therapy of hyperthyroidism. Internist (Berl) 2008;49(12) 1428-1436.

[3] Wang C, Crapo LM. The epidemiology of thyroid disease and implications for screening. Endocrinology and Metabolism Clinics of North America 1997;26(1) 189-218.

[4] Bulow PI, Laurberg P, Knudsen N, Jorgensen T, Perrild H, Ovesen L, Rasmussen LB. Increase in incidence of hyprthyroidism predominantly occurs in young people after iodine fortification of salt in Denmark. J Clin Endocrinol Metab 2006;91(10) 3830-3834.

[5] Brandt F, Green A, Hegedüs L, Brix TH. A critical review and meta-analysis of the association between overt hyperthyroidism and mortality. Eur J Endocrinol 2011;165(4) 491-497.

[6] Petersen P, Hansen JM. Stroke in thyrotoxicosis with atrial fibrillation. 1988;19(1) 15-18.

[7] Bielecka-Dabrowa A, Mikhailidis DP, Rysz J, Banach M. The mechanisms of atrial fibrillation in hyperthyroidism. Thyroid Res. 2009;2(1) 4.

[8] Biondi B, Kahaly GJ. Cardiovascular involvement in patients with different causes of hyperthyroidism. Nat Rev Endocrinol 2010;6(8) 431-443.

[9] Leng X, Bianco J, Tsai SY, Ozato K, O'Malley BW, Tsai MJ. Mechanisms for synergic activation of thyroid hormone receptor and retinoid X receptor on different response elements.J Biol Chem 1994;269(50) 31436-1442.

[10] Tsika RW, Bahl JJ, Leinwand LA, Morkin E. Thyroid hormone regulates expression of a transfected human alpha-myosin heavy chain fusion gene in fetal rat heart cells. Proc Natl Acad Sci USA 1990;87(1) 379-383.

[11] Zarain-Herzberg A, Marques J, Sukovich D, Periasamy M. Thyroid hormone receptor modulates the expression of the rabbit cardiac sarco(endo)plasmic reticulum Ca++-ATPase gene. J Biol Chem 1994;269(2) 1460-1467.

[12] Averyheart-Fullard V, Fraker LD, Murphy AM, Solaro RJ. Differential regulation of slow skeletal and cardiac troponon I mRNA during development and by thyroid hormone in rat heart. J Mol Cell Cardiol 1994;26(5) 609-616.

[13] Morkin E. Regulation of myosin heavy chain genes in the heart. Circulation 1993;87(5) 1451-1460.

[14] Ojamaa K, Klemperer JD, MacGlivray SS. Thyroid hormone and hemodynamic regulation of beta-myosin heavy chain promoter in the heart. Endocrinology 1996;137(3) 802-808.

[15] Izumo S, Nadal-Ginard B, Mahdavi V. All members of the MHC multigene family respond to thyroid hormone in a highly tissue-specific manner. Science 1986;231(4738) 597-600.

[16] Ladenson PW, Sherman SI, Boughman RL. Reversible alterations in myocardial gene expression in a young man with dilated cardiomyopathy and hypothyroidism. Proc natl Acad Sci USA 1992; 89(12) 5251-5255.

[17] Magner J, Clarck W, Allenby P. Congestive heart failure and sudden death in a young woman with thyrotoxicosis. West J Med 1988;149(1) 86-91

[18] Dillman WH. Biochemical basis of thyroid hormone action in the heart. Am J Med 1990;88(6) 626-630.

[19] Kiss E, Jakab G, Kranias EG, et al. Thyroid hormone-induced alteration in phospholamban protein expression:regulatory effects on sarcoplasmic reticulum Ca2+transport and myocardial relaxation.Circ Res 1994;75(2) 245-251.

[20] Kiss E, Brittsan AG, Elds I, et al. Thyroid hormone-induced alterations in phospholamban deficient mouse hearts. Circ Res 1998;83(6) 608-613.

[21] Panagoulis C, Halapas A, Chariatis E, Driva P, Matsakas E. Hyperthyroidism and heart. Hellenic J Cardiol 2008;49(3) 169-175.

[22] Kasturi S, Ismail-Beigi F. Effect of thyroid hormone on the distribution and activity of Na,K ATPase in ventricular myocardium. Arch Biochem Biophys 2008;475(2) 121-127.

[23] Glick GG, Melikian J, Ismail-Beigi F. Thyoid enhancement of rat myocardial Na/K ATPase preferential expression of alpha 2 activity on mRNA abundance. J Membr Biol 1990;115(3) 273-282.

[24] Ojamaa K, Sabet A, Kenessey A, Shenoy R, et al. Regulation of rat cardiac Kv 1.5 gene expression by thyroid hormone is rapid and chamber specific. Endocrinology 1999;140(7) 3170-3176.

[25] Dudley SC Jr, Baumgarten CM. Bursting of cardiac sodium channels after acute exposure to 3,5,3'– triiodo-L-thyronine. Circ Res 1993;73(2) 301-313.

[26] Walker JD, Crawford FA Jr, Mukherjee R, Spinale FG. The direct effects of 3,5,3' – triiodo-L-thyronine (T3) on myocyte contractile processes. Insights into mechanisms of action. J Thorac Cardiovasc Surg 1995;110(5) 1369-1379.

[27] Chen WJ, Yeh YH, Lin KH, Chang GJ, Kuo CT. Molecular characterisation of thyroid hormone-inhibited atrial L-type calcium channel expression : implication for atrial fibrillation in hyperthyroidism. Basic res Cardiol 2011;106(2) 163-174.

[28] Hammond HK, White FC, Buxton IL, Salzstein P, Brunton LL, Longhurst JC. Increased myocardial beta-recepors and adrenergic responses in hyperthyroid pigs. Am J Physiol 1987;252(2 Pt 2) H283-H290.

[29] Levey GS, Klein I. Cathecholamine thyroid hormone interactions and the cardiovascular manifestations of hyperthyroidism. Am J Med 1990;88(6) 642-646.

[30] Hoit BD, Khoury SF, Shao Y, Gabel M, Liggett SB, Walsh RA. Effects of thyroid hormone on cardiac beta-adrenergic responsiveness in conscious baboons. Circulation 1997;96(2) 592-598.

[31] Ojamaa K, Klein I, Sabet A, Steinberg SF. Chnages in adenylyl cyclase isoforms as a mechanism for thyroid hormone modulation of cardiac beta adrenergic receptor responsiveness. Metabolism 2000;49(2) 275-279.

[32] Cacciatori V, Bellavere F, Pessarosa A, et al. Power spectral analysis of heart rate in hyperthyroidism. J Clin End Metab 1996;81(8) 2828-2835

[33] Klein I, Ojamaa K.Thyrotoxicosis and the heart. Endocrinol Metab Clin North Am 1998;27(1) 51-62.

[34] Davis PJ, Davis FB. Acute cellular actions of thyroid hormone and myocardial function. Ann Thorac Surg 1993; 56 (1 Suppl) S16-S23.

[35] Klemperer JD, Klein I, Gomez M, et al. Thyroid hormone treatment after coronary artery by-pass surgery, N Eng J Med. 1995;333(23) 1522-1527

[36] Walker JD, Crawford FA, Kato S, et al. The novel effects of 3,5,3' –triiodo-L-thyronine on myocyte contractile function and beta adrenergic responsiveness in dilated cardiomyopathy. J Thorac Cardiovasc Surg 1994;108(4) 672-679.

[37] Almeida NA, Corderio A, Machado DS, et al. Connexin 40 messenger ribonucleic activity is posotovely regulated by thyroid hormone (TH)acting in cardiac atria via the TH receptor. Endocrinology 2009;150(1) 546-554.

[38] Lin H, Mitasikova M, Dlugosova K, et al. Thyroid hormones suppress epsilon PKC-signalling, downregulate connexin-43 and increase lethal arrhythmia susceptibility in nondiabetic and diabetic rats.J Phsiol Pharm 2008;59(2) 271-285.

[39] Pantos C, Xinaris C, Mourouzis I, Perimenis P, Politi E, Spanau D, Cokkinos DV. Thyroid hormone receptor alpha 1 : a switch to cardiac cell "metamorphosis"? J Physiol Pharmacol 2008;59(2) 253-269.

[40] Suarez J, Scott BT, Suarez-Ramirez JA, Chavira CV, DillmannWH. Thyroid hormone inhibits ERK phosphorylation in pressure overload induced hypertrophied mouse hearts through a receptor-mediated mechanism. Am J Physiol Cll Physiol 2010;299(6) C1524-1529.

[41] Haddad F, Jiang W, Bodell PW, Qin AX, Baldwin KM. Cardiac myosin heavy chain gene regulation by thyroid hormone involves altered histone modifications. Am J Physiol Heart Circ Physiol 2010;299(6) H1968-1980.

[42] Valcavi R, Menozzi C, Roti Elio et al. Sinus node function in hyperthyroid patients. JCEM 1992;75(1) 239-242

[43] Sun ZQ, Ojamaa K,Nakamura TY et al. Thyroid hormone increases pacemaker activity in rat neonatal atrial myocytes. J Moll Cell Cardiol 2001;33(4) 811-824.

[44] Messarah M, Saoudi M, Boulakaud MS, Feki AE. Oxidative stress induced by thyroid dysfunction in rat erythrocytes and heart. Environ Toxicol Pharmacol 2011;31(1) 33-41.

[45] Cacciatori V, Bellavere F, Pezzarossa A, Dellera A, et al. Power spectral analysis of heart rate in hyperthyroidism. J Clin Endocrinol Metab 1996;81(8) 2828-2835.

[46] Bielecka-Dabrowa A, Mikhailidis DP, Rysz J, Banach M. The mechanisms of atrial fibrillation in hyperthyroidism. Thyroid Res 2009;2(1) 4.

[47] Resnick LM, Laragh JH. Plasma rennin activity in syndromes of hyroid hormone excess and deficiency. Life Sci 1982;30(7-8) 58558-6.

[48] Polikar R, Burger AG, Scherrer U, Nicod P. The thyroid and the heart.Circulation 1993;87(5) 1435-1441.

[49] Ojamaa K, Klemperer JD, Klein I. Acute effects of thyroid hormone on vascular smooth muscle. Thyroid 1996;6(5) 505-512.

[50] Klein I, Ojamaa K, Thyroid hormone and the cardiovascular system. N Eng J Med 2001;344(7) 501-509.

[51] Wang YY, Morimoto S, Du CK, et al. up-regulation of type-2 iodothyronine deiodinase in dilated cardiomyopathy. Cardiovasc Res 2010;87(4) 636-646.

[52] Cotomacci G, Sarkis JJ, Fürstenau CR, Barreto-Chaves ML. Thyroid hormones are involved in 5'-nucleotidase modulation in soluble fraction of cardiac tissue. Life Sci. 2012;91(3-4) 137-142.

[53] Carneiro-Ramos MS, Dinis GP, Nadu AP, et al. Blockage of angiotensin-II type 2 receptor prevents thyroxine-mediated cardiac hypertrophy by blocking Akt action. Basic Res cardiol 2010;105(3) 325-335.

[54] Wang YY, Jiao B, Guo WG, Che HL, Zu ZB. Excessive thyroxine enhances susceptibility to apoptosis and decreased contractility of cardiomyocytes. Moll Cell Endocrinol 2010;320(1-2) 65-75.

[55] Maity S, Kar D, De K, Chander V, Bandyopadhyay A. Hyperthyroidism causes cardiac dysfunction by mitochondrial impairment and energy depletion. J Endocrinol. 2013;217(2) 215-228.

[56] Weltman NY, Wang D, Redetzke RA, Gerdes AM. Longstanding hyperthyroidism is associated with normal or enhanced intrinsic cardiomyocyte function despite decline in global cardiac function. PLoS One. 2012;7(10) e46655. www.plosone.org/article/info/Adoi: 10.1371/journal.pone.0046655

[57] Kim BH, Cho KI, Kim SM, Kim JY, Choi BG, Kang JH, Jeon YK, Kim SS, Kim SJ, Kim YK, Kim IJ. Irbesartan prevents myocardial remodeling in experimental thyrotoxic cardiomyopathy. Endocr J. 2012;59(10) 919-929.

[58] Park KW, Dai HB, Ojamaa K, Lowenstein E, Klein I, Sellke FW. The direct vasomotor effect of thyroid hormones on rat skeleteal muscle resistance arteries. Anesth Analog 1997;85(4) 734-738.

[59] Resnick LM, Laragh JH. Plasma renin activity in syndromes of thyroid hormone excess and deficiency. Life Sci 1982;30(7-8) 585-586.

[60] Klein I, Levey GS. Unusual manifestations of hypothyroidism. Arch Intern Med 1984;144(1) 123-128.

[61] Fadel BM, Ellahham S, Ringel MD, Lindsay J, Wartofsky L, Burman KD. Hyperthyroid heart disease. Clin Cardiol 2000;23(6) 402-408.

[62] Kontos HA, Shapiro W, Mauck HP Jr, Richardson DW, Patterson JL Jr, Sharpe AR Jr, Mechanism of certain abnormalities of the circulation to the limbs in thyrotoxicosis. J Clin Invest 1965;44 947-956.

[63] Theilen EO, Wilson WR. Hemodynamic effects of peripheral vasoconstriction in normal and thyrotoxic subjects. J Appl Physiol 1967;22(2) 207-210.

[64] Auer J, Scheibner P, Mische T, et al. Subclinical hyperthyroidism as a risk factor for atrial fibrillation. Am Heart J, 2001;142(5) 838-842.

[65] Vardas PE, Mavrakis HE. Atrial fibrillation : a symptom treated as a disease? Hellenic J Cardiol 2006;47(4) 191-193.

[66] Shenfield GM. Influence of thyroid dysfunction on drug pharmacokinetics. Clin Pharmacokinet 1981;6(4) 275-297.

[67] Nakazawa HK, Sakurai K, Hamada N, Momotani N, Ito K. Management of atrial fibrillation in the post-thyrotoxic state. Am J Med 1982;72(6) 903-906.

[68] Petersen P, Hansen JM. Stroke in thyrotoxicosis with atrial fibrillation. Stroke 1988;19(1) 15-18

[69] Gilligan DM, Ellenbogen KA, Epstein AE. The management of atrial fibrillation. Am J Med 1996;101(4) 413-421.

[70] Chaudhury S, Ismail-Beigi F, Gick GG, Levenson E, Edelman IS. Effect of thyroid hormone on the abundance of Na,K,ATPase alpha subunit messenger ribonucleic acid. Mol Endocrinol 1987;1(1) 83-89.

[71] Klein I, Levey GS: The cardiovascular system in thyrotoxicosis. In Braverman LE, Utiger RD (eds): Werner and Ingbar's the Thyroid : A Fundamental and Clinical Text.8th edition Philadelphia. Lippincott and Williams & Wilkins;2000

[72] Klein I, Ojamaa K. Thyroid hormone and the cardiovascular system. N Eng J Med 2001; 344(7) 501-509.

[73] Kahaly GJ, Kampmann C, Mohr-Kahaly S. Cardiovascular hemodynamics and exercise tolerance in thyroid disease. Thyroid 2002;12(6) 473-481

[74] Dahl P, Danzi S, Klein I. Thyrotoxic cardiac disease. Curr Heart Fail Re 2008;5(3) 170-176.

[75] Yue WS, Chong BH, Zhang XH, et al. Hyperthyroidism-induced left ventricular diastolic dysfunction: implication in hyperthyroidism-related heart failure. Clin Endocrinol (oxf) 2011;74(5) 636-643.

[76] Gu LQ, Zhao L, Zhu W, et al. Relationships between serum levels of thyroid hormones and serum concentrations of symmetric dimethylarginine (ADMA) and N-terminal-pro-B-type natriuretic peptide (NT-proBNP) in patients with Graves' Disease. Endocrine 2011;39(3) 266-271

[77] Mercuro G, Panzuto MG, Bina A, et al. Cardiac function, physical exercise capacity, and quality of life during long-term thyrotropin suppressive therapy with levothyroxine :effect of individual dose tailoring. J Clin Endocrinol Metab 2000;85(1) 159-164.

[78] Patane S, Marte F. Changing axis deviation and paroxysmal atrial flutter associated with subclinical hyperthyroidism. Int J Cardiol 2010;144(2) e31-e33.

[79] Sawin CT, Geller A, Wolf PA, et al. Low serum thyrotropin concentrations as a risk factor for atrial fibrillation in older patients. N Eng j Med 1994;331(19) 1249-1252.

[80] Vigario Pdos S, Chachamovitz DS, Teixeira Pde F, Santos MA, Oliveira FP, Vaisman M. Impaied functional and hemodynamic response to graded exercise testing and its recovery in patients with subclinical hyperthyroidism. Arq Bras Endocrinol Metabol 2011;55(3) 203-212.

[81] Biondi B, Fazio S, Carella C et al. Control of adrenergic overactivity by beta-blockade improves the quality of life in patients receiving long-term suppressive therapy with levothyroxine. J Clin end Metab 1994;78(5) 1028-1033.

[82] Heeringa J, Hoogendoorn EH, van der Deure WM, et al. High-normal thyroid function and risk of atrial fibrillation: the Rotterdam Study. Arch Intern Med 2008;168(20) 2219-2224.

[83] Fazio S, Palmieri EA, Lombardi G, Biondi B. Effects of thyroid hormone on cardiovascular system. Recent Prog Horm Res. 2004;59 31-50.

[84] Garrity JA, Bahn RS. Pathogenesis of Graves Ophthalmopathy: Implications for Prediction, Prevention, and Treatment. American Journal of Ophthalmology. 2006;142(1) 147–153.

[85] Marcocci C, Bartelena L, Bogazzi FM, Panicucci M, Pinchera A. Studies on the occurrence of ophthalmopathy in Graves' disease. Acta Endocrinol (Copenh) 1989;120(4) 473–478.

[86] Bahn RS. Assessment and management of the patient with Graves' ophthalmopathy. Endocr Pract 1995;1(3) 172–178.

[87] Prummel M, Bakker A, Wiersinga W, et al. Multi-center study on the characteristics and treatment strategies of patients with Graves' orbitopathy: the first European Group on Graves' Orbitopathy experience. Eur J Endocrinol. 2003;148(5) 491–495.

[88] Schotthoefer EO, Wallace DK. Strabismus associated with thyroid eye disease. Curr Opin Ophthalmol. 2007;18(5) 361–365.

[89] Mourits MP, Koornneef L, Wiersinga WM, Prummel MF, Berghout A, van der Gaag R. Clinical criteria for the assessment of disease activity in Graves' ophthalmopathy: a novel approach. Br J Ophthalmol. 1989;73(8) 639–644.

[90] Bartalena L, Pinchera A, Marcocci C. Management of Graves' ophthalmopathy: reality and perspectives. Endocr Rev. 2000;21(2) 168–199.

[91] Han R, Smith TJ. T helper type 1 and type 2 cytokines exert divergent influence on the induction of prostaglandin E_2 and hyaluronan synthesis by interleukin-1β in orbital fibroblasts: implications for the pathogenesis of thyroid-associated ophthalmopathy. *Endocrinology*. 2006;147(1) 13–19.

[92] Douglas RS, Gianoukakis AG, Goldberg RA, Kamat S, Smith TJ. Circulating mononuclear cells from euthyroid patients with thyroid-associated ophthalmopathy exhibit characteristic phenotypes. *Clinical & Experimental Immunology*. 2007;148(1) 64–71.

[93] Powell JD. The induction and maintenance of T cell anergy. *Clinical Immunology*. 2006;120(3) 239–246.

[94] Melchers F. Anergic B cells caught in the act. *Immunity*. 2006;25(6) 864–867.

[95] Smith TJ. Insights into the role of fibroblasts in human autoimmune diseases. *Clinical & Experimental Immunology*. 2005;141(3) 388–397.

[96] Koumas L, Smith TJ, Phipps RP. Fibroblast subsets in the human orbit: Thy-1+and Thy-1-subpopulations exhibit distinct phenotypes. *European Journal of Immunology*. 2002;32(2) 477–485.

[97] Sempowski GD, Rozenblit J, Smith TJ, Phipps RP. Human orbital fibroblasts are activated through CD40 to induce proinflammatory cytokine production. *American Journal of Physiology*. 1998;274(3) C707–C714.

[98] Valyasevi RW, Erickson DZ, Harteneck DA, et al. Differentiation of human orbital preadipocyte fibroblasts induces expression of functional thyrotropin receptor. *Journal of Clinical Endocrinology & Metabolism*. 1999;84(7) 2257–2562.

[99] Cao HJ, Han R, Smith TJ. Robust induction of PGHS-2 by IL-1 in orbital fibroblasts results from low levels of IL-1 receptor antagonist expression. *American Journal of Physiology*. 2003;284(6) C1429–C1437.

[100] Smith TJ, Sciaky D, Phipps RP, Jennings TA. CD40 expression in human thyroid tissue: evidence for involvement of multiple cell types in autoimmune and neoplastic diseases. *Thyroid*. 1999;9(8) 749–755.

[101] Feldon SE, John Park DJ, O'Loughlin CW, et al. Autologous T-lymphocytes stimulate proliferation of orbital fibroblasts derived from patients with Graves' ophthalmopathy. *Investigative Ophthalmology & Visual Science*. 2005;46(11) 3913–3921.

[102] Lehmann GM, Garcia-Bates TM, Smith TJ, et al. Regulation of Lymphocyte Function by PPARgamma: Relevance to Thyroid Eye Disease-Related Inflammation. PPAR Res. 2008;2008:895901.

[103] Pritchard J, Han R, Horst N, Cruikshank WW, Smith TJ. Immunoglobulin activation of T cell chemoattractant expression in fibroblasts from patients with Graves' disease is mediated through the insulin-like growth factor I receptor pathway. *Journal of Immunology*. 2003;170(12) 6348–6354.

[104] Smith TJ, Hoa N. Immunoglobulins from patients with Graves' disease induce hyaluronan synthesis in their orbital fibroblasts through the self-antigen, insulin-like growth factor-I receptor. *Journal of Clinical Endocrinology & Metabolism*. 2004;89(10) 5076–5080.

[105] de Carli M, D'Elios MM, Mariotti S, et al. Cytolytic T cells with Th1-like cytokine profile predominate in retroorbital lymphocytic infiltrates of Graves' ophthalmopathy. *Journal of Clinical Endocrinology & Metabolism*. 1993;77(5) 1120–1124

[106] Smith TJ, Sempowski GD, Berenson CS, Cao HJ, Wang H-S, Phipps RP. Human thyroid fibroblasts exhibit a distinctive phenotype in culture: characteristic ganglioside profile and functional CD40 expression. *Endocrinology*. 1997;138(12) 5576–5588.

[107] Zhang Y, Cao HJ, Graf B, Meekins H, Smith TJ, Phipps RP. Cutting edge: CD40 engagement up-regulates cyclooxygenase-2 expression and prostaglandin E2 production in human lung fibroblasts. *Journal of Immunology*. 1998;160(3) 1053–1057.

[108] Antonelli A, Rotondi M, Ferrari SM, et al. Interferon-γ-inducible α-chemokine CXCL10 involvement in Graves' ophthalmopathy: modulation by peroxisome proliferator-activated receptor-γ agonists. *Journal of Clinical Endocrinology & Metabolism*. 2006;91(2) 614–620.

[109] Feldon SE, O'Loughlin CW, Ray DM, Landskroner-Eiger S, Seweryniak KE, Phipps RP. Activated human T lymphocytes express cyclooxygenase-2 and produce proadipogenic prostaglandins that drive human orbital fibroblast differentiation to adipocytes. *The American Journal of Pathology*. 2006;169(4) 1183–1193.

[110] Forman BM, Tontonoz P, Chen J, Brun RP, Spiegelman BM, Evans RM. 15-Deoxy-$\Delta^{12,14}$-prostaglandin J_2 is a ligand for the adipocyte determination factor PPAR-γ. Cell. 1995;83(5) 803–812.

[111] Kliewer SA, Lenhard JM, Willson TM, Patel I, Morris DC, Lehmann JM. A prostaglandin J_2 metabolite binds peroxisome proliferator-activated receptor γ and promotes adipocyte differentiation. Cell. 1995;83:813–819.

[112] Zhang J, Fu M, Cui T, et al. Selective disruption of PPARγ2 impairs the development of adipose tissue and insulin sensitivity. *Proceedings of the National Academy of Sciences of the United States of America*. 2004;101(29) 10703–10708.

[113] Kumar S, Coenen MJ, Scherer PE, Bahn RS. Evidence for enhanced adipogenesis in the orbits of patients with Graves' ophthalmopathy. *Journal of Clinical Endocrinology & Metabolism*. 2004;89(2) 930–935.

[114] Mimura LY, Villares SMF, Monteiro MLR, Guazzelli IC, Bloise W. Peroxisome proliferator-activated receptor-γ gene expression in orbital adipose/connective tissues is increased during the active stage of Graves' ophthalmopathy. *Thyroid*. 2003;13(9) 845–850.

[115] Chen M, Liao S, et al. Role of macrophage infiltration in the orbital fat of patients with Graves' ophthalmopathy. Clin Endocrinol 2008;69(2) 332-337.

[116] Bartalena L, Baldeschi L, Dickinson A, et al. Consensus statement of the European Group on Graves' Orbitopathy (EUGOGO) on management of GO. Eur J Endocrinol 2008;158(3) 273-285.

[117] Yang SR, Chida AS, Bauter MR, Shafiq N, Seweryniak K, Maggirwar SB, Kilty I, Rahman I 2006 *Cigarette smoke induces proinflammatory cytokine release by activation of NF-κB and posttranslational modifications of histone deacetylase in macrophages. Am J Physiol Lung Cell Mol Physiol 2006;291(1) L46–L57*

[118] Metcalfe RA, Weetman AP . *Stimulation of extraocular muscle fibroblasts by cytokines and hypoxia: possible role in thyroid-associated ophthalmopathy.* Clin Endocrinol (Oxf) *1994; 40(1) 67–72.*

[119] Burch HB, Lahiri S, Bahn RS, Barnes S . *Superoxide radical production stimulates retroocular fibroblast proliferation in Graves' ophthalmopathy.* Exp Eye Res *1997;65(2)* 311–*316.*

[120] Mack WP, Stasior GO, Cao HJ, Stasior OG, Smith TJ 1999 The effect of cigarette smoke constituents on the expression of HLA-DR in orbital fibroblasts derived from patients with Graves ophthalmopathy. Ophthal Plast Reconstr Surg 199;15(4) 260–271.

[121] Pfeilschifter J & Ziegler R. Smoking and endocrine ophthalmopathy: impact of smoking severity and current vs lifetime cigarette consumption. Clinical Endocrinology 1996;45(4) 477–481.

[122] Eckstein A, Quadbeck B, Mueller G, Rettenmeier AW, Hoermann R, Mann K, Steuhl P, Esser J. Impact of smoking on the response to treatment of thyroid associatedophthalmopathy.Br J Ophthalmol. 2003 Jun;87(6) 773-776.

[123] Wiersinga WM. Smoking and thyroid. Clin Endocrinol (Oxf). 2013;79(2) 145-151.

[124] Salvi M. Zhang ZG. Haegert D. Woo M. Liberman A. Cadarso L. Wall JR. Patients with endocrine ophthalmopathy not associated with overt thyroid disease have multiple thyroid immunological abnormalities. J Clin Endocrinol Metab. 1990;70 89–94.

[125] Wiersinga WM. Smit T. van der Gaag R. Koornneef L. Temporal relationship between onset of Graves' ophthalmopathy and onset of thyroidal Graves' disease. J Endocrinol Invest. 1988;11(8) 615–619.

[126] Tsai KH, Tsai FJ, Lin HJ, Lin HJ, Liu YH, Liao WL, Wan L. Thymic stromal lymphopoietin gene promoter polymorphisms and expression levels in Graves' disease and Graves' ophthalmopathy. BMC Med Genet. 2012;13 116.

[127] Liao WL, Chen RH, Lin HJ, Liu YH, Chen WC, Tsai Y, Wan L, Tsai FJ. Toll-like receptor gene polymorphisms are associated with susceptibility to Graves' ophthalmopathy in Taiwan males.BMC Med Genet. 2010;11 154.

[128] Liao WL, Chen RH, Lin HJ, Liu YH, Chen WC, Tsai Y, Wan L, Tsai FJ. The association between polymorphisms of B7 molecules (CD80 and CD86) and Graves' ophthalmopathy in a Taiwanese population. Ophthalmology. 2011;118(3) 553-557.

[129] Gianoukakis AG, Jennings TA, King CS, et al. Hyaluronan accumulation in thyroid tissue: evidence for contributions from epithelial cells and fibroblasts. Endocrinology. 2007;148(1) 54–62.

[130] Cawood TJ, Moriarty P, O'Farrelly C, O'Shea D. The effects of tumour necrosis factor-alpha and interleukin1 on an in vitro model of thyroid-associated ophthalmopathy: contrasting effects on adipogenesis. Eur J Endocrinol. 2006;155 395–403.

[131] Liu YH, Chen RH, Wu HH, Liao WL, Chen WC, Tsai Y, Tsai CH, Wan L, Tsai FJ. Association of interleukin-1beta (IL1B) polymorphisms with Graves' ophthalmopathy in Taiwan Chinese patients. Invest Ophthalmol Vis Sci. 2010;51(12) 6238-6246.

[132] Vaidya B. Imrie H. Perros P. Dickinson J. McCarthy MI. Kendall-Taylor P. Pearce SH. Cytotoxic T lymphocyte antigen-4 (CTLA-4) gene polymorphism confers susceptibility to thyroid associated orbitopathy. Lancet. 1999;354(9180) 743–744.

[133] Allahabadia A. Heward JM. Nithiyananthan R. Gibson SM. Reuser TT. Dodson PM. Franklyn JA. Gough SC. MHC class II region, CTLA4 gene, and ophthalmopathy in patients with Graves' disease. Lancet. 2001;358(9286) 984–985.

[134] Daroszewski J. Pawlak E. Karabon L. Frydecka I. Jonkisz A. Slowik M. Bolanowski M. Soluble CTLA-4 receptor an immunological marker of Graves' disease and severity of ophthalmopathy is associated with CTLA-4 Jo31 and CT60 gene polymorphisms. Eur J Endocrinol. 2009;161(5) 787–793.

[135] Alevizaki M, Mantzou E, Cimponeriu A, Saltiki K, Philippou G, Wiersinga W. The Pro 12 Ala PPAR gamma gene polymorphism: possible modifier of the activity and severity of thyroid-associated orbitopathy (TAO).Clin Endocrinol (Oxf). 2009;70(3) 464-468

[136] Huber AK, Jacobson EM, Jazdzewski K, Concepcion ES, Tomer Y. Interleukin (IL)-23 receptor is a major susceptibility gene for Graves' ophthalmopathy: the IL-23/T-helper 17 axis extends to thyroid autoimmunity. J Clin Endocrinol Metab. 2008;93(3) 1077-1081.

[137] Syed AA, Simmonds MJ, Brand OJ, et al. Preliminary evidence for interaction of PTPN12 polymorphism with TSHR genotype and association with Graves' ophthalmopathy. Clin Endocrinol (Oxf) 2007; 67(5) 663–667

[138] Kurylowicz A, Hiromatsu Y, Jurecka-Lubieniecka B, et al. Association of NFKB1-94ins/del ATTG promoter polymorphism with susceptibility to and phenotype of Graves' disease. Genes Immun 2007; 8(7) 532–538.

[139] Weetman A P, Zhang L, Webb S, Shine B. Analysis of HLA-DQB and HLA-DPB alleles in Graves' disease by oligonucleotide probing of enzymatically amplified DNA. Clin. Endocrinol (Oxf) 1990;33(1) 65–71.

[140] Akaishi PM, Cruz AA, Silva FL, Rodrigues Mde L, Maciel LM, Donadi EA. The role of major histocompatibility complex alleles in the susceptibility of Brazilian patients to develop the myogenic type of Graves' orbitopathy. Thyroid. 2008;18(4) 443–7.

[141] Inoue D, Sato K, Enomoto T et al.Correlation of HLA types and clinical findings in Japanese patients with hyperthyroid Graves' disease: evidence indicating the existence of four subpopulations. Clin. Endocrinol (Oxf) 1992;36(1) 75–82.

[142] Inoue D, Sato K, Maeda M et al. Genetic differences shown by HLA typing among Japanese patients with euthyroid Graves' ophthalmopathy, Graves' disease and Ha-

shimoto's thyroiditis: genetic characteristics of euthyroid Graves' ophthalmopathy. Clin. Endocrinol (Oxf) 1991;34(1) 57–62.

[143] Molnar I., Balazs C. High circulating IL-6 level in Graves' ophthalmopathy. Autoimmunity 1997; 25(2) 91-96.

[144] Wakelkamp IM., Gerding MN.,Van Der Meer JW., Prummel MF., Wiersinga WM. Both Th1-and Th2-derived cytokines in serum are elevated in Graves' ophthalmopathy. Clin. Exp. Immunol. 2000; 121(3) 453-457.

[145] Chen B, Tsui S, Smith TJ. IL-1 beta induces IL-6 expression in human orbital fibroblasts: identification of an anatomic-site specific phenotypic attribute relevant to thyroid-associated ophthalmopathy. J Immunol 2005; 175(2) 1310–1319.

[146] Kim SE, Yoon JS, Kim KH, Lee SY. Increased serum interleukin-17 in Graves' ophthalmopathy.Graefes Arch Clin Exp Ophthalmol. 2012;250(10) 1521-1526.

[147] Ujhelyi B, Gogolak P, Erdei A, Nagy V, Balazs E, Rajnavolgyi E, Berta A, Nagy EV. Graves' orbitopathy results in profound changes in tear composition: a study of plasminogen activator inhibitor-1 and seven cytokines. Thyroid. 2012;22(4) 407-414.

[148] Raikow RB, Tyutyunikov A, Kennerdell JS, Kazim M, Dalbow MH, Scalise D. Correlation of serum immunoglobulin E elevations with clinical stages of dysthyroid orbitopathy. Ophthalmology. 1992; 99(3) 361–365.

[149] Cekić S, Stanković-Babić G. Application of ultrasound in diagnosing and follow-up of endocrine orbitopathy. Med Pregl. 2010;63(3-4) 241-248.

[150] Demer JL, Kerman BM. Comparison of standardized echography with magnetic resonance imaging to measure extraocular muscle size. Am J Ophthalmol. 1994;118(3) 351-361.

[151] Casper DS, Chi TL & Trokel SL. Orbital Disease, Imaging and Analysis. Edn 1. Stuttgart: Thieme. 1993. / Pester RG & Hoover ED. Graves' orbiopathy. In Computerized Tomography in Orbital Diseases and Neuroopthalmology. Edn 1. ch 3. pp 97-114. Chicago: Yera Book Medical Publisher. 1984

[152] Nugent RA, Belkin RI, Neigel JM, Rootman J, Robertson WD, Spinelli J, Graeb DA. Graves orbitopathy: correlation of CT and clinical findings. Radiology. 1990;177(3) 675-682.

[153] Barrett L, Glatt HJ, Burde RM, Gado MH. Optic nerve dysfunction in thyroid eye disease: CT. Radiology. 1988;167(2) 503-507.

[154] Feldon SE, Lee CP, Muramatsu SK, Weiner JM. Quantitative computed tomography of Graves' ophthalmopathy. Extraocular muscle and orbital fat in development of optic neuropathy. Arch Ophthalmol. 1985;103(2) 213-215.

[155] Hallin ES, Feldon SE. Graves' ophthalmopathy: II. Correlation of clinical signs with measures derived from computed tomography. Br J Ophthalmol. 1988;72(9) 678-682.

[156] Nishikawa M, Yoshimura M, Toyoda N, Masaki H, Yonemoto T, Gondou A, Kato T, Kurokawa H, Furumura T, Inada M. Correlation of orbital muscle changes evaluated by magnetic resonance imaging and thyroid-stimulating antibody in patients with Graves' ophthalmopathy. Acta Endocrinol (Copenh). 1993;129(3) 213-219.

[157] Yokoyama N, Nagataki S, Uetani M, Ashizawa K, Eguchi K. Role of magnetic resonance imaging in the assessment of disease activity in thyroid-associated ophthalmopathy. Thyroid. 2002;12(3) 223-227.

[158] Wiersinga WM, Gerding MN, Prummel MF, Krenning EP. Octreotide scintigraphy in thyroidal and orbital Graves' disease. Thyroid. 1998;8(5) 433-436.

[159] Krassas G, Dumas A. Octreoscan in Graves' ophthalmopathy. Thyroid. 1997;7(5) 805-806.

[160] Krassas GE, Dumas A, Pontikides N, Kaltsas T. Somatostatin receptor scintigraphy and octreotide treatment in patients with thyroid eye disease. Clin Endocrinol (Oxf) 1995;42(6) 571-580.

[161] Postema PTE, Krenning EP, Wijngaarde R et al. (111In-DTPA-D-Phe1) octreotide scintigraphy in thyroidal and orbital Graves' disease: a parameter for disease activity? J Clin Endocrinol Metab 1994;79(6) 1845-1851.

[162] Krassas GE. Octreoscan in thyroid-associated ophthalmopathy. Thyroid. 2002;12(3) 229-231.

[163] Krassas GE, Kahaly GJ. The role of octreoscan in thyroid eye disease. Eur J Endocrinol. 1999;140(5) 373-375.

[164] Kuo PH, Monchamp T, Deol P. Imaging of inflammation in Graves' ophthalmopathy by positron emission tomography/computed tomography. Thyroid. 2006;16(4) 419–420.

[165] Konuk O, Atasever T, Unal M, Ayvaz G, Yetkin I, Cakir N, Arslan M, Hasanreisoglu B. Orbital gallium-67 scintigraphy in Graves' ophthalmopathy. Thyroid. 2002 ;12(7) 603-608.

[166] Durak H, Söylev M, Durak I, Değirmenci B, Capa Kaya G, Uysal B. Tc-99m polyclonal human immunoglobulin G imaging in Graves' ophthalmopathy. Clin Nucl Med. 2000;25(9) 704-707.

[167] Lopes FP, de Souza SA, Dos Santos Teixeira Pde F, Rebelo Pinho Edos S, da Fonseca LM, Vaisman M, Gutfilen B. 99mTc-Anti-TNF-α scintigraphy: a new perspective within different methods in the diagnostic approach of active Graves ophthalmopathy. Clin Nucl Med. 2012;37(11) 1097-1101.

[168] García-Rojas L, Adame-Ocampo G, Alexánderson E, Tovilla-Canales JL. 18-Fluorodeoxyglucose Uptake by Positron Emission Tomography in Extraocular Muscles of Patients with and without Graves' Ophthalmology. J Ophthalmol. 2013;2013:529187.

[169] Wiersinga WM, Prummel MF, Mourits MP, et al. Classification of the eye changes of Graves' disease. Thyroid 1991;1(4) 357–360.

[170] Dolman PJ, Rootman J. VISA classification for Graves orbitopathy. Ophthal Plast Reconstr Surg 2006;22(5) 319–324.

[171] Bartalena L, Tanda ML. Clinical practice. Graves' ophthalmopathy. N Engl J Med. 2009;360(10) 994-1001

[172] Mourits MP, Prummel MF, Wiersinga WM, Koornneef L. Clinical activity score as a guide in the management of patients with Graves' ophthalmopathy. Clin Endocrinol (Oxf) 1997;47(1) 9-14.

[173] Bartalena L, Marcocci C, Bogazzi F, Manetti L, Tanda ML, Dell'Unto E,Bruno-Bossio G, Nardi M, Bartolomei MP, Lepri A, Rossi G, Martino E, Pinchera A. Relation between therapy for hyperthyroidism and the course of Graves' ophthalmopathy. N Engl J Med. 1998;338(2) 73-78.

[174] Prummel MF, Wiersinga WM, Mourits MP, Koornneef L, Berghout A, van der Gaag R Amelioration of eye changes of Graves' ophthalmopathy by achieving euthyroidism. Acta Endocrinologica 1989; 121(Suppl 2):185–189

[175] Laurberg P, Wallin G, Tallstedt L, Abraham-Nordling M, Lundell G, Tørring O. TSH-receptor autoimmunity in Graves' disease after therapy with anti-thyroid drugs, surgery, or radioiodine: a 5-year prospective randomized study. Eur J Endocrinol. 2008;158(1) 69-75.

[176] Bałdys-Waligórska A, Gołkowski F, Kusnierz-Cabala B, Buziak-Bereza M,Hubalewska-Dydejczyk A. Graves' ophthalmopathy in patients treated with radioiodine 131-I. Endokrynol Pol. 2011;62(3) 214-219.

[177] El-Kaissi S, Bowden J, Henry MJ, Yeo M, Champion BL, Brotchie P, Nicholson GC, Wall JR. Association between radioiodine therapy for Graves' hyperthyroidism and thyroid-associated ophthalmopathy. Int Ophthalmol. 2010;30(4) 397-405.

[178] Wilhelm SM, McHenryCR2010 Total thyroidectomy is superior to subtotal thyroidectomy for management of Graves' disease in the United States. World J Surg 2010;34(6) 1261–1264.

[179] Bartalena L, Marcocci C, Bogazzi F, Bruno-Bossio G, Pinchera A. Glucocorticoid therapy of Graves' ophthalmopathy. Exp Clin Endocrinol 1991;97(2-3) 320–328.

[180] Smith TJ. Dexamethasone regulation of glycosaminoglycan synthesis in cultured human fibroblasts: similar effects of glucocorticoid and thyroid hormone therapy. J Clin Invest 1984;74(6) 2157–2163.

[181] Bartalena L, Marcocci C, Pinchera A. Treating severe Graves' ophthalmopathy. Bailliere's Clin Endocrinol Metab 1997;11(3) 521–536.

[182] Marcocci C, Bartalena L, Tanda ML, et al. Comparison of the effectiveness and tolerability of intravenous or oral glucocorticoids associated with orbital radiotherapy in

the management of severe Graves' ophthalmopathy: results of a prospective, single-blind, randomized study. J Clin Endocrinol Metab 2001;86(8) 3562-3567.

[183] Kahaly GJ, Pitz S, Hommel G, Dittmar M. Randomized, single blind trial of intravenous versus oral steroid monotherapy in Graves' orbitopathy. J Clin Endocrinol Metab 2005;90(9) 5234-5240.

[184] Bartalena L, Krassas GE, Wiersinga W et al; European Group on Graves' Orbitopathy. Efficacy and safety of three different cumulative doses of intravenous methylprednisolone for moderate to severe and active Graves' orbitopathy. J Clin Endocrinol Metab. 2012;97(12) 4454-63.

[185] Gursoy A, Cesur M, Erdogan MF, et al. New-onset acute heart failure after intravenous glucocorticoid pulse therapy in a patient with Graves' ophthalmopathy. Endocrine 2006;29(3) 513–516.

[186] Chang TC, Kao SCS, Huang KM 1992 Octreotide and Graves' ophthalmopathy and pretibial myxoedema. Br Med J 1992;304(6820) 158.

[187] Uysal AR, Corapçioğlu D, Tonyukuk VC, Güllü S, Sav H, Kamel N, Erdoğan G. Effect of octreotide treatment on Graves' ophthalmopathy. Endocr J. 1999;46(4) 573-577.

[188] Stan MN, Garrity JA, Bradley EA, Woog JJ, Bahn MM, Brennan MD, Bryant SC, Achenbach SJ, Bahn RS 2006 Randomized, double-blind, placebo-controlled trial of long-acting release octreotide for treatment of Graves' ophthalmopathy. J Clin Endocrinol Metab 2006;91(12) 4817–4824.

[189] Krassas GE, Doumas A, Kaltsas T, Halkias A, Pontikides N. Somatostatin receptor scintigraphy before and after treatment with somatostatin analogues in patients with thyroid eye disease. Thyroid 1999;9(1) 47-52.

[190] Antonelli A, Saracino A, Alberti B, Canapicchi R, Cartei F, Lepri A, Laddaga M, Baschieri L. High-dose intravenous immunoglobulin treatment in Graves' ophthalmopathy. Acta Endocrinol (Copenh) 1992;126(1) 13-23.

[191] Kahaly G, Pitz S, Muller-Forell W, Hommel G. Randomized trial of intravenous immunoglobulins versus prednisolone in Graves' ophthalmopathy. Clin Exp Immunol 1996;106(2) 197-202.

[192] Seppel T, Schlaghecke R, Becker A, Engelbrecht V, Feldkamp J, Kornely E. High-dose intravenous therapy with 7S immunoglobulins in autoimmune endocrine ophthalmopathy. Clin Exp Immunol 1996;14(Suppl 15) S109-S114.

[193] Weetman AP, McGregor AM, Ludgate M, Beck L, Mills PV, Lazarus JH, Hall R. Cyclosporin improves Graves' ophthalmopathy. Lancet. 1983;2(8348) 486-489.

[194] Prummel MF, Mourits MP, Berghout A, Krenning EP, van der Gaag R, Koornneef L, Wiersinga WM. Prednisone and cyclosporine in the treatment of severe Graves' ophthalmopathy. N Engl J Med 1989;321(20) 1353–1359.

[195] Weissel M, Zielinski CC, Hauff W, Till P. Combined therapy with cyclosporin A and cortisone in endocrine Basedow endocrine orbitopathy: successful use in compressive optic neuropathy. Acta Med Austriaca. 1993;20(1-2) 9-13.

[196] Weetman AP, Wiersinga WM. Current management of thyroid-associated ophthalmopathy in Europe. Results of an international survey. Clin Endocrinol (Oxf) 1998;49(1) 21-8.

[197] Smith JR, Rosenbaum JT. A role of methotrexate in the management of non-infectious orbital inflammatory disease. Br J Ophthalmol 2001;85(10) 1220-1224.

[198] Bouzas EA, Karadimas P, Mastorakos G, Koutras DA 2000 Antioxidant agents in the treatment of Graves' ophthalmopathy. Am J Ophthalmol 2000;129(5) 618-622.

[199] Yoon JS, Chae MK, Lee SY, Lee EJ. Anti-inflammatory effect of quercetin in a whole orbital tissue culture of Graves' orbitopathy. Br J Ophthalmol. 2012;96(8) 1117-1121.

[200] Marcocci C, Kahaly GJ, Krassas GE, Bartalena L, Prummel M, Stahl M, Altea MA, Nardi M, Pitz S, Boboridis K, Sivelli P, von Arx G, Mourits MP, Baldeschi L, Bencivelli W, Wiersinga W; European Group on Graves' Orbitopathy. Selenium and the course of mild Graves' orbitopathy. N Engl J Med. 2011;364(20) 1920-1931.

[201] Chang CC, Chang TC, Kao SC, Kuo YF, Chien LF. Pentoxifylline inhibits the proliferation and glycosaminoglycan synthesis of cultured fibroblasts derived from patients with Graves' ophthalmopathy and pretibial myxoedema. Acta Endocrinol (Copenh). 1993;129(4) 322-327.

[202] Balazs C, Kiss E, Vamos A, Molnar I, Farid NR. Beneficial effect of pentoxifylline on thyroid associated ophthalmopathy (TAO)*: a pilot study. J Clin Endocrinol Metab. 1997;82(6) 1999-2002.

[203] Finamor FE, Martins JR, Nakanami D, Paiva ER, Manso PG, Furlanetto RP. Pentoxifylline (PTX)--an alternative treatment in Graves' ophthalmopathy (inactive phase): assessment by a disease specific quality of life questionnaire and by exophthalmometry in a prospective randomized trial. Eur J Ophthalmol. 2004;14(4) 277-283.

[204] Paridaens D, van den Bosch WA, van der Loos TL, et al. The effect of etanercept on Graves' ophthalmopathy: a pilot study. Eye 2005;19(12) 1286–1289.

[205] Durrani OM, Reuser TQ, Murray PI. Infliximab: a novel treatment for sight-threatening thyroid associated ophthalmopathy. Orbit. 2005;24(2) 117-119.

[206] Komorowski J, Jankiewicz-Wika J, Siejka A, Lawnicka H, Kłysik A, Goś R, Majos A, Stefańczyk L, Stepień H. Monoclonal anti-TNFalpha antibody (infliximab) in the treatment of patient with thyroid associated ophthalmopathy. Klin Oczna. 2007;109(10-12) 457-460.

[207] Salvi M, Vannucchi G, Campi I, et al. Efficacy of rituximab treatment for thyroid-associated ophthalmopathy as a result of intraorbital B-cell depletion in one patient unresponsive to steroid immunosuppression. Eur J Endocrinol 2006; 154:511–517.

[208] Salvi M, Vannucchi G, Campi I et al. Treatment of Graves' disease and associated ophthalmopathy with the anti-CD20 monoclonal antibody rituximab: an open study. Eur J Endocrinol. 2007;156(1) 33-40.

[209] Silkiss RZ, Reier A, Coleman M, Lauer SA. Rituximab for thyroid eye disease. Ophthal Plast Reconstr Surg. 2010;26(5) 310-314.

[210] Chang S, Perry JD, Kosmorsky GS, et al. Rapamycin for treatment of refractory dysthyroid compressive optic neuropathy. Ophthal Plast Reconstr Surg 2007;23(3) 225–226.

[211] Stamato FJ, Maciel RM, Manso PG, Wolosker AM, Paiva ER, Lopes AC, Furlanetto RP. Colchicine in the treatment of the inflammatory phase of Graves' ophthalmopathy: a prospective and randomized trial with prednisone. Arq Bras Oftalmol. 2006;69(6) 811-816.

[212] Zhang C, Zhang X, Ma L, Peng F, Huang J, Han H. Thalidomide inhibits adipogenesis of orbital fibroblasts in Graves' ophthalmopathy. Endocrine. 2012;41(2) 248-255.

[213] Han Hui, Huang Jiao, Zhang Xian-Feng et al. The immunoregulatory effect of thalidomide on peripheral blood mononuclear cells in patients with thyroid-associated ophthalmopathy. Chin J End Met. 2013;29(7) 584-585.

[214] Valyasevi RW, Harteneck DA, Dutton CM, Bahn RS. Stimulation of adipogenesis, peroxisome proliferator-activated receptor-gamma (PPARgamma), and thyrotropin receptor by PPARgamma agonist in human orbital preadipocyte fibroblasts. J Clin Endocrinol Metab. 2002;87(5) 2352-2358.

[215] Starkey K, Heufelder A, Baker G, Joba W, Evans M, Davies S, Ludgate M. Peroxisome proliferator-activated receptor-gamma in thyroid eye disease: contraindication for thiazolidinedione use? J Clin Endocrinol Metab. 2003;88(1) 55–59.

[216] Thiazolidinedione induced thyroid associated orbitopathy.BMC Ophthalmol. 2007;7 8.

[217] Antonelli A, Rotondi M, Ferrari SM, Fallahi P, Romagnani P, Franceschini SS, Serio M, Ferrannini E. Interferon-gamma-inducible alpha-chemokine CXCL10 involvement in Graves' ophthalmopathy: modulation by peroxisome proliferator-activated receptor-gamma agonists. J Clin Endocrinol Metab. 2006;91(2) 614-620.

[218] Antonelli A, Ferrari SM, Fallahi P, Frascerra S, Santini E, Franceschini SS, Ferrannini E. Monokine induced by interferon gamma (IFNgamma) (CXCL9) and IFNgamma inducible T-cell alpha-chemoattractant (CXCL11) involvement in Graves' disease and ophthalmopathy: modulation by peroxisome proliferator-activated receptor-gamma agonists. J Clin Endocrinol Metab. 2009;94(5) 1803-1809.

[219] Bartalena L, Marcocci C, Manetti L, Tanda ML, Dell'Unto E, Rocchi R, Cartei F, Pinchera A. Orbital radiotherapy for Graves' ophthalmopathy. Thyroid 1998;8(5) 439–441.

[220] Kahaly G, Beyer J. Immunosuppressant therapy of thyroid eye disease. Klin Wochenschr 1988;66(21) 1049–1059.

[221] Viani GA, Boin AC, De Fendi LI, Fonseca EC, Stefano EJ, de Paula JS. Radiation therapy for Graves' ophthalmopathy: a systematic review and meta-analysis of randomized controlled trials. Arq Bras Oftalmol. 2012;75(5) 324-332.

[222] Petersen IA, Kriss JP, McDougall IR, Donaldson SS 1990 Prognostic factors in the radiotherapy if Graves' ophthalmopathy. Int J Radiat Oncol Biol Phys 1190;19(2) 259–264.

[223] Wei RL, Cheng JW, Cai JP. The use of orbital radiotherapy for Graves' ophthalmopathy: quantitative review of the evidence. Ophthalmologica 2008; 222(1) 27–31.

[224] Schaefer U, Hesselmann S, Micke O, Schueller P, Bruns F, Palma C, Willich N. A long-term follow-up study after retro-orbital irradiation for Graves' ophthalmopathy. Int J Radiat Oncol Biol Phys. 2002;52(1) 192-197.

[225] Wakelkamp IM, Tan H, Saeed P, Schlingemann RO, Verbraak FD, Blank LE, Prummel MF,Wiersinga WM. Orbital irradiation for Graves' ophthalmopathy: Is it safe? A long-term follow-up study. Ophthalmology. 2004;111(8) 1557-1562.

[226] Haenssle HA, Richter A, Buhl T, Haas E, Holzkamp R, Emmert S, Schön MP. Pigmented basal cell carcinomas 15 years after orbital radiation therapy for Graves ophthalmopathy. Arch Dermatol. 201;147(4) 511-522.

[227] Dandona P, Marshall NJ, Bidey SP, Nathan A, Havard CW. Successful treatment of exophthalmos and pretibial myxoedema with plasmapheresis. Br Med J. 1979;1(6160) 374-376.

[228] Glinoer D, Etienne-Decerf J, Schrooyen M, Sand G, Hoyoux P, Mahieu P, Winand R. Beneficial effects of intensive plasma exchange followed by immunosuppressive therapy in severe Graves' ophthalmopathy. Acta Endocrinol (Copenh). 1986;111(1) 30-38.

[229] Sawers JSA, Irvine WJ, Toft AD, Urbaniak SJ, Donaldson AA. Plasma exchange in conjunction with immunosuppressive drug therapy in the treatment of endocrine exophthalmos. J Clin Lab Immunol 1981;6(3) 245–250.

[230] Kelly W, Longson D, Smithard D, Fawcitt R, Wensley R, Noble J, Keeley J. An evaluation of plasma exchange for Graves' ophthalmopathy. Clin Endocrinol (Oxf) 1983;18(5) 485–493.

[231] Burch HB, Wartofsky L. Graves' ophthalmopathy: current concepts regarding pathogenesis and management. Endocr Rev 1993;14(6) 747-793.

[232] Bartalena L, Marcocci C, Pinchera A. Graves' ophthalmopathy: a preventable disease? Eur J Endocrinol. 2002;146(4) 457-461.

[233] Wiersinga WM, Bartalena L. Epidemiology and prevention of Graves' ophthalmopathy. Thyroid. 2002;12(10) 855-860.

[234] Pacini F, Mariotti S, Formica N, Elisei R, Anelli S, Capotorti E, Pinchera A. Thyroid autoantibodies in thyroid cancer: incidence and relation with tumour outcome. Acta Endocrinol (Copenh) 1988;119(3) 373-380.

[235] Spinelli C, Bertocchini A, Lima M, Miccoli P. Graves-Basedow's disease in children and adolescents: total vs subtotal thyroidectomy. Pediatr Med Chir. 2002;24(5) 383-386.

[236] De Bellis A, Conzo G, Cennamo G, Pane E, Bellastella G, Colella C, Iacovo AD, Paglionico VA, Sinisi AA, Wall JR, Bizzarro A, Bellastella A. Time course of Graves' ophthalmopathy after total thyroidectomy alone or followed by radioiodine therapy: a 2-year longitudinal study. Endocrine. 2012;41(2) 320-326.

[237] Burch HB, Wartofsky L. Graves' ophthalmopathy: current concepts regarding pathogenesis and management. Endocr Rev 1993;14(6) 747–793.

[238] Garrity JA, Fatourechi V, Bergstralh EJ, Bartley GB, Beatty CW, DeSanto LW, Gorman CA. Results of transantral orbital decompression in 428 patients with severe Graves' ophthalmopathy. Am J Ophthalmol 1993;116(5) 533–547

[239] Wojcicka A, Bassett JH, Williams GR. Mechanisms of action of thyroid hormones in the skeleton. Biochim Biophys Acta. 2013;1830(7) 3979-3986.

[240] Manicourt D, Demeester-Mirkine N, Brauman H, Corvilain J. Disturbed mineral metabolism in hyperthyroidism: good correlation with tri-iodothyronine. Clin Endocrinol (Oxf). 1979;10(4) 407-412.

[241] Mosekilde L, Eriksen EF, Charles P. Effects of thyroid hormones on bone and mineral metabolism. Endocrinol Metab Clin North Am. 1990;19(1) 35-63.

[242] Lee MS, Kim SY, Lee MC, Cho BY, Lee HK, Koh CS, Min HK. Negative correlation between the change in bone mineral density and serum osteocalcin in patients with hyperthyroidism. J Clin Endocrinol Metab. 1990;70(3) 766-770.

[243] Franklyn, J. A. & Sheppard, M. C. The thyroid and osteoporosis. Trends Endocrinol. Metab. 1992;3: 113-116.

[244] Mundy GR, Shapiro JL, Bandelin JG. Direct stimulation of bone resorption by thyroid hormones. J Clin Invest. 1976;58(3) 529–534.

[245] Rizzoli R, Poser J, Bürgi U. Nuclear thyroid hormone receptors in cultured bone cells. Metabolism. 1986;35(1) 71–74.

[246] Abu EO, Bord S, Horner A. The expression of thyroid hormone receptors in human bone. Bone. 1997;21(2) 137–142.

[247] Britto JM, Fenton AJ, Holloway WR, Nicholson GC. Osteoblasts mediate thyroid hormone stimulation of osteoclastic bone resorption. Endocrinology. 1994;134(1) 169–176.

[248] Lakatos P, Foldes J, Horvath C. Serum interleukin-6 and bone metabolism in patients with thyroid function disorders. J Clin Endocrinol Metab. 1997;82(1) 78–81.

[249] Lakatos P, Foldes J, Nagy Z, Takacs I, Speer G, Horvath C, Mohan S, Baylink DJ, Stern PH. Serum insulin-like growth factor-I, insulin-like growth factor binding proteins, and bone mineral content in hyperthyroidism. Thyroid. 2000;10(5) 417-423.

[250] Stevens DA, Harvey CB, Scott AJ, O'Shea PJ, Barnard JC, Williams AJ, Brady G, Samarut J, Chassande O, Williams GR. Thyroid hormone activates fibroblast growth factor receptor-1 in bone. Mol Endocrinol. 2003;17(9) 1751-1766.

[251] FOLLIS RH Jr. Skeletal changes associated with hyperthyroidism.Bull Johns Hopkins Hosp. 1953;92(6) 405-421.

[252] Mosekilde L, Melsen F. A tetracycline-based histomorphometric evaluation of bone resorption and bone turnover in hyperthyroidism and hyperparathyroidism.Acta Med Scand. 1978;204(1-2) 97-102.

[253] Mosekilde L, Christensen MS. Decreased parathyroid function in hyperthyroidism: inter relationship between serum parathyroid hormone, calcium phosphorus metabolism and thyroid function. Acta Endocrinol (Copenh) 1977;84: 566–75.

[254] Baxter JD, Bondy PK. Hypercalcemia of thyrotoxicosis. Ann Intern Med. 1966;65(3) 429–442.

[255] Bouillon, R., Muls, E. & De Moor, P. Influence of thyroid function on the serum concentration of 1,25-dihydroxyvitamin D3. J. Clin. Endocrinol. Metab.1980;51(4) 793-797.

[256] Skrabanek P. Catecholamines cause the hypercalciuria and hypercalcaemia in pheochromocytoma and in hyperthyroidism. Med Hypotheses. 1977;3(2) 59–62.

[257] Bouillon R, DeMoor P. Parathyroid function in patients with hyper or hypothyroidism. J Clin Endocrinol Metab. 1974;38(6) 999–1004.

[258] Giovanella L, Suriano S, Keller F, Borretta G, Ceriani L. Evaluation of serum parathyroid hormone-related peptide in hyperthyroid patients. Eur J Clin Invest. 201;41(1) 93-97.

[259] Macfarlane IA, Mawer EB, Berry J, Hann J. Vitamin D metabolism in hyperthyroidism. Clin Endocrinol (Oxf) 1982;17(1) 51–59.

[260] Velentzas C, Orepoulos DB, From G, Porret B, Rapopart A. Vitamin D levels in thyrotoxcosis. Lancet. 1977;1(8007) 370–371.

[261] Yamashita H, Nognchi S, Takatsu K, Koike E, Murakami T, Watanabe S, et al. High prevalence of vitamin D deficiency in Japanese female patients with Graves' disease. Endocr J. 2001;48(1) 63–69.

[262] Karsenty G, Bouchard P, Ulmann A, Schaison G. Elevated metabolic clearance rate of 1 alpha,25-dihydroxyvitamin D3 in hyperthyroidism. Acta Endocrinol (Copenh). 1985;110(1) 70-74.

[263] Mosekilde L, Christensen MS, Melsen F, Sorensen NS. Effect of anti-thyroid treatment on calcium phosphorus metabolism in hyperthyroidism.1: Chemical quantities in serum and urine. Acta Endocrinol (Copenh) 1978;87(4) 743–50.

[264] Tibi L, Patrick AW, Leslie P, Toft AD, Smith AF. Alkaline phosphatase isoenzymes in plasma in hyperthyroidism.Clin Chem. 1989;35(7) 1427-1430.

[265] Harvey RD, McHardy KC, Reid IW, Paterson F, Bewsher PD, Duncan A, Robins SP. Measurement of bone collagen degradation in hyperthyroidism and during thyroxine replacement therapy using pyridinium cross-links as specific urinary markers. J Clin Endocrinol Metab. 1991;72(6) 1189-1194.

[266] Ohishi T, Takahashi M, Kushida K, Horiuchi K, Ishigaki S, Inoue T. Quantitative analyses of urinary pyridinoline and deoxypyridinoline excretion in patients with hyperthyroidism. Endocr Res. 1992;18(4) 281-290.

[267] Pandolfi C, Montanari G, Mercantini F, Sbalzarini G. Osteocalcin and hyperthyroidism. Minerva Endocrinol. 1992;17(2) 75-78.

[268] Miyakawa M, Tsushima T, Demura H. Carboxy-terminal propeptide of type 1 procollagen (P1CP) and carboxy-terminal telopeptide of type 1 collagen (1CTP) as sensitive markers of bone metabolism in thyroid disease. Endocr J. 1996;43(6) 701-708.

[269] Garrel DR, Delmas PD, Malaval L, Tourniaire J. Serum bone Gla protein: a marker of bone turnover in hyperthyroidism. J Clin Endocrinol Metab. 1986;62(5) 1052-1055.

[270] Amato G, Mazziotti G, Sorvillo F, Piscopo M, Lalli E, Biondi B, Iorio S, Molinari A, Giustina A, Carella C. High serum osteoprotegerin levels in patients with hyperthyroidism: effect of medical treatment. Bone. 2004;35(3) 785-791.

[271] Wakasugi M, Wakao R, Tawata M, Gan N, Koizumi K, Onaya T. Bone mineral density in patients with hyperthyroidism measured by dual energy X-ray absorptiometry. Clin Endocrinol (Oxf). 1993;38(3) 283-286.

[272] Ben-Shlomo A, Hagag P, Evans S, Weiss M. Maturitas. Early postmenopausal bone loss in hyperthyroidism. 2001;39(1) 19-27.

[273] Boonya-Ussadorn T, Punkaew B, Sriassawaamorn N. A comparative study of bone mineral density between premenopausal women with hyperthyroidism and healthy premenopausal women. J Med Assoc Thai. 2010;93 (Suppl 6) S1-5.

[274] Majima T, Komatsu Y, Doi K, Takagi C, Shigemoto M, Fukao A, Morimoto T, Corners J, Nakao K. Negative correlation between bone mineral density and TSH receptor antibodies in male patients with untreated Graves' disease. Osteoporos Int. 2006;17(7) 1103-1110.

[275] Foldes J, Tarjan G, Szathmary M, Varga F, Krasznai I & Horvath C. Bone mineral density in patients with endogenous subclinical hyperthyroidism: is the thyroid status a risk factor for osteoporosis? Clinical Endocrinology 1993;39(5) 521–527.

[276] Muddle AH, Houben AJ & Nieuwenhuijzen Kruseman AC. Bone metabolism during anti-thyroid drug treatment of endogenous subclinical hyperthyroidism. Clinical Endocrinology 1994;41(4) 421–424.

[277] Lemke J, Bogner U, Felsenber D, Peters H & Schleusener H. Determination of bone mineral density by quantitative computed tomography and single photon absorptiometry in subclinical hyperthyroidism: a risk of early osteopenia in post-menopausal women. Clinical Endocrinology 1992;36(5) 511–517.

[278] Gurlek A & Gedik O. Effect of endogenous subclinical hyperthyroidism on bone metabolism and bone mineral density in premenopausal women. Thyroid 1999;9(6) 539–543.

[279] Földes J, Tarján G, Szathmari M, Varga F, Krasznai I, Horvath C. Bone mineral density in patients with endogenous subclinical hyperthyroidism: is this thyroid status a risk factor for osteoporosis? Clin Endocrinol (Oxf). 1993;39(5) 521-527.

[280] Adlin EV, Maurer AH, Marks AD, Channick BJ. Bone mineral density in postmenopausal women treated with L-thyroxine. Am J Med. 1991;90(3) 360-366.

[281] De Rosa G, Testa A, Giacomini D, Carrozza C, Astazi P, Caradonna P. Prospective study of bone loss in pre-and post-menopausal women on L-thyroxine therapy for non-toxic goitre. Clin Endocrinol (Oxf). 1997;47(5) 529-535.

[282] Giannini S, Nobile M, Sartori L, Binotto P, Ciuffreda M, Gemo G, Pelizzo MR, D'Angelo A, Crepaldi G. Bone density and mineral metabolism in thyroidectomized patients treated with long-term L-thyroxine. Clin Sci (Lond). 1994;87(5) 593-597.

[283] Jódar E, Martínez-Díaz-Guerra G, Azriel S, Hawkins F. Bone mineral density in male patients with L-thyroxine suppressive therapy and Graves disease. Calcif Tissue Int. 2001;69(2) 84-87.

[284] Hanna FW, Pettit RJ, Ammari F, Evans WD, Sandeman D, Lazarus JH. Effect of replacement doses of thyroxine on bone mineral density.Clin Endocrinol (Oxf). 1998;48(2) 229-234.

[285] Nuzzo V, Lupoli G, Esposito Del Puente A, Rampone E, Carpinelli A, Del Puente AE, Oriente P. Bone mineral density in premenopausal women receiving levothyroxine suppressive therapy. Gynecol Endocrinol. 1998;12(5) 333-337.

[286] Heijckmann AC, Huijberts MS, Geusens P, de Vries J, Menheere PP, Wolffenbuttel BH. Hip bone mineral density, bone turnover and risk of fracture in patients on long-term suppressive L-thyroxine therapy for differentiated thyroid carcinoma. Eur J Endocrinol. 2005;153(1) 23-29.

[287] Földes J, Lakatos P, Zsadányi J, Horváth C. Decreased serum IGF-I and dehydroepiandrosterone sulphate may be risk factors for the development of reduced bone mass in postmenopausal women with endogenous subclinical hyperthyroidism. Eur J Endocrinol. 1997;136(3) 277-281.

[288] Obermayer-Pietsch BM, Frühauf GE, Chararas K, Mikhail-Reinisch S, Renner W, Berghold A, Kenner L, Lackner C. Association of the vitamin D receptor genotype BB with low bone density in hyperthyroidism. J Bone Miner Res. 2000;15(10) 1950-1955.

[289] Mysliwiec J, Zbucki R, Nikolajuk A, Mysliwiec P, Kaminski K, Bondyra Z, Dadan J, Gorska M, Winnicka MM. Estrogens modulate RANKL-RANK/osteoprotegerin mediated interleukin-6 effect on thyrotoxicosis-related bone turnover in mice. Horm Metab Res. 2011;43(4) 236-240.

[290] Udayakumar N, Chandrasekaran M, Rasheed MH, Suresh RV, Sivaprakash S. Evaluation of bone mineral density in thyrotoxicosis. Singapore Med J. 2006;47(11) 947-950.

[291] Njeh CF, Fuerst T, Diessel E, Genant HK. Is quantitative ultrasound dependent on bone structure? A reflection. Osteoporos Int. 2001;12(1) 1-15.

[292] Gómez Acotto C, Schott AM, Hans D, Niepomniszcze H, Mautalen CA, Meunier PJ. Hyperthyroidism influences ultrasound bone measurement on the Os calcis. Osteoporos Int. 1998;8(5) 455-459.

[293] Allain TJ, McGregor AM. Thyroid hormones and bone. J Endocrinol. 1993;139(1) 9-18.

[294] Kung AWC, Yeung SSC. Prevention of bone loss induced by thyroxine suppressive therapy in postmenopausal women: The effect of calcium and calcitonin. J Clin Endocrinol Metab. 1996;81(3) 1232–1236.

[295] Franklyn JA, Betteridge J, Holder R, Sheppard MC. Effect of estrogen replacement therapy upon bone mineral density in thyroxine-treated postmenopausal women with a past history of thyrotoxicosis. Thyroid. 1995;5(5) 359-363.

[296] Schneider DL, Barrett-Connor EL, Morton DJ. Thyroid hormone use and bone mineral density in elderly women. Effect of estrogen. JAMA. 1994;271(16) 1245–1249.

[297] Rossouw JE, Anderson GL, Prentice RL et al; Writing Group for the Women's Health Initiative Investigators.Risks and benefits of estrogen plus progestin in healthy post-

menopausal women. Principal results from the Women's Health Initiative randomized controlled trial. JAMA. 2002;288(3) 321–333.

[298] Guo CY, Weetman AP, Eastell R. Longitudinal changes of bone mineral density and bone turnover in postmenopausal women on thyroxine. Clin Endocrinol. 1997;46(3) 301–307.

[299] Bayley TA, Harrison JE, McNeill KG, Mernagh JR. Effect of thyrotoxicosis and its treatment on bone mineral and muscle mass. J Clin Endocrinol Metab. 1980;50(5) 916-922.

[300] Toh SH, Claunch BC, Brown PH. Effect of hyperthyroidism and its treatment on bone mineral content. Arch Intern Med. 1985;145(5) 883-886.

[301] Rosen CJ, Adler RA. Longitudinal changes in lumbar bone density among thyrotoxic patients after attainment of euthyroidism (Abstract). In: Program of the 74th Annual Meeting of the Endocrine Society, San Antonio, Texas, 1992:436.

[302] Lupoli GA, Fittipaldi MR, Fonderico F, Panico A, Colarusso S, Di Micco L, Cavallo A, Costa L, Paglione A, Lupoli G. Methimazole versus methimazole and diphosphonates in hyperthyroid and osteoporotic patients. Minerva Endocrinol. 2005;30(2) 89-94

[303] Yang LJ, Shen FX, Zheng JC, Zhang HL. Clinical application of alendronate for osteoporosis/osteopenia secondary to hyperthyroidism. Zhongguo Gu Shang. 2012;25(2) 133-137.

[304] Majima T, Komatsu Y, Doi K, Takagi C, Shigemoto M, Fukao A, Morimoto T, Corners J, Nakao K. Clinical significance of risedronate for osteoporosis in the initial treatment of male patients with Graves' disease. J Bone Miner Metab. 2006;24(2) 105-113.

[305] Kung AWC, Yeung SSC. Prevention of bone loss induced by thyroxine suppressive therapy in postmenopausal women: The effect of calcium and calcitonin. J Clin Endocrinol Metab. 1996;81(3) 1232–1236.

[306] Jódar E, Muñoz-Torres M, Escobar-Jiménez F, Quesada M, Luna JD, Olea N. Antiresorptive therapy in hyperthyroid patients: longitudinal changes in bone and mineral metabolism. J Clin Endocrinol Metab. 1997;82(6) 1989-1994.

[307] Akçay MN, Akçay G, Bilen H. The effects of calcitonin on bone resorption in hyperthyroidism: a placebo-controlled clinical study. J Bone Miner Metab. 2004;22(2) 90-93.

[308] Chong HW, See KC, Phua J. Thyroid storm with multiorgan failure. Thyroid. 2010;20(3) 333–336.

[309] Bhasin S, Ballani P, Mac RP. Endocrine problems in critically ill. In: Bongard FS, Sue DY, Vintch JR, editors. Current diagnosis and treatment critical care. New York: McGraw-Hill; 2008. pp. 566–80.

[310] Pimentel L, Hansen K. Thyroid disease in the emergency department: A clinical and laboratory review. J Emerg Med. 2005;28(2) 201–209.

[311] Preziati D, La Rosa L, Covini G, Marcelli R, Rescalli S, Persani L, Del Ninno E, Meroni PL, Colombo M, Beck-Peccoz P. Autoimmunity and thyroid function in patients with chronic active hepatitis treated with recombinant interferon alpha-2a. Eur J Endocrinol. 1995;132(5) 587-593.

[312] Mammen JS, Ghazarian SR, Rosen A, Ladenson PW. Patterns of Interferon-Alpha-Induced Thyroid Dysfunction Vary with Ethnicity, Sex, Smoking Status, and Pretreatment Thyrotropin in an International Cohort of Patients Treated for Hepatitis C. Thyroid. 2013;23(9) 1151-1158

[313] Carroll R, Matfin G. Endocrine and metabolic emergencies: thyroid storm. Ther Adv Endocrinol Metab. 2010;1(3) 139-145.

[314] Goldberg PA, Inzucchi SE. Critical issues in endocrinology. Clin Chest Med. 2003;24(4) 583–606.

[315] Burch, H.B. and Wartofsky, L.Life-threatening thyrotoxicosis. Thyroid storm. Endocrinol Metab Clin North Am 1993;22(2) 263-277.

[316] Izumi K, Kondo S, Okada T. A case of atypical thyroid storm with hypoglycemia and lactic acidosis. Endocr J. 2009;56(6) 747-752.

[317] Deng Y, Zheng W, Zhu J. Successful treatment of thyroid crisis accompanied by hypoglycemia, lactic acidosis, and multiple organ failure. Am J Emerg Med. 2012;30(9) 2094.e5-6.

[318] Nayak, B. and Burman, K.Thyrotoxicosis and thyroid storm. Endocrinol Metab Clin N Am 2006;35(4) 663-686.

[319] Malozowski, S. and Chiesa, A. Propylthiouracil-Induced Hepatotoxicity and Death. Hopefully, Never More. J. Clin. Endocrinol. Metab 2010;95(7) 3161–3163.

[320] Andrioli M, Pecori Giraldi F, Cavagnini F. Isolated corticotrophin deficiency. Pituitary. 2006;9(4) 289-295.

[321] Erdogan MF, Güleç S, Tutar E, Başkal N, Erdogan G. A stepwise approach to the treatment of amiodarone-induced thyrotoxicosis. Thyroid. 2003;13(2) 205-209.

[322] Tsai, W.C., Pei, D., Wang, T., Wu, D.A., Li, J.C., Wei, C.L. et al. The effect of combination therapy with propylthiouracil and cholestyramine in the treatment of Graves' hyperthyroidism. Clin Endocrinol (Oxf) 2005;62(5) 521-524.

[323] Carhill A, Gutierrez A, Lakhia R, Nalini R. Surviving the storm: two cases of thyroid storm successfully treated with plasmapheresis. BMJ Case Rep. 2012;2012.

[324] Jha S, Waghdhare S, Reddi R, Bhattacharya P. Thyroid storm due to inappropriate administration of a compounded thyroid hormone preparation successfully treated with plasmapheresis. Thyroid. 2012;22(12) 1283-1286.

[325] Koball S, Hickstein H, Gloger M, Hinz M, Henschel J, Stange J, Mitzner S. Treatment of thyrotoxic crisis with plasmapheresis and single pass albumin dialysis: a case report. Artif Organs. 2010;34(2) E55-8.

[326] Kreisner E, Lutzky M, Gross JL. Charcoal hemoperfusion in the treatment of levothyroxine intoxication. Thyroid. 2010;20(2) 209-212.

[327] Tinker TD, Vannatta JB. Thyrotoxic hypokalemic periodic paralysis: report of four cases and review of the literature (1). J Okla State Med Assoc. 1987;80(1) 11-15.

[328] Hawkins BR, Ma JT, Lam KS, Wang CC, Yeung RT. Association of HLA antigens with thyrotoxic Graves' disease and periodic paralysis in Hong Kong Chinese. Clin Endocrinol (Oxf). 1985;23(3) 245-252.

[329] Tamai H, Tanaka K, Komaki G, Matsubayashi S, Hirota Y, Mori K, Kuma K, Kumagai LF, Nagataki S. HLA and thyrotoxic periodic paralysis in Japanese patients. J Clin Endocrinol Metab. 1987;64(5) 1075-1078.

[330] Pandolfi C, Pellegrini L, Vitelli E, Sbalzarini G. Thyrotoxic periodic paralysis and Graves' disease. Description of an HLA-CW7-positive case. Minerva Endocrinol. 1991;16(3) 153-155.

[331] Ahlawat SK, Sachdev A. Hypokalaemic paralysis. Postgrad Med J. 1999;75(882) 193-197.

[332] Manoukian, M.A., Foote, J.A. & Crapo, L.M. Clinical and metabolic features of thyrotoxic periodic paralysis in 24 episodes. Archives of Internal Medicine 199;159(6) 601–606.

[333] Silva, M.R., Chiamolera, M.I., Kasamatsu, T.S., Cerutti, J.M. & Maciel, R.M. Thyrotoxic hypokalemic periodic paralysis, an endocrine emergency: clinical and genetic features in 25 patients. Arquivos Brasileiros de Endocrinologia e Metabologia 2004;48(1) 196–215.

[334] Sanyal D, Bhattacharjee S. Thyrotoxic hypokalemic periodic paralysis as the presenting symptom of silent thyroiditis. Ann Indian Acad Neurol. 2013;16(2) 218-220.

[335] Ozaki H, Mori K, Nakagawa Y, Hoshikawa S, Ito S, Yoshida K. Autonomously functioning thyroid nodule associated with thyrotoxic periodic paralysis. Endocr J. 2008;55(1) 113-119.

[336] Ghosh S, Sahoo R, Rao S, Rath D. Pituitary macroadenoma: a rare cause of thyrotoxic hypokalaemic periodic paralysis. BMJ Case Rep. 2013;2013.

[337] Pappa T, Papanastasiou L, Markou A, Androulakis I, Kontogeorgos G, Seretis A, Piaditis G. Thyrotoxic periodic paralysis as the first manifestation of a thyrotropin-secreting pituitary adenoma. Hormones (Athens). 2010;9(1) 82-86.

[338] Hannon MJ, Behan LA, Agha A. Thyrotoxic periodic paralysis due to excessive L-thyroxine replacement in a Caucasian man. Ann Clin Biochem. 2009;46(Pt 5) 423-5.

[339] Akinyemi E, Bercovici S, Niranjan S, Paul N, Hemavathy B. Thyrotoxic hypokalemic periodic paralysis due to dietary weight-loss supplement. Am J Ther. 201;18(3) e81-3.

[340] Tran, H.A. Inadvertent iodine excess causing thyrotoxic hypokalemic periodic paralysis. Archives of Internal Medicine 2005;165(21) 2536.

[341] Laroia, S.T., Zaw, K.M., Ganti, A.K., Newman, W. & Akinwande, A.O. Amiodarone-induced thyrotoxicosis presenting as hypokalemic periodic paralysis. Southern Medical Journal 202;95(11) 1326–1328.

[342] Cesur, M., Gursoy, A., Avcioglu, U., Erdogan, M.F., Corapcioglu, D. & Kamel, N. Thyrotoxic hypokalemic periodic paralysis as the first manifestation of interferon-alpha-induced Graves' disease. Journal of Clinical Gastroenterology 2006;40(9) 864–865.

[343] Akar, S., Comlekci, A., Birlik, M., Onen, F., Sari, I., Gurler, O., Bekis, R. & Akkoc, N. Thyrotoxic periodic paralysis in a Turkish male; the recurrence of the attack after radioiodine treatment. Endocrine Journal 2005;52(1) 149–151.

[344] Cesur M, Bayram F, Temel MA, Ozkaya M, Kocer A, Ertorer ME, Koc F, Kaya A, Gullu S. Thyrotoxic hypokalaemic periodic paralysis in a Turkish population: three new case reports and analysis of the case series. Clin Endocrinol (Oxf). 2008;68(1) 143-152.

[345] Lin, S.H. Thyrotoxic periodic paralysis. Mayo Clinic Proceedings, 2005;80: 99–105.

[346] Mellgren, G., Bleskestad, I.H., Aanderud, S. & Bindoff, L. Thyrotoxicosis and paraparesis in a young woman. case report and review of the literature. Thyroid 2002;12(1) 77–80.

[347] Cesur M, Ilgin SD, Baskal N, Gullu S. Hypokalemic paralysis is not just a hypokalemic paralysis. Eur J Emerg Med. 2008;15(3) 150-153.

[348] Kung, A.W. Clinical review: Thyrotoxic periodic paralysis: a diagnostic challenge. Journal of Clinical Endocrinology and Metabolism 2006;91(7) 2490–2495.

[349] Ober, K.P. Thyrotoxic periodic paralysis in the United States. Report of 7 cases and review of the literature. Medicine 1992;71(3) 109–120.

[350] Liu YC, Tsai WS, Chau T, Lin SH. Acute hypercapnic respiratory failure due to thyrotoxic periodic paralysis. Am J Med Sci 2004;327(5) 264–267.

[351] Gonzalez-Trevino, O. & Rosas-Guzman, J. Normokalemic thyrotoxic periodic paralysis: a new therapeutic strategy. Thyroid 1999;9(1) 61–63.

[352] Wu, C.C., Chau, T., Chang, C.J. & Lin, S.H. An unrecognized cause of paralysis in ED: thyrotoxic normokalemic periodic paralysis. American Journal of Emergency Medicine 2003;21(1) 71–73.

[353] Randall, B.B. Fatal hypokalemic thyrotoxic periodic paralysis presenting as the sudden, unexplained death of a Cambodian refugee. American Journal of Forensic Medicine and Pathology 1992;13(3) 204–206.

[354] Loh KC, Pinheiro L, Ng KS. Thyrotoxic periodic paralysis complicated by near-fatal ventricular arrhythmias. Singapore Med J. 2005;46(2) 88-89.

[355] Singhal, P.C., Abramovici, M., Venkatesan, J. & Mattana, J. Hypokalemia and rhabdomyolysis. Mineral and Electrolyte Metabolism 1991;17(5) 335–339.

[356] Amanzadeh, J. & Reilly, R.F. Jr. Hypophosphatemia: an evidencebased approach to its clinical consequences and management. Nature Clinic Practice Nephrology 2006;2(3) 136–148.

[357] Lichtstein, D.M., Arteaga, R.B. Rhabdomyolysis associated with hyperthyroidism. American Journal of Medical Science 2006;332(2) 103–105.

[358] Sabau, I., Canonica, A. Hypokalaemic periodic paralysis associated with controlled thyrotoxicosis. Schweizerische Medizinische Wochenschrift 2000;130(44) 1689–1691.

[359] Ee, B., Cheah, J.S. Electrocardiographic changes in thyrotoxic periodic paralysis. Journal of Electrocardiology 1979;12(3) 263–279.

[360] Hsu, Y.J., Lin, Y.F., Chau, T., Liou, J.T., Kuo, S.W., Lin, S.H. Electrocardiographic manifestations in patients with thyrotoxic periodic paralysis. American Journal of Medical Science 2003;326(3) 128–132.

[361] Lu KC, Hsu YJ, Chiu JS, Hsu YD, Lin SH. Effects of potassium supplementation on the recovery of thyrotoxic periodic paralysis. Am J Emerg Med 2004;22(7) 544–547.

[362] Lin SH, Lin YF. Propranolol rapidly reverses paralysis, hypokalemia, and hypophosphatemia in thyrotoxic periodic paralysis. Am J Kidney Dis 2001;37(3) 620–623.

[363] Tigas S, Papachilleos P, Ligkros N, Andrikoula M, Tsatsoulis A. Hypokalemic paralysis following administration of intravenous methylprednisolone in a patient with Graves' thyrotoxicosis and ophthalmopathy. Hormones (Athens). 2011;10(4) 313-316.

[364] Shulkin D, Olson BR, Levey GS. Thyrotoxic periodic paralysis in a Latin-American taking acetazolamide. Am J Med Sci 1989;297(5) 337–338.

[365] Chen YC, Fang JT, Chang CT, Chou HH. Thyrotoxic periodic paralysis in a patient abusing thyroxine for weight reduction. Ren Fail 2001;23(1) 139–142.

[366] Bunevicius R, Prange AJ Jr. Psychiatric manifestations of Graves' hyperthyroidism: pathophysiology and treatment options. CNS Drugs 2006;20(11) 897-909.

[367] Stern RA, Prange AJ. Neuropsychiatric aspects of endocrine disorders. In: Kaplan HI, Sadock BJ, eds. Comprehensive Textbook of Psychiatry. 6th ed. Baltimore: Wiliams & Wilkins, 1995:241-251.

[368] Whybrow PC, Prange AJ Jr. A hypothesis of thyroid-catecholamine-receptor interaction: its relevance to affective illness. Arch Gen Psychiatry 1981;38(1) 106-113.

[369] Hall RC. Psychiatric effects of thyroid hormone disturbance. Psychosomatics 1983; 24(1) 7–11, 15–18.

[370] Aszalós Z. Some neurologic and psychiatric complications in endocrine disorders: the thyroid gland. Orv Hetil 2007;148(7) 303-310.

[371] Hughes JR. A review of sleepwalking (somnambulism): the enigma of neurophysiology and polysomnography with differential diagnosis of complex partial seizures. Epilepsy Behav 2007;11(4) 483-491.

[372] Greer S & Parsons V. Schizophrenia-like psychosis in thyroid crisis. British Journal of Psychiatry 1968;114(516) 1357–1362.

[373] Taylor JW. Depression in thyrotoxicosis. Americal Journal of Psychiatry 1975;132(5) 552–553.

[374] Lee S, Chow CC, Wing YK, Leung CM, Chiu H, Chen CN. Mania secondary to thyrotoxicosis. British Journal of Psychiatry 1991;159 712–713.

[375] Khuan TC. Psychoses associated with thyrotoxicosis: a retrospective study of twenty cases. Medical Journal of Malaysia 1985;40(3) 247–251.

[376] Jane P. Gagliardi, Greg L. Clary. Treatment of Thyrotoxicosis – Induced Psychosis. Psychopharmacology Bulletin 2002;36(4) 7-13.

[377] Rizvi AA. "Thyrotoxic psychosis" associated with subacute thyroiditis. South Med J. 2007;100(8) 837-840.

[378] Lee KA, Park KT, Yu HM, Jin HY, Baek HS, Park TS. Subacute thyroiditis presenting as acute psychosis: a case report and literature review. Korean J Intern Med. 2013;28(2) 242-246.

[379] Bokhari R, Bhatara VS, Bandettini F, McMillin JM. Postpartum psychosis and postpartum thyroiditis. Psychoneuroendocrinology 1998;23(6) 643-650.

[380] Carta MG, Loviselli A, Hardoy MC, Massa S, Cadeddu M, Sardu C, Carpiniello B, Dell'Osso L, Mariotti S. The link between thyroid autoimmunity (antithyroid peroxidase autoantibodies) with anxiety and mood disorders in the community: a field of interest for public health in the future. BMC Psychiatry 2004;4:25.

[381] Roca RP, Blackman MR, Ackerley MB, et al. Thyroid hormone elevations during acute psychiatric illness: relationship to severity and distinction from hyperthyroidism. Endocr Res 1990;16(4) 415–447.

[382] Spratt DI, Pont A, Miller MB, McDougall IR, Bayer MF, McLaughlin WT. Hyperthyroxinemia in patients with acute psychiatric disorders. Am J Med 1982;73(1) 41-48.

[383] Trzepacz PT, McCue M, Klein I, et al. Psychiatric and neuropsychological response to propranolol in Graves' disease. Biol Psychiatry 1988; 23(7) 678-88.

[384] Kathol RG, Turner R, Delahunt J. Depression and anxiety associated with hyperthyroidism: response to antithyroid therapy. Psychosomatics 1986; 27(7) 501-5.

[385] Lazarus A, Jaffe R. Resolution of thyroid-induced schizophreniform disorder following subtotal thyroidectomy: case report.Gen Hosp Psychiatry. 1986;8(1) 29-31.

[386] De Leu N, Unuane D, Poppe K, Velkeniers B. Seizures and postictal stupor in a patient with uncontrolled Graves' hyperthyroidism. BMJ Case Rep. 2012;2012.

[387] Hecht T, Brand J, Vlaho S. Encephalopathy and sinustachycardia in childhood--a possible differential diagnosis. J Pediatr Endocrinol Metab. 2012;25(1-2) 149-151.

[388] Vergely N, Garnier P, Guy C, Khalfallah Y, Estour B. Seizure during Graves' disease. Epileptic Disord. 2009;11(2) 136-137.

[389] Ho J, Jackson R, Johnson D. Massive levothyroxine ingestion in a pediatric patient: case report and discussion. CJEM. 2011;13(3) 165-168.

[390] Sundaram MB, Hill A, Lowry N. Thyroxine-induced petit mal status epilepticus. Neurology 1985;35(12) 1792-1793.

[391] Obeid T, Awada A, al Rajeh S, Chaballout A. Thyroxine exacerbates absence seizures in juvenile myoclonic epilepsy. Neurology 1996;47(2) 605-606.

[392] Scorza FA, Arida RM, Cysneiros RM, Terra VC, de Albuquerque M, Machado HR, Cavalheiro EA. Subclinical hyperthyroidism and sudden unexpected death in epilepsy. Med Hypotheses. 2010;74(4) 692-694.

[393] Sakurai T, Tanaka Y, Koumura A, Hayashi Y, Kimura A, Hozumi I, Yoneda M, Inuzuka T Case report of a patient with Hashimoto's encephalopathy associated with Basedow's disease mimicking Creutzfeldt-Jakob disease. Brain Nerve. 2008;60(5) 559-565.

[394] Li Voon Chong JS, Lecky BR, Macfarlane IA. Recurrent encephalopathy and generalised seizures associated with relapses of thyrotoxicosis. Int J Clin Pract. 2000;54(9) 621-622.

[395] Dai A, Wasay M, Dubey N, Giglio P, Bakshi R. Superior sagittal sinus thrombosis secondary to hyperthyroidism. J Stroke Cerebrovasc Dis. 2000;9(2) 89-90.

[396] Siegert CE, Smelt AH, de Bruin TW. Superior sagittal sinus thrombosis and thyrotoxicosis. Possible association in two cases. Stroke. 1995;26(3) 496-497.

[397] Ra CS, Lui CC, Liang CL, Chen HJ, Kuo YL, Chen WF. Superior sagittal sinus thrombosis induced by thyrotoxicosis. Case report. J Neurosurg. 2001;94(1) 130-132.

[398] Song TJ, Kim SJ, Kim GS, Choi YC, Kim WJ. The prevalence of thyrotoxicosis-related seizures. Thyroid. 2010;20(9) 955-958.

[399] Philips S, Kuan C C, Hsu M C, Lue H C. Thyroid hormone-induced seizures a case report and review of literature. Pediat Therapeut 2012;2(5) 1000129

[400] Su YH, Izumi T, Kitsu M, Fukuyama Y. Seizure threshold in juvenile myoclonic epilepsy with Graves' disease. Epilepsia 1993;34(3) 488-492.

[401] Jabbari B, Huott AD. Seizures in thyrotoxicosis. Epilepsia 1980;21:91-96.

[402] Atterwill CK, Kingsbury AE, Balázs R. Effect of thyroid hormone on neural development in vitro. Monogr Neural Sci 1983;9:50-61.

[403] Timiras PS, Woodbury DM, Ag SL. Effect of thyroxine and triiodothyronine on brain function and electrolyte distribution in intact and adrenalectomized rats. J Pharmacol Exp Ther 1955;115(2) 154-171.

[404] Woodburry DM, Hurley RE, Lewis NG, Mcarthur MW, Coprland WW, et al. Effect of thyroxin, thyroidectomy and 6-n-propyl-2-thiouracil on brain function. J Pharmacol Exp Ther 1952;106(3) 331-340.

[405] Lin CS, Yiin KT, Lin WH, Huang SY. Thyrotoxicosis accompanied with periodic seizure attacks a case report and review of literature. Zhonghua Yi Xue Za Zhi (Taipei). 1992;50(4) 335-337.

[406] Zander Olsen P, Stoier M, Siersbaek-Nielsen K, Molholm Hansen J, Scholer M, et al. Electroencephalographic findings in hyperthyroidism. Electroencephalogr Clin Neurophysiol 1972;32(2) 171-177.

[407] Wohl MG, Shuman CR. Atypical syndromes in hyperthyroidism. Ann Intern Med 1957;46(5) 857-867.

[408] Isojärvi JI, Turkka J, Pakarinen AJ, Kotila M, Rättyä J, et al. Thyroid function in men taking carbamazepine, oxcarbazepine, or valproate for epilepsy. Epilepsia 2001;42(7) 930-934.

[409] Gul Mert G, Horoz OO, Herguner MO, Incecik F, Yildizdas RD, Onenli Mungan N, Yuksel B, Altunbasak S. Hashimoto's Encephalopathy: Four Cases and Review of Literature. Int J Neurosci. 2013 Oct 2. [Epub ahead of print]

[410] Hernán Martínez J, Torres O, Mangual MM, Palermo C, Figueroa C, Santiago M, Miranda Mde L, González E. Hashimoto's encephalopathy: an underdiagnosed clinical entity. Bol Asoc Med P R. 2013;105(1) 57-61.

[411] Resmini E, Minuto F, Colao A, Ferone D. Secondary diabetes associated with principal endocrinopathies: the impact of new treatment modalities. Acta Diabetol. 2009;46(2) 85-95.

[412] Vondra K, Vrbíková J, Sterzl L, Bílek R, Vondrova M, Zamrazil V: Thyroid autoantibodies and their clinical relevance in young adults with type 1 diabetes during the first 12 years after diabetes onset. J Endocrinol Invest 2004, 27(8) 728-732.

[413] Greco D, Pisciotta M, Gambina F, Maggio F. Graves' disease in subjects with type 1 diabetes mellitus: a prevalence study in western Sicily (Italy). Prim Care Diabetes. 2011;5(4) 241-244.

[414] Lambadiari V, Mitrou P, Maratou E, Raptis AE, Tountas N, Raptis SA, Dimitriadis G. Thyroid hormones are positively associated with insulin resistance early in the development of type 2 diabetes. Endocrine. 2011;39(1) 28-32.

[415] Komiya I, et al : Studies on the association of NIDDM in Japanese patients with hyperthyroid Graves' disease. Horm Res. 1992;38(5-6) 264-268.

[416] Huber A, Menconi F, Corathers S, Jacobson EM, Tomer Y. Joint genetic susceptibility to type 1 diabetes and autoimmune thyroiditis: from epidemiology to mechanisms. Endocr Rev. 2008;29(6) 697-725.

[417] Chidakel A, Mentuccia D, Celi FS. Peripheral metabolism of thyroid hormone and glucose homeostasis. Thyroid 2005;15(8) 899-903.

[418] Mitrou P, Raptis SA, Dimitriadis G: Insulin action in hyperthyroidism: a focus on muscle and adipose tissue. Endocr Rev 2010;31(5) 663-679.

[419] Ikeda T, Fujiyama K, Hoshino T, Takeuchi T, Tominaga M, Mashiba H. Glucose tolerance and gastric emptying in thyrotoxic rats. Metabolism. 1989;38(9) 874-877.

[420] Pfaffenbach B, Adamek RJ, Hagelmann D, Schaffstein J, WegenerM. Effect of hyperthyroidism on antral myoelectrical activity, gastric emptying and dyspepsia in man. Hepatogastroenterology 1997;44(17) 1500–1508

[421] Barczynski M, Thor P. Reversible autonomic dysfunction in hyperthyroid patients affects gastric myoelectrical activity and emptying. Clin Auton Res 2001;11(4) 243–249

[422] Wegener M, Wedmann B, Langhoff T, Schaffstein J, AdamekR. Effect of hyperthyroidism on the transit of a caloric solid-liquid meal through the stomach, the small intestine, and the colon in man. J Clin Endocrinol Metab 192;75(3) 745–749

[423] Jonderko K, Jonderko G, Marcisz C, GołabT. Gastric emptying in hyperthyroidism. AmJ Gastroenterol 1997;92(5) 835–838

[424] Brenta G. Why can insulin resistance be a natural consequence of thyroid dysfunction? J Thyroid Res. 2011;2011:152850.

[425] Klieverik LP, Janssen SF, Van Riel A, et al. Thyroid hormone modulates glucose production via a sympathetic pathway from the hypothalamic paraventricular nucleus

to the liver. *Proceedings of the National Academy of Sciences of the United States of America*. 2009;106(14) 5966–5971.

[426] Laville M, Rio JP, Bougneres PF, Mornex R. Glucose metabolism in experimental hyperthyroidism: intact in vivo sensitivity to insulin with abnormal binding and increased glucose turnover. *Journal of Clinical Endocrinology & Metabolism*. 1984;58(6) 960–965.

[427] Bratusch-Marrain PR, Gasić S, Waldhäusl WK. Triiodothyronine increases splanchnic release and peripheral uptake of glucose in healthy humans. *The American Journal of Physiology*. 1984;247(5, part 1) E681–E687.

[428] Dimitriadis GD, Baker B, Marsh H, et al. Effect of thyroid hormone excess on action, secretion, and metabolism of insulin in humans. *The American Journal of physiology*. 1985;248(5) E593–E601.

[429] Randin J, Scarriga B, Jequier F, Felber J. Studies of glucose and lipid metabolism and continues indirect calorimetry in Graves' disease: effect of an oral glucose load. *Journal of Clinical Endocrinology & Metabolism*. 1985;61(6) 1165–1171.

[430] McCulloch AJ, Nosadini R, Pernet A, et al. Glucose turnover and indices of recycling in thyrotoxicosis and primary thyroid failure. *Clinical Science*. 1983;64(1) 41–47.

[431] Sandler MP, Robinson RP, Rabin D, Lacy WW, Abumrad NN. The effect of thyroid hormones on gluconeogenesis and forearm metabolism in man. *Clinical Endocrinology & Metabolism*. 1983;56(3) 479–485.

[432] Celsing F, Blomstrand E, Melichna J, et al. Effect of hyperthyroidism on fibre-type composition, fibre area, glycogen content and enzyme activity in human skeletal muscle. *Clinical Physiology*. 1986;6(2) 171–181.

[433] Foss MC, Paccola GMGF, Saad MJA, Pimenta WP, Piccinato CE, Iazigi N. Peripheral glucose metabolism in human hyperthyroidism. *Journal of Clinical Endocrinology & Metabolism*. 1990;70(4) 1167–1172.

[434] Dimitriadis GD, Leighton B, Vlachonikolis IG, et al. Effects of hyperthyroidism on the sensitivity of glycolysis and glycogen synthesis to insulin in the soleus muscle of the rat. *Biochemical Journal*. 1988;253(1) 87–92.

[435] Parry-Billings M, Dimitriadis GD, Leighton B, et al. Effects of hyperthyroidism and hypothyroidism on glutamine metabolism by skeletal muscle of the rat. *Biochemical Journal*. 1990;272(2) 319–322.

[436] Leighton B, Dimitriadis GD, Oarry-Billings M, Bond J, Kemp P, Newsholme EA. Thyroid hormone analogue SKF L-94901: effects on amino acid and carbohydrate metabolism in rat skeletal muscle in vitro. *Biochemical Pharmacology*. 1990;40(5) 1161–1164.

[437] Dimitriadis GD, Mitrou P, Lambadiari V, Boutati E, Maratou E, Koukkou E, Tzanela M, Thalassinos N, Raptis SA. Glucose and lipid fluxes in the adipose tissue after meal ingestion in hyperthyroidism. J Clin Endocrinol Metab 2006;91(3) 1112–1118.

[438] Taylor R, McCulloch AJ, Zeuzem S, Gray P, Clark F, Alberti KG. Insulin secretion, adipocyte insulin binding and insulin sensitivity in thyrotoxicosis. Acta Endocrinol 1985;109(1) 96–103.

[439] Hales CN, Hyams DE. Plasma concentrations of glucose non-esterified fatty acid, and insulin during oral glucose tolerance tests in thyrotoxicosis. Lancet 1964;2(7350) 69–71.

[440] Cavagnini F, Peracchi M, Raggi U, Bana R, Pontiroli AE, Malinverni A, Pinto M. Impairment of growth hormone and insulin secretion in hyperthyroidism. Eur J Clin Invest 1974;4(1) 71–77.

[441] Roubsanthisuk W, Watanakejorn P, Tunlakit M, Sriussadaporn S. Hyperthyroidism induces glucose intolerance by lowering both insulin secretion and peripheral insulin sensitivity. J Med Assoc Thai 2006;89(Suppl 5) S133–S140.

[442] Holness MJ, GreenwoodGK, SmithND,SugdenMC. PPAR-α activation and increased dietary lipid oppose thyroid hormone signaling and rescue impaired glucose-stimulated insulin secretion in hyperthyroidism. Am J Physiol Endocrinol Metab 2008;295(6) E1380–E1389.

[443] Kabadi U, Eisenstein A. Impaired pancreatic a-cell response in hyperthyroidism. J Clin Endocrinol Metab 1980;51(3) 478–482

[444] J. P. Randin, L. Tappy, and B. Scazziga. Insulin sensitivity and exogenous insulin clearance in Graves' disease. Measurement by the glucose clamp technique and continuous indirect calorimetry. Diabetes 1986;35(2) 178-181

[445] Nijs HG, Radder JK, Foolich M, Krans HM. Increased insulin action and clearance in hyperthyroid newly diagnosed IDDM patient. Restoration to normal with antithyroid treatment. Diabetes Care 1989;12(5) 319-324.

[446] Malaisse WJ, Malaisse-Lagae F, McCraw EF. Effects of thyroid function upon insulin secretion. Diabetes 1967;16(9) 643–646.

[447] S. Lenzen and H. Kucking. Inhibition of insulin secretion by L-thyroxine and thyroxine treatment in rats under the influence of drugs affecting the adrenergic nervous system. Acta Endocrinologica 1982;100(4) 527–533.

[448] H. M. Ximenes, S. Lortz, A. J°orns, and S. Lenzen. Triiodothyronine (T3)-mediated toxicity and induction of apoptosis in insulin-producing INS-1 cells. Life Sciences 2007;80(22) 2045–2050

[449] Dimitriadis G, Hatziagelaki E, Mitrou P, Lambadiari V, Maratou E, Raptis AE, Gerich JE, Raptis SA. Effect of hyperthyroidism on clearance and secretion of glucagon in man. Exp Clin Endocrinol Diabetes. 2011;119(4) 214-217.

[450] Maratou E, Hadjidakis DJ, Peppa M, Alevizaki M, Tsegka K, Lambadiari V, Mitrou P, Boutati E, Kollias A, Economopoulos T, Raptis SA, Dimitriadis G. Studies of insulin resistance in patients with clinical and subclinical hyperthyroidism. Eur J Endocrinol. 2010;163(4) 625-630.

[451] Rezzonico J, Niepomniszcze H, Rezzonico M, Pusiol E, Alberto M, Brenta G. The association of insulin resistance with subclinical thyrotoxicosis. Thyroid. 2011;21(9) 945-949.

[452] Yavuz DG, Yüksel M, Deyneli O, Ozen Y, Aydin H, Akalin S. Association of serum paraoxonase activity with insulin sensitivity and oxidative stress in hyperthyroid and TSH-suppressed nodular goitre patients. Clinical Endocrinology 2004;61(4) 515–521.

[453] Yavuz DG, Yazici D, Toprak A, Deyneli O, Aydin H, Yuksel M, Akalin S. Exogenous subclinical hyperthyroidism impairs endothelial function in nodular goiter patients. Thyroid 2008;18(4) 395–400.

[454] Heemstra KA, Smit JW, Eustatia-Rutten CF, Heijboer AC, Fro°lich M, Romijn JA, Corssmit EP. Glucose tolerance and lipid profile in longterm exogenous subclinical hyperthyroidism and the effects of restoration of euthyroidism, a randomised controlled trial. Clinical Endocrinology 2006;65(6) 737–744.

[455] Wu, P. Thyroid Disease and Diabetes. Clinical Diabetes 2000; 18(1).

[456] Yeo KF, et Simultaneous presentation of thyrotoxicosis and diabetic ketoacidosis resulted in sudden cardiac arrest. Endocr J. 2007;54(6) 991-993.

[457] Moon SW et al. A case of hyperglycemic hyperosmolar state associated with Graves' a case report. J Korean Med Sci. 2006;21(4) 765-767.

Chapter 5

Graves' Ophthalmopathy Imaging Evaluation

Miłosz P. Kawa, Anna Machalińska,
Grażyna Wilk and Bogusław Machaliński

Additional information is available at the end of the chapter

1. Introduction

Graves' ophthalmopathy (GO), known as Graves' orbitopathy or thyroid eye disease (TED), is an autoimmune disorder and the main extrathyroidal expression of Graves' disease (GD). GO occurs mainly, but not exclusively, in patients with Graves' disease (up to 50% of GD patients have clinically apparent ophthalmopathy). The major clinical risk factor for developing thyroid eye disease is smoking. Moreover, radioactive iodine used to treat hyperthyroidism can worsen GO. There is an age-specific and gender-related distribution of GO, and the annual incidence is 0.4% for women and 0.1% for men but this largely reflects the increased incidence of GD in women [1]. In addition to GD, thyroid eye disease can also be seen in chronic autoimmune thyroiditis, albeit is far less common and occurs in 2–5% of these patients [2]. Although the link between GD and GO is still not totally clear, the close association between onset of GD and the development of GO suggests that both disorders would have common pathogenic mechanisms [3]. The ocular involvement of GD is explained by the expression of receptor for thyroid-stimulating hormone (TSH-R) present not only in the thyroid follicular cells but also in adipocytes, and fibroblasts located in the orbit, and lymphocytes infiltrating orbit tissues [3]. Likewise, the signs and symptoms of GO occur due to inflammatory reaction and subsequent fibrosis of the orbital components, including orbital connective tissue, and the extraocular muscles [4]. Inflammatory cell infiltration of extraocular muscles is associated with increased secretion of glycosaminoglycans and osmotic retention of water. The muscles become enlarged, sometimes up to eight times their normal size, and may compress the optic nerve. Subsequent degeneration of muscle fibers eventually leads to fibrosis, which exerts a tethering effect on the involved muscle resulting in the muscle dysfunction and ophthalmoplegia. Infiltration of interstitial tissues, orbital fat and lacrimal glands with lymphocytes, plasma cells, macrophages and mast cells along with accumulation of glycosaminoglycans and retention of fluid cause an increase in the volume of orbital content and secondary elevation of intraorbital pressure, which may itself cause further fluid retention within the orbit [4].

In general, GO can be divided into two clinical stages: the earlier inflammatory (congestive) stage and the late fibrotic (quiescent) stage. The inflammatory stage is marked by edema and deposition of glycosaminoglycans in the extraocular muscles. This results in the clinical manifestations of orbital swelling, proptosis (exophthalmos), diplopia due to restricted ocular motility, periorbital edema, and lid retraction. At this stage the eyes are red and painful. This tends to remit within 3 years and only 10% of patients develop serious long-term ocular problems. The fibrotic stage is a convalescent phase and may result in further restrictive myopathy and lid retraction. The most serious complication of GO is optic neuropathy, caused by compression of the optic nerve or its blood supply at the orbital apex by the congested and enlarged recti. Such compression, which may occur in the absence of significant proptosis, may lead to severe but preventable visual impairment.

The first step in diagnosis of thyroid-associated ophthalmopathy in an individual patient is the ophthalmological examination performed by ophthalmologist. Then, dedicated specialized imaging methods need to be employed in selected clinical situations in GO patients. For example, muscle enlargement, and not retrobulbar fat accumulation, is associated with an increased risk for development of dysthyroid optic neuropathy, which may lead to partial/total loss of vision [5]. As shown by computer tomography (CT) and magnetic resonance imaging (MRI), the swelling of extraocular muscles and disappearance of adipose tissue in the apex of the orbit is suggestive for active development of dysthyroid optic neuropathy [6]. Also, a stretched optic nerve is associated with an increased risk for visual loss [6], thus it should be confirmed with particular imaging modality and the therapy should be immediately provided. In principle, thyroid-associated ophthalmopathy is a bilateral condition, but it can occur unilaterally in about 20% of all GO patients [7]. Indeed, Graves' disease is the most common cause (20–30%) of unilateral exophthalmos [8]. Since a variety of other neuro-ophthalmic disorders require consideration when the unilateral proptosis or malposition of the eyelid are detected, including a retrobulbar tumors, myasthenia gravis, myositis, lymphoma, metastasis, arterio-venous malformation, carotid-sinus cavernous fistula, infection, diffuse or focal idiopathic orbital inflammation with mass effect, or illusory ptosis of the opposite eyelid, the comprehensive neuroimaging should be implicated. Therefore, all patients with unilateral eye disease suspected to GO development should undergo broad orbital imaging, involving several diagnostic methods, to exclude an alternative diagnosis. Apart from the comprehensive diagnosing of GO, clinical imaging is also indicated for the control checkup in the course of the thyroid-associated ophthalmopathy, especially for examination of the disease activity, what may predict the onset and response to therapy.

In this chapter, we will highlight the use of different imaging techniques, such as ultrasonography, computer tomography, magnetic resonance, and nuclear medicine-based examinations in the assessment of patients with Graves' ophthalmopathy for diagnostic purposes and to provide information about the optimal indications for use of each imaging method in the clinical setting.

2. Orbital imaging evaluation in Graves' ophthalmopathy

Radiological neuroimaging of Graves' ophthalmopathy plays an important role in the differential diagnosis and interdisciplinary management of patients with GO. Orbital imaging especially can be helpful in establishing the diagnosis of GO, because it objectively describes the morphological abnormalities of the orbital structures. Likewise, it is estimated that orbital imaging reveals anomalies in 90% of patients with Graves' disease [9]. Based on the selected imaging techniques, it is possible to establish the degree of extraocular muscle and orbital fat enlargement, exclude other coexisting orbital pathology, clarify a confusing clinical set of symptoms, and perform surgical planning [10]. Importantly, the signs and symptoms of thyroid ophthalmopathy usually develop within one year after the thyroid gland dysfunction onset, but up to 20% of subjects with exophthalmos may exhibit euthyroidism [11]. Moreover, the widespread availability of CT and MRI have made early detection of exophthalmos possible, and the imaging presentation of GO may even precede clinical signs of hyperthyroidism and significant changes in related laboratory tests. Therefore, it is postulated that abnormal imaging findings may be a sign of early thyroid disease that subsequently need to be diagnosed in detail [12-13]. Consequently, it is important to provide accurate diagnosis based on specific radiological findings and to propose the following testing to rule out the thyroid dysfunction in yet euthyroid patients.

Certainly, the commonly used imaging modalities posses the selected advantages and disadvantages for their use in specific clinical situations in case of GO patients. Some selected techniques have been reserved for patient examination in different phases of the disease activity. For example, the assessing of vascularity around extraocular muscles is achieved with the contrast-based CT and MR imaging techniques. On the contrary, the assessment of local tissue edema is accomplished with the dedicated MRI sequences, and quantitative monitoring of inflammation activity may require the radionuclide scintigraphy. Nevertheless, the search for optimal method to characterize the selected GO features necessary for different diagnostic and therapeutic purposes is not yet completed.

2.1. Ultrasound-based imaging evaluation of Graves' ophthalmopathy

Ultrasonography (US) is a non-invasive, well-established imaging modality, that is widely used in clinical practice and it enables the evaluation and measurement of extraocular muscles, general assessment of the optic nerve status, detection of the existing gross edema or the enlargement of lacrimal glands [14-16]. Especially, US may be conveniently used to investigate some of the orbital muscle parameters. First ultrasonography-based evidence that extraocular muscle enlargement can be documented directly by US was given by Werner and coworkers in 1974 [17]. From this time, several groups have proposed selected methods for detection and analysis of the thickness of the extraocular muscles and it was determined that their thickness expands with increasing disease severity [18]. However, this technique has also been found by several groups to have limited accuracy and not to be as effective as CT and MRI studies [19-22]. Especially, ultrasound investigation do not include all the extraocular muscles, thus sensitivity and specificity of this imaging modality is getting lower. Moreover, US examination of the orbit is not enough detailed in delineating the relationship of orbital pathology with soft-tissue structures located in the orbits, nor is it reliable in imaging lesions of the posterior part of the orbit, where compression of the optic nerve often occurs. Likewise, US has strong limitations in imaging of the bone elements of the orbit. In addition, the accuracy of measurements in US examination is strongly dependent on investigator's experience and qualifications. In the concise analysis of differences between orbital MRI and US imaging that was performed in 43 patients with orbitopathy and developed diplopia, the US has not provided sufficient degree of information on muscles and connective tissue that, in contrast, was obtainable by MRI [21]. Nevertheless, US permits to some extent for differential diagnosis of proptosis due to the high degree of similarity between the right and left eye, and the diagnosis of symmetric muscle enlargement is valuable in distinguishing the GO from other similar but often unilateral ophthalmologic disorders [18].

Changes in ocular blood flow may alter the functions of the retina and retinal pigment epithelium and may affect the prognosis of different ophthalmological disorders, including TED. Ocular hemodynamic changes have been reported in GO by several authors using different techniques, including Heidelberg retina flowmeter, ocular blood flow tonography, and oculodynamometry [23-25]. In general, the numerous factors may cause alterations in ocular blood flow in patients with Graves' disease. It is assumed that in hyperthyroidism, increased systemic blood pressure, increased intraocular pressure, and orbital inflammation may affect ocular blood flow [26]. Color Doppler imaging (CDI) is a sonographic imaging technique that permits for non-invasive assessment of blood flow velocity in orbital vessels, and thus, it has been used to study the ocular blood flow in patients with GO. Importantly, it allows for simultaneous imaging of the anatomic structures by B-mode ultrasonography with superimposed color-coded vascular flow. The orbital venous congestion and decreased flow velocity in the superior ophthalmic vein measured with CDI have been found in GO subjects by several groups [26-28]. Similarly, Li et al. and Alp et al. found independently the significantly lower value of the peak systolic velocity (PSV) of blood flow in the central retinal artery in GO patients compared to controls [26,29]. Additionally, Li et al. observed in the same vessel the decreased end diastolic velocity (EDV) of blood flow and the resistance indexes (RIs) significantly increased [29]. Besides, Perez-Lopez et al. measured the changes in retrobulbar blood flow parameters in 14 GO patients before and after decompression surgery and found that in inactive moderate-to-severe GO, the RIs of central retinal artery and ophthalmic artery were preoperatively significantly higher compared to healthy subjects. After decompression surgery, the authors observed a significant decrease of calculable US parameters, such as resistive index (RI), which occurred in both ocular arteries mentioned above. These results may indicate that increased RI of inactive GO might be due to orbital extrinsic compression of vascular structures and decompression surgery leads to significant decreases of the RIs of different orbital arteries [30]. Moreover, Doppler ultrasound parameters of the retrobulbar arteries have been related to the clinical activity score, suggesting increased arterial blood flow velocity in patients with active GO due to inflammation of the orbital tissues [31]. Some studies have showed that evaluation of the impaired arterial vascularization of the orbit and the optic nerve in inactive GO may indicate the necessity of performing the earlier decompression surgery to prevent dysthyroid optic neuropathy in these patients. Altogether, these findings raise the possibility that CDI measurements represent a clinically useful tool in adjunction to basic ultrasonography for diagnosis and follow-up of GO and, to some extent, for the evaluation of its activity. However, it is necessary to take into account that there are certain limitations that need to be recognized, when interpreting data obtained by retrobulbar CDI measurements. As expected, there is a high intraobserver variability, and even higher the interobserver variability, when the consecutive measurements are performed by two observers in one patient. Therefore, the adequate training is mandatory to allow reproducible CDI measurements. In addition, another limitation of retrobulbar CDI measurements is that it can be influenced by proximal carotid artery stenosis and this abnormality should be excluded prior to retrobulbar CDI. Finally, the resolution of CDI is insufficient up until today to provide reliable volumetric vascular flow measurements. Hence, a high flow velocity in an artery supplying the eyeball does not necessarily reflect the high flow, but may also reflect a stenosis or constriction at the site of measurement. Despite the mentioned limitations, CDI has an important advantage over the other imaging techniques as it is noninvasive, it requires no contrast or radiation, and is available in almost every hospital setting. Nevertheless, according to authors of the recent report on the use of colour Doppler imaging for assessment of retrobulbar blood flow, it is not relevant for routine use in current clinical practice [32].

2.2. Computer tomography-based imaging evaluation of Graves' ophthalmopathy

Computer tomography imaging can distinguish abnormal structures of different tissue density based on their differing X-ray absorption properties. Generally, CT is the preferred imaging modality for the diagnosis of patients with GO because of its ability to visualize bone and soft tissues of the orbit. The orbital fat that acts as a natural contrast medium allows for good spatial and density resolution of orbital structures [33]. As analyzed on the large GO patient cohort, the extraocular muscles most frequently affected are the medial and inferior recti followed by superior and lateral recti, which were involved less frequently and less severely. Importantly, the two or more muscles were enlarged in 70% of patients with ocular involvement [34-35]. The extraocular muscles affected by GO appear to be enlarged in a fusiform fashion with sharp borders [36]. The attempts to establish normative measurements of thickness of the extraocular muscles have been performed by several groups based on national and international cohorts of patients [37-39]. However, the assessment of muscle enlargement is often subjective and requires comparison with the opposite orbit and prior qualitative experience in CT imaging analysis.

Clinical symptoms of GO derive from the discrepancy between limited space of the orbit and expansion of pathologically affected orbital tissues. CT permits to evaluate the differences in orbital soft tissue volumes and densities that are different in GO patients compared to healthy controls. For example, studies using three dimensional CT showed the increase in volume of extra-ocular muscles alone in 20% of 40 subjects with GO, and 28% of GO patients presented only the increased orbital fat tissue volume, however, almost half of the patients had augmented volume of both analyzed structures of the orbit, i.e. muscles and fat [40]. These results indicate that orbital changes might be presented separately as the myogenic and the lipogenic abnormal forms. Furthermore, Regensburg et al. determined by CT imaging that orbital fat density was significantly higher in GO patients than in the normal population and it negatively correlated to orbital fat volume. They also found a positive correlation between orbital fat density and muscle volume or muscle density [38]. The same group proposed the useful method for calculating orbital soft tissue volume using a manual segmentation technique for CT scans. Based on their results, this technique seems to be reliable and might be an accurate tool for diagnostic follow-up evaluation of GO patients [41]. A decade ago, Nishida et al. hypothesized that orbital fat volume has larger influence on proptosis induction than increased extraocular muscle volume [42]. Recently, Fang et al. observed in CT imaging that orbital fat changes were more important in mild proptosis than in severe one [11]. Imaging-based studies are not only important for the diagnosis of GO, but they can aid in the evaluation of disease activity. Changes observed in sequential measurements of the extraocular muscles obtained with CT may be related to clinical activity of the disease as muscular involvement occurs early in GO and it may correlate with other clinical signs [43]. Other abnormal findings in the orbits that may be determined by CT are a dilated superior ophthalmic vein and abrupt angulations of the posterior muscle belly [44].

Computer tomography is also valuable for the evaluation of the orbital bone wall structures and their remodeling. For example, in long-lasting GO a spontaneous bony orbit decompression could be noted with an impression of the normally parallel laminae papyraceae, which create the medial orbital walls, and then leading to the so-called "Coca Cola sign", when GO has bilateral occurrence and forms the shape typical for internationally-known bottle of Coca-Cola [45]. Orbital CT is the modality of choice to particularly examine the osseous structures of the orbital apex, the sinus, and the intra-orbital elements for the orbital decompression surgery planning. In this notion, CT imaging is recommended pre-and postoperatively in order to define the site and extent of the bony decompression.

Compressive optic neuropathy, which occurs in approximately 5% of patients with thyroid eye disease, is caused by direct compression of the optic nerve at the orbital apex. Such compression in general occurs due to enlarged extraocular muscles [46]. However, optic nerve function in thyroid eye disease may be also compromised by other mechanisms. There have been described several cases of dysthyroid optic neuropathy without apparent orbital apex congestion in which the combination of increased orbital fat volume, shallow orbits, and/or outbowing of the medial orbital wall caused sufficient anterior ocular displacement to allow linear antero-posterior stretching of the optic nerve [47]. As the CT-based examination in patients with dysthyroid optic neuropathy often reveals crowding of the optic nerve at the orbital apex by enlarged extraocular muscles [46], thus several methods have been proposed to delineate the degree of crowding of the optic nerve at the orbital apex using CT imaging that comprised the radiologist-based subjective judgment of the appearance of the apex, quantization of the total extraocular muscle volume by using an image analyzer [48], or just the linear measurements of the amount of orbital height or width occupied by the extraocular muscles at a selected point in the orbit (e.g. the middle between the posterior surface of the globe and the orbital apex) [49]. As a result, every of the above-mentioned methods has shown independently that optic nerve dysfunction is more common in crowded orbit and less common in uncrowded orbit. Birchall et al. described an additional CT sign that has a high correlation with the presence of optic nerve dysfunction in patients with dysthyroid optic neuropathy, which is the hernia of orbital fat raising out 2-4 mm from the superior orbital fissure [50].

The muscles are usually involved bilaterally in GO and they present a "fusiform" appearance due to characteristic sparing of the muscle tendons. The enlarged muscles produce not only the apical crowding in the orbit, but also venous congestion what can be clearly noticeable in the CT scans performed with intravenous contrast enhancement. As the inflammation starts naturally in the extraocular muscles, it has a crisp, well-defined border within the affected muscle, and thus can be distinguished from pseudotumors. The another characteristic sign, helping in differential diagnosis of Graves' orbitopathy versus orbital myositis, is lack of the involvement of the muscle tendon into the inflammatory process. In the later, the tendon should present swelling and enlargement. Consequently, the inflammatory process leaks from the intramuscular tissue into the intraorbital fat and produces streaking within the fat giving a characteristic 'dirty fat' sign inside the orbit. Concurrently, the medial rectus muscle enlargement may produce the deformation or even the breakage of delicate lamina papyracea of the orbital bony wall. These imaging features are efficiently diagnosed and monitored with CT, especially obtained in the coronal plane [51]. However, the apical crowding is assessed better on coronal planes of MRI scans.

Altogether, CT scanning of the orbits is non-invasive, simple, fast, and cost-effective imaging technique. Findings such as spindle-shaped thickness >4 mm of more than one of the extraocular muscles without involvement of the corresponding tendon, with preferential involvement of the inferior and medial rectus, followed by the superior and lateral rectus muscles, apparent increase in orbital fat volume and the compression of the optic nerve at the orbital apex ("crowded orbital apex syndrome") are the most important morphological diagnostic criteria of GO, when analyzing the axial and coronal CT scans [52]. For the above reasons, and especially because of lower costs and better availability than the MR equipment, the CT imaging should be considered first imaging step in diagnostic evaluation of GO and other thyroid-associated diseases. Moreover, CT provides precise imaging of the osseous periorbital structures, therefore this is the method of choice to plan CT-guided orbital decompression surgery in the inactive phase of GO. To the limitations of this imaging modality belong the radiation exposure to the organism, and especially to the eye lenses. Moreover, CT does not reveal information on the disease activity in most cases. It is also important to be aware that there is a risk for thyrotoxicosis development due to the performance of CT with commonly used iodinated contrast agents.

2.3. Magnetic resonance-based imaging evaluation of Graves' ophthalmopathy

The main advantages of MRI are the excellent soft-tissue contrast, obtainable with a great spatial tissue resolution, compared even to a high-resolution CT imaging and absence of ionizing radiation during the examination. Therefore, MRI is the preferred modality for soft tissue imaging. In orbital MR imaging, slices ranging from 3 to 5 mm are used, normally oriented in the transverse and coronal direction and, along to the optic nerve, in the parasagittal plane. One of the neuroimaging protocols proposed in the literature for examination of the orbits with MRI is comprised of spin-echo T1-weighted sequences in the axial and coronal planes with 3-mm-slice thickness, multi-echoes T2-weighted sequence in the coronal plane, and short time inversion recovery (STIR) sequence in the coronal plane. Paramagnetic contrast-enhanced images are acquired with T1-weighted sequence with fat-suppression in the axial, coronal and sagittal oblique planes [53]. Our currently used MRI protocol for examination of GO patients is given in Table 1.

Sequence Number	Sequence Name	TR / TE ms	Resolution	Slice Thickness mm	Slice Spacing mm	FOV cm	Contrast Medium
1	3-plane, Gradient Echo, 3-pl T2* FGRE, whole brain	3000 ms / 102 ms	512 x 512	5	5	30.0	No
2	Oblique, Ax T2 Propeller, bulbus	3000 ms / 102 ms	512 x 512	5	15	24.0	No
3	Oblique, Ax T2 FRFSE, bulbus	3000 ms / 102 ms	512 x 512	3	0.3	16.0	No
4	Oblique, Ax T1 FSE, bulbus	575 ms / Minimal Full	512 x 512	3	0.3	16.0	No
5	Oblique, R-SAG T1 FSE, bulbus	475 ms / Minimal Full	512 x 512	2	0.2	14.0	No
6	Oblique, L-SAG T1 FSE, bulbus	475 ms / Minimal Full	512 x 512	2	0.2	14.0	No
7	Oblique, COR T1 FSE, bulbus	575 ms / Minimal Full	512 x 512	3	0.3	14.0	No
8	Oblique, COR STIR, bulbus	2975 ms / 68 ms	512 x 512	3	0.3	14.0	No

Table 1. MR-imaging protocol used in GE Signa HDxt MR apparatus with 8-channel HR head coil for patients with thyroid-associated ophthalmopathy.

Importantly, the T1-weighted MRI sequence offers a better contrast resolution for evaluating the orbit structures and measurement of the thickness of the intra-orbital muscles [54]. In contrast, the pathophysiological conditions of the muscles could be better evaluated on T2-weighted MRI sequences [55]. Moreover, the STIR sequences suppress the fatty signal and allow a more adequate assessment of pathological tissues. Not affected extraocular muscles are defined with a low signal intensity on T1-weighted sequences and low to intermediate signal intensity on T2-weighted sequences, with evident and clear edges. Due to the immense vascular supply of the orbital muscles the strong contrast enhancement is observed during the examination with paramagnetic contrast mediums (e.g. gadolinium containing agents).

Morphological imaging criteria, suggestive for GO on MRI are a bilateral, spindle-like thickening of normally multiple extraocular recti muscles over 5 mm and an increase of intra- and extra-conal fat, both leading to exophthalmos (Figure 1A-C). MRI imaging is specifically advantageous for clinical diagnosis of exophthalmos, because it depicts a clear outline of the eye globe that allows precise measurements. In the clinical setting, exophthalmos is usually measured manually with a Hertel exophthalmometer. The average measurement is around 13.5 mm, and the difference between bilateral eye protrusions should be within 2 mm. However, this manual diagnostic method has poor reproducibility due to the orbital interval, variance of eye diameter as a result of ametropia, exophthalmometer variance and instrument operator bias. In contrast, on axial T1-weighted sequences, the level of proptosis can be measured very precisely, compared to the clinically measured Hertel-index [56]. On imaging, a interzygomatic line is drawn between the right and left ventral zygomatic border. From there, a perpendicular line, representing the value of Hertel-index in mm, is taken to the apex of each globe, thus depicting the measurement of proptosis. Physiologically, 1⁄3 of the globe is located behind the interzygomatic line and a Hertel-index of ≥ 22 mm is pathological and indicates exophthalmos (Figure 1A).

Although changes in extraocular muscle size and increased amounts of orbital fat can be assessed with CT, the orbital soft tissue edema and water content changes in the extraocular muscles can be only assessed by MRI imaging. There are several studies indicating the specific applications of MRI imaging in establishing of the disease phase due to the ability to estimate the water content in orbital tissues. Especially, the images from strong T2-weighted and fat suppressed sequences have been found to be useful in detecting tissue edema [44]. Inflammatory process of the extra-ocular muscles can be detected in MRI independently from the size of the muscles [21]. Young and colleagues proposed to employ in GO patients the MRI turbo inversion recovery magnitude (TIRM) sequences used with short inversion times (80–150 ms). These strong T2-weighted and fat-suppressed images have been found to be useful in detecting edema and therefore, TIRM sequences can be used to define inflammation in extra-ocular muscles [57]. Specifically, the STIR signal intensity, which is directly related to the raise of relaxation in T2 time caused by increased abnormal content in the analyzed tissue, correlates with the inflammatory activity in GO [58]. STIR-sequence MRI may also detect peri-muscular inflammation [59]. Importantly, Kirsch et al. reported that the difference in T2-STIR versus T1-STIR would be helpful to distinguish inflammatory edema of the extra-ocular muscles from intra-orbital congestion due to reduced venous outflow [60]. Therefore, the results of MRI examination have a great therapeutic impact, identifying inflammatory and edematous alterations in orbital muscles that are critical to achieve a good outcome of the anti-inflammatory treatment, which is effective only in the active phase of the disease. Likewise, increase in the signal intensity on T2-weighted sequences was associated with a good response to methylprednisolone pulse therapy [61]. Also, longer T2 relaxation times in the extraocular muscles before treatment were associated with a good response to orbital irradiation [62]. Moreover, individual STIR imaging was useful for predicting the outcome of immunosuppressive therapy [61]. On the other hand, the T1-weighted images with contrast enhancement and in combination with fat saturation are helpful to detect intense signal enhancement of the eyelid, which is also affected in the inflammatory GO stage [63]. Interestingly, the decrease of

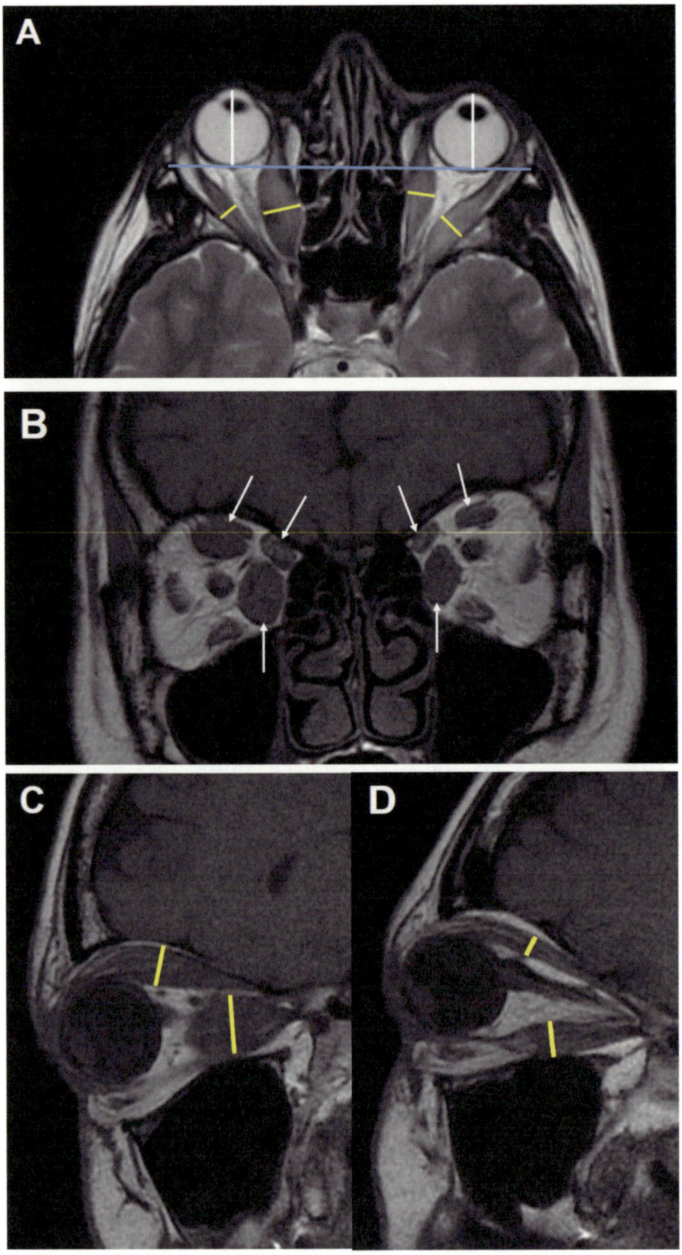

Figure 1. 59-year-old female patient with diagnosis of clinically active Graves' orbitopathy. (A) Axial T2 FRFSE MR image of orbits without contrast shows marked bilateral exophthalmos as indicated by interzygomatic line (blue line) and Hertel-index (perpendicular white lines). This image shows also the largest diameters (yellow lines) perpendicular to long axis of medial and lateral rectus muscles in both orbits. (B) Unenhanced T1 FSE coronal image of orbits shows the transverse sections of the thickest extraocular muscles in both orbits (arrows). (C) and (D) Unenhanced T1 FSE sagittal images parallel to optic nerve show corresponding maximal diameters (yellow lines) for inferior rectus muscle and for superior muscle group of right (C) and left (D) orbit.

T2 relaxation times of the extraocular muscles in response to immunosuppressive therapy occurs even in spite of unchanged laboratory markers during and after the treatment [64]. Nagy et al. found that T2 relaxation times on MRI provided more diagnostic and prognostic information than other applied eleven clinical and laboratory factors [21]. In summary, the major result of the above studies is the relationship between response to therapy and pre-therapeutic value of the T2 times of relaxation in MRI sequences. Consequently, the measurement of T2 before giving the therapy might play a role in the prediction of the reversibility of orbital tissue abnormalities (e.g. muscle thickening, increased fat volume), and favors the choice of anti-inflammatory therapy regimens in GO patients.

MRI is also a valuable tool that can be used to detect other features of the active inflammatory phase of the disease that include lacrimal gland hypertrophy, palpebral edema, anterior displacement of the orbital septum and optic nerve stretching. On the contrary, gradual decreasing of signal intensity of intra-orbital muscles on T1-and T2-weighted sequences suggests the presence of chronic fibrotic alterations that clinically correspond to chronic phase at the Rundle's curve of disease activity [65]. Hyper-intense intramuscular foci on T1-and T2-weighted sequences are suggestive of chronic fat degeneration [66]. Of note, chronic fat degeneration may also be identified at CT imaging through hypodense areas corresponding to fat infiltration of muscle tissue [53]. The above-mentioned findings indicate the presence of the non-congestive phase of the disease with restricted ocular motion secondary to extraocular muscle fibrosis and subsequent loss of elasticity in association with volume reduction of the muscles [66]. Recently, the dynamic contrast-enhanced MRI (DCE-MRI) technique that is used for assessment of microcirculation was able to establish the correlation between disease activity and the microcirculation characteristics of extraocular muscles in patients with GO [63, 67-68]. The natural consequence of the pressure at the orbital apex by increased volume of orbital contents, and resulting overcrowding and stretching of the optic nerve is the compressive optic neuropathy, in which the nerve diameter at the orbital apex has been found to be significantly reduced in MRI imaging. The high-resolution volume acquisition (T1-w-3D) with curved multiplanar reformatting process can be used to measure the optic nerve diameter along its entire length, and thus it can be used to predict possible optic nerve compression. The group of Dodds et al. has demonstrated in MRI modality a reproducible decrease in mean nerve diameter as it extends posterior from the globe in patients with chronic GO [69]. Importantly, this situation may occur even in orbits without increased muscle indices but with clinical signs of optic neuropathy. An additional sign of nerve compression is intracranial fat prolapse in the orbital apex [44].

In conclusion, MRI remains a valuable tool in the care of patients with GO, despite its limited usage due to the time-consuming and a relatively high cost, as well as the still reduced availability, and magnetism contraindicated in patients with certain types of implants. MRI offers extraordinary images of orbital anatomy, except for bony structures, and has an ability to quantify muscle enlargement that outperforms the results obtained from other modalities such as the US and CT imaging. MRI modality is the most effective tool not only in establishing the initial diagnosis but also in diagnosing of the disease stage and immune activity of GO for predicting therapeutic efficacy and of the potential harmful disease complications (damage to the optic nerve), what makes it a unique instrument in determining the proper treatment and monitoring of the therapeutic response.

2.4. Radionuclide-based imaging evaluation of Graves' ophthalmopathy

Direct neuroimaging methods (US, CT and MRI) play currently a significant role as an aid in the diagnostic process and clinical evaluation of patients with endocrine ophthalmopathy, however, there is no sufficient imaging modality that could be applied to determine with a high sensitivity and specificity the GO activity. It is suggested that intervention using immunosuppressive drugs will be most successful, if applied in the phase of active inflammation. Therefore, to decide, when the treatment should be given, it is important to determine the phase of the disease in an individual patient. One of such imaging possibilities gives octreotide scintigraphy so-called "octreoscan". Previously, it was observed that accumulation of octreotide, a somatostatin analogue labelled with radioisotope indium-111, binds in the thyroid and the orbit to the somatostatin receptor in patients with active GO [70]. Octreotide uptake was significantly higher in patients with active GO compared to those with non-active GO, and the observed high orbital radionuclide activity decreased after therapy. Postema and colleagues have also performed thyroid octreoscan in patients with confirmed Graves' disease and in controls [71]. In this study, the thyroidal octreotide accumulation was increased in thyrotoxicosis, and was almost absent after radioiodine-induced hypothyroidism. The cause of specific orbital and thyroid uptake of octreotide is not well known yet. Most probably, the orbital uptake of octreotide in GO is caused by the expression of somatostatin receptors on the surface of both activated T lymphocytes and fibroblasts, which infiltrate the orbital and thyroid tissues in patients with GO [72-73]. Radio-labeled octreotide accumulated within the orbits can be detected via single-photon emission CT (SPECT), and may serve as a marker of disease activity [70]. On the other hand, the octreoscan does not provide information on inactive patients nor gives any anatomical and morphologic information on the orbit. Importantly, although several studies have found a relation between octreoscan uptake and severity of GO [74-76], the others did not find such a correlation [77-78]. Due to the above-mentioned results indicating substantial limitations of octreoscan (i.e. high demand of the technique in terms of accuracy needed for prediction, inter-observer variance, significant price, modest availability, a non-negligible radiation burden of patients, long acquisition protocol and relative lack of specificity), it is not recommended by some specialists to use it as a routine imaging procedure in a regular clinical practice with GO patients [79-80].

In contrast to octreotide labeled with In-111, the orbital SPECT with other radionuclide tracers has been proposed as clinically suitable protocols for activity evaluation of Graves' ophthalmopathy and differential diagnosis of GO cases sensitive or resistant to the immune suppressive therapy. Indeed, the diethylenetriamine pentaacetic acid labeled with technetium-99 (Tc-99m DTPA) has been indicated as suitable radiopharmaceutical for such examination [81]. The theoretical basis of this method is that the high capillarisation in the orbit and edematous swelling of orbital tissues may be reflected on SPECT images, as the Tc-99m DTPA uptake has been reported as related to the inflammatory process, and signal disappearing with the resolution of the inflammation. The Tc-99m DTPA complex (molecular weight 492 Da), administered intravenously, marks the high capillarization of inflammation sites leaving the vascular bed through damaged capillary walls. It goes out into the interstitial fluid and binds to polypeptides present in the extracellular fluid at inflammation sites [82]. This may explain the high DTPA uptake in GO since the orbital inflammation is a basic pathophysiological process in GO. The determination of periorbital inflammation tissue by testing with intravenously given Tc-99m DTPA may identify the patients that will benefit from anti-inflammatory treatment. This protocol was clinically tested by Galuska et al., who was able to visualize the active retrobulbar inflammation in GO patient by Tc-99m DTPA SPECT [83]. Moreover, Ujhelyi et al. found that the mean retrobulbar Tc-99m DTPA uptake is useful to estimate GO activity and may predict the effectiveness of immunosuppressive therapy with corticosteroids in GO patients [84]. Especially, patients included in this study with Tc-99m DTPA uptake score above 12.28MBq/cm^3 were more likely to respond to corticosteroid treatment. Another promising method for the diagnosis of inflammatory state is SPECT technique, which uses polyclonal and monoclonal antibodies labeled with technetium-99 (Tc-99m). This technique was previously reported to allow the use of polyclonal human immunoglobulin gamma labeled with Tc-99m (Tc-99m HIG) as a radiopharmaceutical tool in the evaluation of the disease activity in GO [85]. Recently, Lopes and colleagues proposed Tc-99m anti-TNF-alpha scintigraphy based on labeling of a human monoclonal antibody directed against TNF-alpha molecule, commercially known as adalimumab, with technetium-99, as a promising method for the diagnosis of active ocular disease [86]. This method is based on the demonstration of TNF-alpha as one of the cytokines involved in the initial active phase of GO development. They reported the successful use of Tc-99m-anti-TNF-alpha scintigraphy in case of unilateral exophthalmos in which intense uptake of anti-TNF-alpha antibody was observed, indicating the development of active retrobulbar inflammation that may be related with active phase of GO.

Concurrently, the positron emission tomography (PET) appears also as promising tool for diagnosing of active phase of GO. PET is a noninvasive diagnostic method that has been used as a mean for differential diagnosis of inflammatory and malignant processes and it offers the ability to perform functional and metabolic assessment in cases of the absence of any tissue structural alteration [87]. One of its main advantages over other methods is its ability to detect early inflammatory stages prior to structural changes in the tissue [88]. Recently, García-Rojas et al. demonstrated in PET combined with CT (PET/CT) imaging a significant correlation between extraocular muscle uptake of 18-fluorodeoxyglucose (18-FDG) radiotracer and GO developed in hyperthyroid patients [89]. These studies indicate that modern PET/CT imaging modality may provide the valuable clinical information and may be a helpful tool in detecting, localizing, and quantifying the GO inflammation. Ultimately, in the same line of work, Pichler et al. reported the case of subclinical hyperthyroidism due to Graves' disease without presenting exophthalmos in a 53-year-old woman. Application of specific radiotracer Ga-68-DOTA-NOC for high-resolution hybrid PET/CT imaging comprised of gallium-68 radionuclide demonstrated marked accumulation at the thyroid and the right rectus inferior muscle in this patient. Therefore, this specific imaging modality revealed active Graves' orbitopathy in a single extraorbital muscle. The authors concluded that the Ga-68 labeled PET tracers may provide the possibility to evaluate the status of activity in any single extraorbital muscle in hybrid imaging of PET with CT [90]. Whether novel radiopharmaceutical, such as Ga-68-DOTA-NOC, which has a stronger discriminative capability for detecting active endocrine orbitopathy than octreotide will achieve clinical applicability similar to technetium-99-labelled tracers, it remains to be demonstrated in the future.

In conclusion, the nuclear medicine-based imaging continues to be important in the diagnosis and management of thyroid-associated ophthalmopathy. Although, the previously used SPECT technique known as octreoscan presents nowadays the restricted clinical application [91] due to its high costs, relative lack of specificity (i.e., the number of false positives in other inflammatory or non-inflammatory orbital disorders), and a non-negligible radiation burden, some other SPECT-based methods including technetium-related scintigraphy with the new target-based modalities (i.e. antibodies against selected pro-inflammatory molecules), can be used in the reliable evaluation of patients with unilateral/bilateral active GO. Particularly, the better image quality due to the high energy of technetium, the lower radiation dose for patients and personnel, and the short acquisition protocol favor scintigraphy with Tc-99m-over In-111-labeled compounds [92]. In the near future, the modern PET/CT imaging technique may still improve significantly the process of the treatment selection and the outcome in patient with GO. The results of the currently reported studies demonstrated that PET/CT imaging modalities are able to recognize the early active phase from the late stable stage of the disease and to predict the response to anti-inflammatory treatment in majority of GO patients. Especially, the hybrid PET/CT imaging modality provides valuable and useful information for the diagnosis, characterization, and therapeutic decision in cases, where clinical doubts and uncertainties exist.

3. Predicting therapeutic efficacy and disease activity based on orbital neuroimaging

The activity and severity are important pathophysiological characteristics in Graves' orbitopathy and have implications for the treatment, although the biologic activity of ophthalmopathy is neither synonymous nor coincident with the clinical severity of the eye disease. Severity of GO is defined by the functional impairment and should be categorized using an examination form and a photographic color atlas, which includes the clinical signs of the disease [5]. The European Group of Graves' Orbitopathy (EUGOGO) suggests classifying the GO severity, based on subjective symptoms and objective signs, into three categories: sight-threatening, moderate-to-severe, and mild GO [93]. On the other hand, the activity of GO is related to the presence of inflammatory signs in the orbits. It can be measured using the *Clinical Activity Score* (CAS) classification that is based on the classical features of inflammation (pain, redness, swelling, and impaired function). In the CAS ten-point scoring system, which was developed by Mourits et al., one point is given for each of the following 10 items: painful, oppressive feeling on and behind the globe during the past 4 weeks; pain attempted up, side, or down gaze during the past 4 weeks; redness of the eyelid; diffuse redness of conjunctiva covering at least one quadrant; swelling of the eyelid; chemosis; swollen caruncle; increase of proptosis of ≥ 2 mm during a period of 1–3 months; decrease of eye movements in any direction ≥ 5° during a period of 1–3 months; and decrease of visual acuity of ≥ 1 line(s) on the Snellen chart during a period of 1–3 months. A score ≥ 3 defines an active GO [94]. The second classification, *NOSPECS* mnemonic, is a useful alternative reminder of what should be assessed in patients with Graves' orbitopathy regarding severity, but it is of lesser practical value [5]. Importantly, the clinical problem in GO is not the establishing of the diagnosis of the disease, because this is quite obvious from the clinical presentation, but the treatment of the eye symptoms in an individual patient. Patients with the immunologically-active ophthalmopathy need the anti-inflammatory treatment, and patients with inactive disease require a completely different treatment course, including rehabilitative surgery (strabismus surgery, eyelid surgery, etc.). In general, the decision for anti-inflammatory treatment with steroids or irradiation is based on objective findings of detailed ophthalmological examination. However, it is important to be able to predict, if the patient will benefit from immunosuppression, as some patients might improve without such therapy, whereas in some patients with a severe course of the disease the initial choice of immunosuppressive steroid dosage may be too low. In contrast, patients with the immunologically inactive orbit will only suffer from the serious adverse reactions of otherwise ineffective immunosuppressive therapy given to them. Furthermore, there are always the questions demanding the rapid answer that include the decision whether to continue or to stop the anti-inflammatory therapy in patients with mild but persisting inflammation, and when is the right moment for surgical rehabilitation, which should not be done in patients at risk for further deterioration due to the high disease activity. The clinical decisions in GO patients are often difficult, and it is extremely important for the clinicians to be able to distinguish the specific phases of Graves' orbitopathy. Of note, in the last decade as many as one-third of patients did not respond to given immunosuppressive treatment [95]. Most of these cases were due to lack of the active stage of disease in the course of the therapy. In such scenarios, more discriminative information of better quality is needed to establish the activity phase of the disease and to make the best treatment decision. For this reason, several groups have assessed the predictive value of several potential activity parameters to predict response to therapy including duration of the eye disease, the CAS score, urinary glycosaminoglycan (GAG) excretion, serum cytokine levels, serum levels of TSH-receptor autoantibodies [91,94,96-98]. Lastly, even genetic factors might influence treatment outcome as several HLA markers have been shown to indicate good or bad response to immune therapy [99]. Notwithstanding, some of these parameters could predict a response to treatment only to some extent, while others could predict to some extent a lack of the therapeutic response. This means that probably a combination of different parameters may be necessary to accurately predict the response to the treatment in the particular patient. In this notion, several recent clinical and experimental studies have found evidences that the selected neuroimaging modalities would be valuable in measuring the disease activity to predict therapeutic outcomes in GO patients. Especially, there are two imaging modalities that seem to be highly supportive to detect disease activity, including MRI and radionuclide-based imaging.

MRI has currently emerged as a valuable tool in the evaluation of disease activity in patients with GO as it can illustrate in detail the inflamed regions of orbits. More than two decades ago, Just *et al.* described that in MRI sequences an increased T2 time in the eye muscles before treatment was associated with a good response to orbital irradiation [62]. This first report was confirmed by two others indicating that the T2 time decreases after immunosuppressive therapy, what suggests a transition from an edematous and inflammatory state into a fibrotic chronic stage [100]. In particular, there was established strong positive correlation between the clinical activity score of GO and the T2 relaxation time and ratio of signal intensity in STIR sequences in T2-weighted and fat suppressed images [61]. Moreover, Mayer et al. found, that the area of highest signal intensity within the most inflamed extra-ocular muscle, and the average cross-sectional signal intensity of the most inflamed extra-ocular muscle reliably correlated with CAS, and this was maintained as disease activity changed over time [59]. Recently, the correlation between disease activity and the microcirculation characteristics of extraocular muscles has been demonstrated in GO using sophisticated dynamic contrast-enhanced MR imaging [68]. This novel technique is based on the hypothesis that the pathological changes occurring at different stages of GO might impact the microcirculatory status of extraocular muscles differently, and therefore induce distinct contrast-enhancement characteristics on DCE-MRI images, which might serve as indicators for activity estimation. Furthermore, to improve the sensitivity of detection of active phase of the disease and therefore the prediction of the response to immunosuppressive therapy, over CAS alone, the combination of the orbital MR imaging and CAS estimation was proposed by Tachibana et al. [101]. They reported that the orbital MR imaging combined with CAS could improve the sensitivity of differentiation between the active and inactive GO form and especially the CAS and the maximum of T2 relaxation times of extraocular muscles (maxT2RT) showed significant positive correlation. Interestingly, 40% of GO patients included in this study were positive by only MR imaging and all these GO patients presented significant improvement after intravenous immunosuppressive therapy due to active GO diagnosis by MRI classification, what indicates the importance of the orbital MR imaging for the diagnosis of active GO. Recently, Le Moli et al. determined positive correlation between CAS score and ratio of extraocular muscles area to the total orbit area measured in CT imaging modality [43].

Similarly, several radionuclide-based imaging methods have been proposed recently to evaluate disease activity in GO. Importantly, the obtained image evaluation and orbital uptake fraction calculation of the selected radiotracers could provide the qualitative (image-based) and quantitative (numerical) information on disease activity. Historically, the imaging of orbital uptake of In-111-labeled octreotide detected by scintigraphy was presented as a sensitive method to estimate immunologic disease activity in GO patients [70]. However, further studies indicated the low specificity for this method, therefore, its clinical applicability is strongly limited nowadays [33,40]. Subsequently, SPECT imaging of the orbits using Tc-99m-labeled DTPA have been proposed by several reports [102-103]. This method has been accepted for evaluation of GO disease activity allowing a rapid imaging at an acceptable cost, and in addition, the successful management of GO has been associated with the decrease in orbital uptake of radiotracer [84]. In addition, to improve the sensitivity of detection of active GO phase, and therefore the prediction of the response to immunosuppressive therapy, over clinical activity score (CAS) alone, the combination of Tc-99m DTPA SPECT imaging and CAS estimation was proposed by Galuska et al. [104]. They reported that Tc-99m DTPA SPECT imaging provides essential supplementary information to traditional CAS evaluation in assessing GO activity. Likewise, Szabados et al. reported recently the results of the study in which they measured the inflammatory activity in the retrobulbar region using Tc-99m DTPA SPECT before and after external radiation to determine whether this method is suitable for predicting the effectiveness of the anti-inflammatory therapy [105]. They found in the group comprised of thirty-two patients with suspected active GO that a high initial DTPA uptake may predict the response to orbital radiation therapy, therefore the orbital SPECT with Tc-99m DTPA may be a suitable technique for the selection of GO patients for radiation therapy [105].

Furthermore, the different imaging methods, which were developed recently, applying scintigraphy of Tc-99m-labeled compounds, including polyclonal and monoclonal antibodies against inflammatory-related molecules (e.g. TNF-alpha), gave a new perspective in the diagnostic approach of active GO, which could be diagnosed with high sensitivity and specificity [85-86]. The preliminary results obtained from the group of 25 GO patients with different CAS score suggest that scintigraphy with Tc-99m-labeled anti-TNF-alpha might be a promising procedure for the evaluation of active orbital inflammation in GO [106]. Lately, the high-resolution PET/CT have been introduced to clinical practice for improved detection, disease grading, and follow-up of patients with GO in order to optimize the treatment in the inflammatory GO phase. Several novel radiotracers have been employed in PET/CT imaging, including gallium-68 and fluor-18 to supply valuable information on localizing and quantifying of GO-related inflammation in retrobulbar tissues [89-90]. Importantly, the availability of novel PET tracers for high-resolution and hybrid imaging in PET/CT enables to evaluate selectively the actual status of immune activity in any single extraorbital muscle.

Altogether, the precise quantitative evaluation of clinical disease activity and prediction of the outcome of immunosuppressive therapy in GO are reserved nowadays for only selected orbital neuroimaging modalities such as MRI and nuclear medicine-based imaging using gallium or technetium scintigraphy. Importantly, there are some limitations to the imaging studies of GO activity. For example, as the histological validation by extraocular muscle biopsy, which is the "golden standard" in diagnosis evaluation, is not available on regular basis in case of the orbits, the discussion about morphology-related changes observed in images obtained by different imaging modalities are speculative to some extent. Moreover, although MRI and radionuclide-based imaging may show increased edema in the muscles and inflammatory process in the orbital tissues during the active phase, however both modalities tend to be less helpful in therapeutic surgical planning since no detail about bone architecture is provided in these techniques.

4. Conclusion

Diagnosis of Graves' orbitopathy is usually given by careful ophthalmological examination when clinical manifestations occur. The main symptoms of the orbitopathy derive from the discrepancy between limited space of the orbit and expansion of pathologically affected orbital tissues. Therefore, in most patients, CT and MRI of the orbit confirm diagnosis by showing enlarged extraocular muscles (without involvement of the tendon) and/or increased orbital fibroadipose tissue. Although extra-ocular muscle enlargement can be documented directly by ultrasonography, the CT scan or MRI highly improve the measurements (i.e. thickness and volume) by direct visualizing the retro-bulbar muscles in their entire length and at the apex of the orbit, where their augmentation is responsible for dysthyroid optic neuropathy. The orbital neuroimaging is especially required in asymmetrical or, particularly, unilateral forms of GO, to rule out that exophthalmos, swelling of periorbital tissue, inflammation, or diplopia exist due to disorders other than GO. The MRI is the preferred modality for soft tissue imaging. As a basic rule, T1-weighted images are best for anatomic details, while T2 images give more information about the different tissue composition. Compared with MRI, computer tomography is less expensive, more available in the national health system and faster to perform, however, is less efficient in the evaluation of soft tissue changes and might not reveal details that could be important in the assessment of disease activity. In addition, the iodinated contrast medium usage for CT imaging should be limited in patients with Graves' disease. On the other hand, MRI provides a precise quantitative evaluation of clinical disease activity and may predict the outcome of immunosuppressive therapy for GO. As a consequence, there is potential for MRI in the evaluation of the therapeutic outcomes of new drugs for GO [45].

The history of the disease, physical examination, and neuroimaging findings can all provide important data on the actual phase of the disease process. But they can also be equivocal or confusing. The orbital cavity is a particularly difficult area for quantitative analysis. It contains various anatomical structures, which are small in size and have significantly different densities, structures, and shapes as well as complicated spatial relationships. This leads to various artifacts that can significantly affect the final results of applied neuroimaging. In addition to this, individual variability strongly affects the established range of standard parameters important for correct disease diagnosis [55]. Diagnostic uncertainties have to be weighed against the benefits and risks of therapy with systemic immunosuppressive treatment, radiation, or surgical orbital decompression.

Author details

Miłosz P. Kawa[1*], Anna Machalińska[2], Grażyna Wilk[3] and Bogusław Machaliński[1]

*Address all correspondence to: kawamilosz@gmail.com

1 Department of General Pathology, Pomeranian Medical University of Szczecin, Szczecin, Poland

2 Department of Ophthalmology, Pomeranian Medical University of Szczecin, Szczecin, Poland

3 Department of General and Dental Radiology, Pomeranian Medical University of Szczecin, Szczecin, Poland

References

[1] Bahn RS Graves' ophthalmopathy. N Engl J Med. 2010;362(8):726-38.

[2] Lazarus JH, Marino M. Orbit–thyroid relationship. In: W.M. Wiersinga, G.J. Kahaly (Eds.), Graves' orbitopathy: a multidisciplinary approach – questions and answers (2nd ed.). Basel: Karger AG; 2010. p26–32.

[3] Khoo TK, Bahn RS. Pathogenesis of Graves' ophthalmopathy: the role of autoantibodies. Thyroid. 2007;17(10):1013-8.

[4] Eckstein AK, Johnson KT, Thanos M, Esser J, Ludgate M. Current insights into the pathogenesis of Graves' orbitopathy. Horm Metab Res. 2009;41(6):456-64.

[5] Dickinson AJ, Perros P. Controversies in the clinical evaluation of active thyroid-associated orbitopathy: use of a detailed protocol with comparative photographs for objective assessment. Clin Endocrinol (Oxf). 2001;55(3):283-303.

[6] Regensburg NI, Wiersinga WM, Berendschot TT, Potgieser P, Mourits MP Do subtypes of graves' orbitopathy exist? Ophthalmology. 2011;118(1):191-6.

[7] Pitz S. Orbital Imaging. In: Wiersinga WM, Kahaly GJ (eds): Graves' Orbitopathy: A Multidisciplinary Approach. Basel: Karger AG; 2007. p57-65.

[8] von Arx G. Atypical manifestations. In: Wiersinga WM, Kahaly GJ, eds. Graves' Orbitopathy. A multidisciplinary approach. Basel: Karger AG; 2007. p212–220.

[9] Müller-Forell W, Pitz S, Mann W, Kahaly GJ. Neuroradiological diagnosis in thyroid-associated orbitopathy. Exp Clin Endocrinol Diabetes. 1999;107 Suppl 5:S177-83.

[10] Kazim M, Trokel SL, Acaroglu G, Elliott A. Reversal of dysthyroid optic neuropathy following orbital fat decompression. Br J Ophthalmol. 2000;84(6):600-5.

[11] Fang ZJ, Zhang JY, He WM. CT features of exophthalmos in Chinese subjects with thyroid-associated ophthalmopathy. Int J Ophthalmol. 2013;6(2):146-149.

[12] Salvi M, Zhang ZG, Haegert D, Woo M, Liberman A, Cadarso L, Wall JR Patients with endocrine ophthalmopathy not associated with overt thyroid disease have multiple thyroid immunological abnormalities. J Clin Endocrinol Metab. 1990;70(1):89-94.

[13] Barbesino G, Tomer Y Clinical review: Clinical utility of TSH receptor antibodies. J Clin Endocrinol Metab. 2013;98(6):2247-55.

[14] Prummel MF, Suttorp-Schulten MS, Wiersinga WM, Verbeek AM, Mourits MP, Koornneef L. A new ultrasonographic method to detect disease activity and predict response to immunosuppressive treatment in Graves ophthalmopathy. Ophthalmology. 1993;100(4):556-61.

[15] Sabetti L, Toscano A, Specchia G, Balestrazzi E. Alterations of the internal reflectivity of extra-ocular muscles associated with several clinical stages of Graves' ophthalmopathy. Ophthalmologica 1998;212 Suppl 1:107-9.

[16] Gerding MN, Prummel MF, Wiersinga WM Assessment of disease activity in Graves' ophthalmopathy by orbital ultrasonography and clinical parameters. Clin Endocrinol (Oxf). 2000;52(5):641-6.

[17] Werner SC, Coleman DJ, Franzen LA. Ultrasonographic evidence of a consistent orbital involvement in Graves's disease. N Engl J Med. 1974;290(26):1447-50.

[18] Willinsky RA, Arenson AM, Hurwitz JJ, Szalai J. Ultrasonic B-scan measurement of the extra-ocular muscles in Graves' orbitopathy. J Can Assoc Radiol. 1984;35(2):171-3.

[19] Demer JL, Kerman BM. Comparison of standardized echography with magnetic resonance imaging to measure extraocular muscle size. American Journal of Ophthalmology 1994;118:351-361

[20] Villadolid MC, Yokoyama N, Izumi M, Nishikawa T, Kimura H, Ashizawa K, Kiriyama T, Uetani M, Nagataki S. Untreated Graves' disease patients without clinical ophthalmopathy demonstrate a high frequency of extraocular muscle (EOM) enlargement by magnetic resonance. J Clin Endocrinol Metab. 1995;80(9):2830-3.

[21] Nagy EV, Toth J, Kaldi I, Damjanovich J, Mezosi E, Lenkey A, Toth L, Szabo J, Karanyi Z, Leovey A. Graves' ophthalmopathy: eye muscle involvement in patients with diplopia. Eur J Endocrinol. 2000;142(6):591-7.

[22] Imbrasienė D, Jankauskienė J, Stanislovaitienė D. Ultrasonic measurement of ocular rectus muscle thickness in patients with Graves' ophthalmopathy. Medicina (Kaunas). 2010;46(7):472-6.

[23] Perri P, Campa C, Costagliola C, Incorvaia C, D'Angelo S, Sebastiani A. Increased retinal blood flow in patients with active Graves' ophthalmopathy. Curr Eye Res. 2007;32(11):985-90.

[24] Alimgil ML, Benian O, Esgin H, Erda S. Ocular pulse amplitude in patients with Graves' disease: a preliminary study. Acta Ophthalmol Scand. 1999;77(6):694-6.

[25] Hartmann K, Meyer-Schwickerath R. Measurement of venous outflow pressure in the central retinal vein to evaluate intraorbital pressure in Graves' ophthalmopathy: a preliminary report. Strabismus. 2000;8:187-93.

[26] Alp MN, Ozgen A, Can I, Cakar P, Gunalp I Colour Doppler imaging of the orbital vasculature in Graves' disease with computed tomographic correlation. Br J Ophthalmol. 2000;84(9):1027-30.

[27] Monteiro ML, Angotti-Neto H, Benabou JE, Betinjane AJ Color Doppler imaging of the superior ophthalmic vein in different clinical forms of Graves' orbitopathy. Jpn J Ophthalmol. 2008;52(6):483-8.

[28] Konuk O, Onaran Z, Ozhan Oktar S, Yucel C, Unal M. Intraocular pressure and superior ophthalmic vein blood flow velocity in Graves' orbitopathy: relation with the clinical features. Graefes Arch Clin Exp Ophthalmol. 2009;247(11):1555-9.

[29] Li H, Liu YH, Li DH, Zhang Y. Value of measurements of blood flow velocity in central retinal artery in thyroid-associated ophthalmopathy. Zhongguo Yi Xue Ke Xue Yuan Xue Bao. 2004;26:460–462.

[30] Pérez-López M, Sales-Sanz M, Rebolleda G, Casas-Llera P, González-Gordaliza C, Jarrín E, Muñoz-Negrete FJ. Retrobulbar ocular blood flow changes after orbital decompression in Graves' ophthalmopathy measured by color Doppler imaging. Invest Ophthalmol Vis Sci. 2011;52(8):5612-7.

[31] Yanik B, Conkbayir I, Acaroglu G, Hekimoglu B. Graves' ophthalmopathy: comparison of the Doppler sonography parameters with the clinical activity score. J Clin Ultrasound. 2005;33(8):375-80.

[32] Stalmans I, Vandewalle E, Anderson DR, Costa VP, Frenkel RE, Garhofer G, Grunwald J, Gugleta K, Harris A, Hudson C, Januleviciene I, Kagemann L, Kergoat H, Lovasik JV, Lanzl I, Martinez A, Nguyen QD, Plange N, Reitsamer HA, Sehi M, Siesky B, Zeitz O, Orgül S, Schmetterer L. Use of colour Doppler imaging in ocular blood flow research. Acta Ophthalmol. 2011;89(8):e609-30.

[33] Kirsch E, von Arx G, Hammer B. Imaging in Graves' orbitopathy. Orbit. 2009;28(4): 219-25.

[34] Enzmann DR, Donaldson SS, Kriss JP. Appearance of Graves' disease on orbital computed tomography. J Comput Assist Tomogr. 1979;3(6):815-9.

[35] Yoshikawa K, Higashide T, Nakase Y, Inoue T, Inoue Y, Shiga H. Role of rectus muscle enlargement in clinical profile of dysthyroid ophthalmopathy. Jpn J Ophthalmol. 1991;35(2):175-81.

[36] Dabbs CB, Kline LB. Big muscles and big nerves. Surv Ophthalmol. 1997;42(3):247-54.

[37] Ozgen A, Ariyurek M. Normative measurements of orbital structures using CT. AJR Am J Roentgenol. 1998;170(4):1093-6.

[38] Regensburg NI, Wiersinga WM, Berendschot TT, Saeed P, Mourits MP. Densities of orbital fat and extraocular muscles in graves orbitopathy patients and controls. Ophthal Plast Reconstr Surg. 2011;27(4):236-40.

[39] Regensburg NI, Wiersinga WM, van Velthoven ME, Berendschot TT, Zonneveld FW, Baldeschi L, Saeed P, Mourits MP. Age and gender-specific reference values of orbital fat and muscle volumes in Caucasians. Br J Ophthalmol. 2011;95(12):1660-3.

[40] Prummel MF. Graves' ophthalmopathy: diagnosis and management. Eur J Nucl Med. 2000 Apr;27(4):373-6.

[41] Regensburg NI, Kok PH, Zonneveld FW, Baldeschi L, Saeed P, Wiersinga WM, Mourits MP. A new and validated CT-based method for the calculation of orbital soft tissue volumes. Invest Ophthalmol Vis Sci. 2008;49(5):1758-62.

[42] Nishida Y, Tian S, Isberg B, Hayashi O, Tallstedt L, Lennerstrand G. Significance of orbital fatty tissue for exophthalmos in thyroid-associated ophthalmopathy. Graefes Arch Clin Exp Ophthalmol. 2002;240(7):515-20.

[43] Le Moli R, Pluchino A, Muscia V, Regalbuto C, Luciani B, Squatrito S, Vigneri R. Graves' orbitopathy: extraocular muscle/total orbit area ratio is positively related to the Clinical Activity Score. Eur J Ophthalmol. 2012;22(3):301-8.

[44] Kahaly GJ. Imaging in thyroid-associated orbitopathy. Eur J Endocrinol. 2001;145(2): 107-18.

[45] Müller-Forell W, Kahaly GJ Neuroimaging of Graves' orbitopathy. Best Pract Res Clin Endocrinol Metab. 2012;26(3):259-71.

[46] Nugent RA, Belkin RI, Neigel JM, Rootman J, Robertson WD, Spinelli J, Graeb DA. Graves orbitopathy: correlation of CT and clinical findings. Radiology. 1990;177(3): 675-82.

[47] Anderson RL, Tweeten JP, Patrinely JR, Garland PE, Thiese SM Dysthyroid optic neuropathy without extraocular muscle involvement. Ophthalmic Surg. 1989;20(8): 568-74.

[48] Feldon SE, Lee CP, Muramatsu SK, Weiner JM. Quantitative computed tomography of Graves' ophthalmopathy. Extraocular muscle and orbital fat in development of optic neuropathy. Arch Ophthalmol. 1985;103(2):213-5.

[49] Barrett L, Glatt HJ, Burde RM, Gado MH. Optic nerve dysfunction in thyroid eye disease: CT. Radiology. 1988;167(2):503-7.

[50] Birchall D, Goodall KL, Noble JL, Jackson A. Graves ophthalmopathy: intracranial fat prolapse on CT images as an indicator of optic nerve compression. Radiology. 1996;200(1):123-7.

[51] Aviv RI, Miszkiel K. Orbital imaging: Part 2. Intraorbital pathology. Clin Radiol. 2005;60(3):288-307.

[52] Neigel JM, Rootman J, Belkin RI, Nugent RA, Drance SM, Beattie CW, Spinelli JA. Dysthyroid optic neuropathy. The crowded orbital apex syndrome. Ophthalmology. 1988;95(11):1515-21.

[53] Machado KFS, Garcia MM. Thyroid ophthalmopathy revisited. Radiol Bras. 2009;42(4):261-266.

[54] Lennerstrand G, Tian S, Isberg B, Landau Högbeck I, Bolzani R, Tallstedt L, Schworm H. Magnetic resonance imaging and ultrasound measurements of extraocular mus-

cles in thyroid-associated ophthalmopathy at different stages of the disease. Acta Ophthalmol Scand. 2007;85(2):192-201.

[55] Majos A, Pajak M, Grzelak P, Stefańczyk L Magnetic Resonance evaluation of disease activity in Graves' ophthalmopathy: T2-time and signal intensity of extraocular muscles. Med Sci Monit. 2007;13 Suppl 1:44-8.

[56] Kirsch E, Hammer B, von Arx G. Graves' orbitopathy: current imaging procedures. Swiss Med Wkly. 2009;139(43-44):618-23.

[57] Young IR, Bydder GM, Hajnal JV Contrast properties of the inversion recovery sequence. In: Bradley WG Jr, Bydder GM (eds) Advanced MR Imaging Techniques. London: Martin Dunitz Ltd; 1997. p143–162.

[58] Mayer E, Herdman G, Burnett C, Kabala J, Goddard P, Potts MJ. Serial STIR magnetic resonance imaging correlates with clinical score of activity in thyroid eye disease. Eye 2001;15:313–8.

[59] Mayer E, Fox DL, Herdman G, Hsuan J, Kabala J, Goddard P, Potts MJ, Lee RW. Signal intensity, clinical activity and cross-sectional areas on MRI scans in thyroid eye disease. Eur J Radiol. 2005;56(1):20-4.

[60] Kirsch E, Kaim A, Gregorio De Oliveira M, von Arx G Correlation of signal intensity ratio on orbital MRI-TIRM and clinical activity score as a possible predictor of therapy response in Graves' orbitopathy—a pilot study at 1.5 T. Neuroradiology 2010;52:91–97.

[61] Hiromatsu Y, Kojima K, Ishisaka N, Tanaka K, Sato M, Nonaka K, Nishimura H, Nishida H. Role of magnetic resonance imaging in thyroid-associated ophthalmopathy: its predictive value for therapeutic outcome of immunosuppressive therapy. Thyroid. 1992;2(4):299-305.

[62] Just M, Kahaly G, Higer HP, Rösler HP, Kutzner J, Beyer J, Thelen M. Graves ophthalmopathy: role of MR imaging in radiation therapy. Radiology. 1991;179(1):187-90.

[63] Cakirer S, Cakirer D, Basak M, Durmaz S, Altuntas Y, Yigit U. Evaluation of extraocular muscles in the edematous phase of Graves ophthalmopathy on contrast-enhanced fat-suppressed magnetic resonance imaging. J Comput Assist Tomogr. 2004;28(1):80-6.

[64] Utech CI, Khatibnia U, Winter PF, Wulle KG. MR T2 relaxation time for the assessment of retrobulbar inflammation in Graves' ophthalmopathy. Thyroid. 1995;5(3): 185-93.

[65] Dolman PJ. Evaluating Graves' orbitopathy. Best Pract Res Clin Endocrinol Metab. 2012 Jun;26(3):229-48.

[66] Yokoyama N, Nagataki S, Uetani M, Ashizawa K, Eguchi K.Role of magnetic resonance imaging in the assessment of disease activity in thyroid-associated ophthalmopathy. Thyroid. 2002;12(3):223-7.

[67] Taoka T, Sakamoto M, Nakagawa H, Fukusumi A, Iwasaki S, Taoka K, Kichikawa K. Evaluation of extraocular muscles using dynamic contrast enhanced MRI in patients with chronic thyroid orbitopathy. J Comput Assist Tomogr. 2005;29(1):115-20

[68] Jiang H, Wang Z, Xian J, Li J, Chen Q, Ai L. Evaluation of rectus extraocular muscles using dynamic contrast-enhanced MR imaging in patients with Graves' ophthalmopathy for assessment of disease activity. Acta Radiol. 2012;53(1):87-94.

[69] Dodds NI, Atcha AW, Birchall D, Jackson A. Use of high-resolution MRI of the optic nerve in Graves' ophthalmopathy. Br J Radiol. 2009;82(979):541-4.

[70] Krassas GE, Kahaly GJ. The role of octreoscan in thyroid eye disease. Eur J Endocrinol. 1999;140(5):373-5.

[71] Postema PT, Krenning EP, Wijngaarde R, Kooy PP, Oei HY, van den Bosch WA, Reubi JC, Wiersinga WM, Hooijkaas H, van der Loos T [111-In-DTPA-D-Phe1] octreotide scintigraphy in thyroidal and orbital Graves' disease: a parameter for disease activity? J Clin Endocrinol Metab. 1994;79(6):1845-51.

[72] Pasquali D, Vassallo P, Esposito D, Bonavolontà G, Bellastella A, Sinisi AA Somatostatin receptor gene expression and inhibitory effects of octreotide on primary cultures of orbital fibroblasts from Graves' ophthalmopathy. J Mol Endocrinol 2000;25:63-71.

[73] Pasquali D, Notaro A, Bonavolontà G, Vassallo P, Bellastella A, Sinisi AA Somatostatin receptor genes are expressed in lymphocytes from retroorbital tissues in Graves' disease. J Clin Endocrinol Metab 2002;87:5125-5129.

[74] Krassas GE, Dumas A, Pontikides N, Kaltsas T. Somatostatin receptor scintigraphy and octreotide treatment in patients with thyroid eye disease. Clin Endocrinol (Oxf). 1995;42(6):571-80.

[75] Kahaly G, Görges R, Diaz M, Hommel G, Bockisch A. Indium-111-pentetreotide in Graves' disease. J Nucl Med. 1998;39(3):533-6.

[76] Gerding MN, van der Zant FM, van Royen EA, Koornneef L, Krenning EP, Wiersinga WM, Prummel MF. Octreotide-scintigraphy is a disease-activity parameter in Graves' ophthalmopathy. Clin Endocrinol (Oxf). 1999;50(3):373-9.

[77] Durak I, Durak H, Ergin M, Yürekli Y, Kaynak S. Somatostatin receptors in the orbits. Clin Nucl Med. 1995;20(3):237-42.

[78] Moncayo R, Baldissera I, Decristoforo C, Kendler D, Donnemiller E. Evaluation of immunological mechanisms mediating thyroid-associated ophthalmopathy by radio-

nuclide imaging using the somatostatin analog 111In-octreotide. Thyroid. 1997;7(1): 21-9.

[79] Kirsch E, von Arx G, Hammer B. Graves' ophthalmopathy: diagnosis and management. Eur J Nucl Med. 2000;27(4):373-6

[80] Prummel MF. Imaging in Graves' orbitopathy. Orbit. 2009;28(4):219-25.

[81] Piciu D. Orbital Single Photon Emission Computed Tomography (SPECT) with Tc-99m DTPA for the Evaluation of Graves' Ophthalmopathy. In: Piciu D., Nuclear Endocrinology. Berlin, Heidelberg: Springer-Verlag; 2012. p122-123.

[82] Rinderknecht J, Shapiro L, Krauthammer M, Taplin G, Wasserman K, Uszler JM, Effros RM. Accelerated clearance of small solutes from the lungs in interstitial lung disease. Am Rev Respir Dis. 1980;121(1):105-17.

[83] Galuska L, Varga J, Szucs Farkas Z, Garai I, Boda J, Szabo J, Leovey A, Nagy EV. Active retrobulbar inflammation in Graves ophthalmopathy visualized by Tc-99m DTPA SPECT. Clin Nucl Med. 2003;28(6):515-6.

[84] Ujhelyi B, Erdei A, Galuska L, Varga J, Szabados L, Balazs E, Bodor M, Cseke B, Karanyi Z, Leovey A, Mezosi E, Burman KD, Berta A, Nagy EV. Retrobulbar 99mTc-diethylenetriamine-pentaacetic-acid uptake may predict the effectiveness of immunosuppressive therapy in Graves' ophthalmopathy. Thyroid. 2009;19(4):375-80.

[85] Ortapamuk H, Hoşal B, Naldöken S. The role of Tc-99m polyclonal human immunoglobulin G scintigraphy in Graves' ophthalmopathy. Ann Nucl Med. 2002;16(7): 461-5.

[86] Lopes FP, de Souza SA, Dos Santos Teixeira Pde F, Rebelo Pinho Edos S, da Fonseca LM, Vaisman M, Gutfilen B 99mTc-Anti-TNF-α scintigraphy: a new perspective within different methods in the diagnostic approach of active Graves ophthalmopathy. Clin Nucl Med. 2012;37(11):1097-101.

[87] Alavi A, Kung JW, Zhuang H. Implications of PET based molecular imaging on the current and future practice of medicine. Semin Nucl Med. 2004;34(1):56-69.

[88] Gotthardt M, Bleeker-Rovers CP, Boerman OC, Oyen WJ. Imaging of inflammation by PET, conventional scintigraphy, and other imaging techniques. J Nucl Med. 2010;51(12):1937-49

[89] García-Rojas L, Adame-Ocampo G, Alexánderson E, Tovilla-Canales JL 18-Fluorodeoxyglucose Uptake by Positron Emission Tomography in Extraocular Muscles of Patients with and without Graves' Ophthalmology. Journal of Ophthalmology 2013;e529187:1-4.

[90] Pichler R, Sonnberger M, Dorninger C, Assar H, Stojakovic T. Ga-68-DOTA-NOC PET/CT reveals active Graves' orbitopathy in a single extraorbital muscle. Clin Nucl Med. 2011;36(10):910-1.

[91] Prummel MF, Wiersinga WM, Mourits, MP Assessment of disease activity of Graves' ophthalmopathy. In: M.F. Prummel ed. Recent Developments in Graves' Ophthalmopathy. Boston: Kluwer; 2000. p59–80.

[92] Burggasser G, Hurtl I, Hauff W, Lukas J, Greifeneder M, Heydari B, Thaler A, Wedrich A, Virgolini I. Orbital scintigraphy with the somatostatin receptor tracer 99mTc-P829 in patients with Graves' disease. J Nucl Med. 2003;44(10):1547-55.

[93] Bartalena L, Baldeschi L, Dickinson A, Eckstein A, Kendall-Taylor P, Marcocci C, Mourits M, et al. European Group on Graves' Orbitopathy (EUGOGO). Consensus statement of the European Group on Graves' orbitopathy (EUGOGO) on management of GO. Eur J Endocrinol. 2008;158(3):273-85.

[94] Mourits MP, Prummel MF, Wiersinga WM, Koornneef L. Clinical activity score as a guide in the management of patients with Graves' ophthalmopathy. Clin Endocrinol (Oxf). 1997;47(1):9-14.

[95] Terwee CB, Prummel MF, Gerding MN, Kahaly GJ, Dekker FW, Wiersinga WM. Measuring disease activity to predict therapeutic outcome in Graves' ophthalmopathy. Clin Endocrinol (Oxf). 2005;62(2):145-55.

[96] Kahaly G, Förster G, Hansen C. Glycosaminoglycans in thyroid eye disease. Thyroid. 1998;8(5):429-32.

[97] Wakelkamp IM, Gerding MN, Van Der Meer JW, Prummel MF, Wiersinga WM Both Th1-and Th2-derived cytokines in serum are elevated in Graves' ophthalmopathy.C lin Exp Immunol. 2000;121(3):453-7.

[98] Gerding MN, van der Meer JW, Broenink M, Bakker O, Wiersinga WM, Prummel MF. Association of thyrotrophin receptor antibodies with the clinical features of Graves' ophthalmopathy. Clin Endocrinol (Oxf). 2000;52(3):267-71.

[99] van der Gaag R, Wiersinga WM, Koornneef L, Mourits MP, Prummel MF, Berghout A, de Vries RR, Schreuder GM, D'Amaro J. HLA-DR4 associated response to corticosteroids in Graves' ophthalmopathy patients. J Endocrinol Invest. 1990;13(6):489-92.

[100] Nakahara H, Noguchi S, Murakami N, Morita M, Tamaru M, Ohnishi T, Hoshi H, Jinnouchi S, Nagamachi S, Futami S, Graves ophthalmopathy: MR evaluation of 10-Gy versus 24-Gy irradiation combined with systemic corticosteroids. Radiology. 1995;196(3):857-62.

[101] Tachibana S, Murakami T, Noguchi H, Noguchi Y, Nakashima A, Ohyabu Y, Noguchi S. Orbital magnetic resonance imaging combined with clinical activity score can improve the sensitivity of detection of disease activity and prediction of response to immunosuppressive therapy for Graves' ophthalmopathy. Endocr J. 2010;57(10): 853-61.

[102] Galuska L, Leovey A, Szucs-Farkas Z, Garai I, Szabo J, Varga J, Nagy EV. SPECT using 99mTc-DTPA for the assessment of disease activity in Graves' ophthalmopathy: a comparison with the results from MRI. Nucl Med Commun. 2002;23(12):1211-6.

[103] Galuska L, Varga J, Szucs Farkas Z, Garai I, Boda J, Szabo J, Leovey A, Nagy EV. Active retrobulbar inflammation in Graves' ophthalmopathy visualized by Tc-99m DTPA SPECT. Clin Nucl Med. 2003;28(6):515-6.

[104] Galuska L, Leovey A, Szucs-Farkas Z, Szabados L, Garai I, Berta A, Balazs E, Varga J, Nagy EV. Imaging of disease activity in Graves' orbitopathy with different methods: comparison of (99m)Tc-DTPA and (99m)Tc-depreotide single photon emission tomography, magnetic resonance imaging and clinical activity scores. Nucl Med Commun. 2005;26(5):407-14.

[105] Szabados L, Nagy EV, Ujhelyi B, Urbancsek H, Varga J, Nagy E, Galuska L. The impact of 99mTc-DTPA orbital SPECT in patient selection for external radiation therapy in Graves' ophthalmopathy. Nucl Med Commun. 2013;34(2):108-12.

[106] Rebelo Pinto E, Lopes FP, de Souza SA, da Fonseca LM, Vaisman M, Gutfilen B, dos Santos PF. A pilot study evaluating 99mTc-anti-TNF-alpha scintigraphy in graves' ophtalmopathy patients with different clinical activity score. Horm Metab Res. 2013;45(10):765-8.

Chapter 6

Thyrotoxic Periodic Paralysis – Clinical Diagnosis and Management

Ana Luiza R. Rolim and Magnus R. Dias da Silva

Additional information is available at the end of the chapter

http://dx.doi.org/10.5772/58475

1. Introduction

1.1. Definition

Periodic paralysis comprises a group of neuromuscular diseases in which the patients present with paroxysmal muscle weakness of the limbs. [1] The most common causes are *thyrotoxic hypokalemic periodic paralysis* (TPP) and familial hypokalemic periodic paralysis (FPP). [1]

Thyrotoxic periodic paralysis (TPP) is a medical emergency characterized by an acute and reversible attack of muscle weakness associated with the *hypokalemia*. [1, 2] TPP is the most common form of acquired flaccid paralysis in adults with *hyperthyroidism* and can occur in patients of any ethnicity, [3, 4] although it is more frequent in Asian populations. [5] TPP is the newest form of endocrine channelopathy included in the large group of periodic paralysis and should be included in the differential diagnosis of acute muscle weakness in patients seeking emergency care.

2. Epidemiology

The association of loss of limb muscle strength and Graves' disease was first published by Rosenfeld in the German literature at the beginning of the last century. [6] In English, the first report was made by Dunlap and Kepler in 1931, describing four patients. [7] In 1968, the first case of TPP diagnosed in Brazil was described by Pereira *et al.* [8]

TPP is more frequently described in Asian descendants, [5] but it can occur in patients of other ancestries. [3, 4] This aspect is particularly important because TPP should not be excluded in the differential diagnosis of paralysis based only on the patient's ethnicity. Although thyrotoxicosis has a higher incidence in women, the paralysis affects predominantly men, with a male:female ratio of approximately 30:1. [2]

TPP symptoms occur in young adults, in contrast to FPP, in which the paralysis crises begin at an earlier age, usually before puberty. [1] TPP is more common between the third and fifth decades of life, which coincides with the peak incidence of thyrotoxicosis [9]. In a study performed with 35 Brazilian patients, the age at diagnosis ranged from 19 to 51 years, [2] similar to the international literature. [9, 10] Unlike the familial form, TPP appears as a sporadic disease. [11] However, rare cases of TPP with a family history of paralysis and thyrotoxicosis have been reported. [12, 13]

3. Etiology and genetic susceptibility

The paralysis crises occur only in the presence of the thyrotoxic state, regardless of its etiology. Several causes of thyrotoxicosis with paralysis have been reported, including Graves' disease (GD), toxic adenoma, toxic multinodular goiter, amiodarone-induced thyrotoxicosis, TSH-producing pituitary tumor, lymphocytic thyroiditis, and factitious thyrotoxicosis. [2] In most of the cases, TPP is associated with the hyperthyroidism in GD, [9, 14] and the paralysis crisis may be an atypical form of initial presentation of the disease. In our studies, there are also a report of TPP in a patient who used formulations containing levothyroxine to lose weight. [2]

The methodological approach to determining the genetic susceptibility to TPP is difficult. This is due in part to the absence of a familial pattern of inheritance that allows linkage analysis by polymorphic allele markers, as almost all of the cases described in the literature are sporadic. Second, the number of cases is relatively small, making an association study to identify genetic susceptibility difficult. Thus, the first genes to be studied were the ones most commonly related to FPP (*CACN1AS* and *SCN4A*) [15], a clinical condition physiopathologically similar to the TPP. However, the investigation of these genes revealed that patients with TPP were negative for these mutations [17, 18]. Several other genes were subsequently studied, and although there were reports of patients bearing the *KCNE3* mutation [18, 19], these patients were later proven to have only a polymorphic variant. [20]

More recently, after the study of Plaster *et al.* [21] on a familial paralysis form associated with facial dysmorphism and arrhythmias called Andersen-Twail Syndrome, a new group of candidate genes arose. Thus, the *KCNJ12* gene (potassium channel Kir2.2) was included in the screening for TPP mutations. Kir2.2 became the candidate of greatest interest because of its expression in the skeletal muscle and the presence of the consensus elements (*cis*), the Thyroid Response Elements (TRE), in its regulatory region. Although no mutation has been found in this group of genes in TPP, during the study of the *KCNJ12* gene, a novel paralog gene was discovered and called *KCNJ18* (Kir2.6). [22] Four different mutations were identified, including two missense (T354M & K366R) and two nonsense (R399X & Q407X) mutations that combined are present in 33% of patients with TPP. [22] These mutations result in a defect in muscle repolarization. The high K^+levels in the muscular system keep the cell in a partially *depolarized*

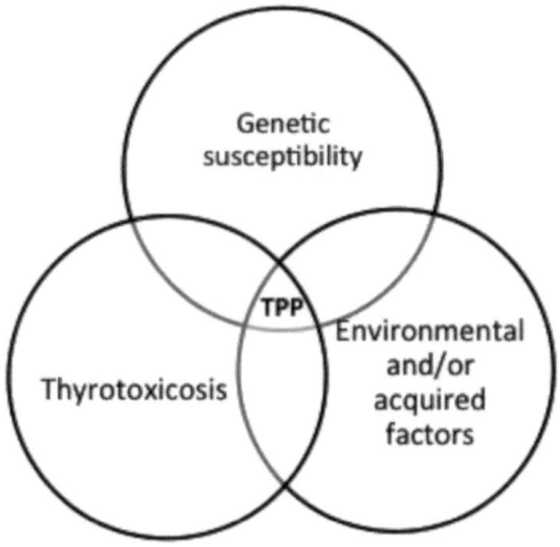

Figure 1. Theoretical model of multifactorial interaction in TPP. Modified from Ref. [1]

state, and the membrane becomes unable to trigger a new muscle excitation-contraction coupling, resulting in flaccid paralysis. [22]

4. Physiopathology

The physiopathology of TPP remains incompletely understood. Evidence suggests that TPP results from a combination of three factors: genetic, environmental, and thyrotoxicosis [1]. From this association, we hypothesized that the interaction of these factors would alter the channel dynamics of the cell membrane at the neuromuscular junction, triggering the *paralysis crises* only in patients genetically susceptible. [2] There are reports of a patient with history of TPP who suffered a paralysis crisis after taking excessive doses of thyroid hormone, [23, 24] which supports this hypothesis. [25]

In Figure 1, we described a theoretical model of multifactorial interactions in TPP. The genetic factors could include a defect in one of the ion channels involved in excitation-contraction coupling (Ca^{2+}, Na^+, and K^+) or a defect in one of the channel's regulatory subunits (ß, ∂, or SUR, for example). Alterations in one of these genes would be responsible for the generation of non-functional ion channels, which would define the TPP as an endocrine channelopathy. [26, 27]

The environmental factors include the excessive consumption of carbohydrate-rich foods, alcohol, or resting after intense exercise. Thyrotoxicosis would be the limiting factor and essential for the paralysis crisis. [1] In addition, several other studies have demonstrated that the activity of the Na^+/K^+-ATPase pump is increased in thyrotoxicosis and is more exacerbated in patients with TPP. [28, 29] The hypokalemia observed in these cases is due to the increased K^+influx into a cell secondary to the increase in the activity of the Na^+/K^+-ATPase pump and by the hyperinsulinemic response to carbohydrate intake in patients susceptible to TPP. [25,

30] Androgens also can increase the activity of the Na^+/K^+-ATPase pump, which explains the higher incidence of the disease in young males. [30]

According to the mechanism illustrated in the Figure 2, we believe that during the TPP crisis, the mutated Kir2.6 potassium channel retains potassium in the sarcolemma, causing hypokalemia and flaccid paralysis.

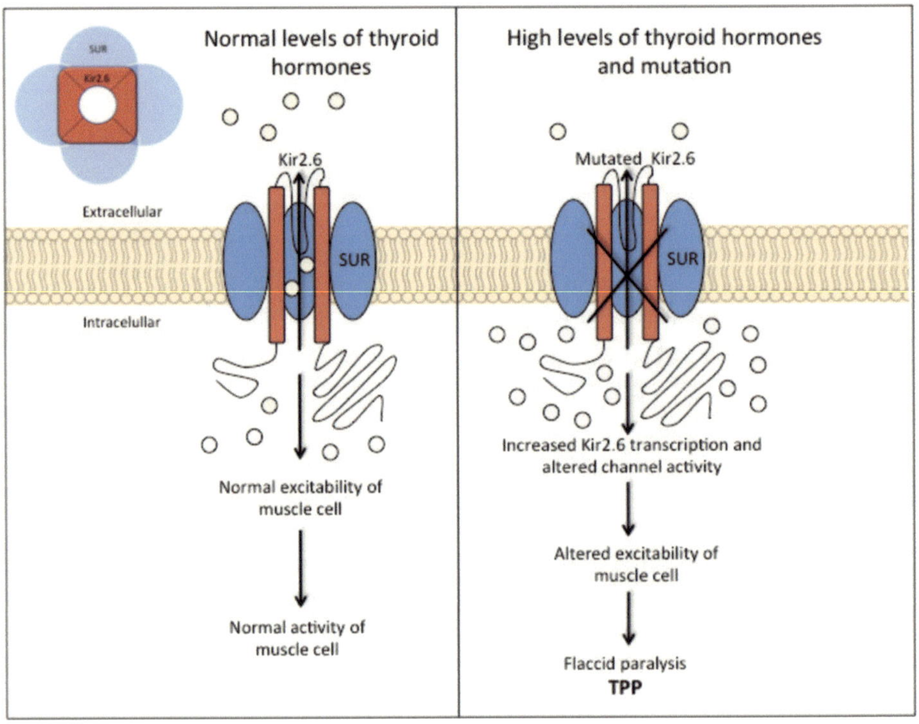

Figure 2. Physiological regulation of Kir2.6 by thyroid hormone and when mutated.

5. Clinical presentation

Illustrative case report of TPP:

A 32-year-old mulatto male patient was brought to the emergency room at 5:00 am by relatives in a wheelchair. He reported being healthy until six months prior to presentation when episodes of muscle weakness in his lower limbs began to develop and kept him from getting out of bed and walking. He also complained of weakness of lower intensity in upper limbs. He denied pain or loss of sensation. All episodes spontaneously resolved without motor sequelae. During physical examination, a decreased in strength, especially in the lower limbs, and hypoactive deep tendon reflexes were noted. In addition, the patient also exhibited diffuse goiter, ocular proptosis, and thyrotoxicosis symptoms (tachycardia, excessive sweating, tremor of the extremities, and 10 kg weight loss). Eating several slices of pizza and soda in a restaurant was identified by the patient as the triggering factor for the crisis the following the next day.

The laboratory tests at the time of the crisis demonstrated hypokalemia (K=1.9 mEq/L; Normal Range: 3.5 to 5.1 mEq/L). The ECG demonstrated the presence of "U" waves and decreased amplitude of the T wave, and oral and intravenous potassium replacement was initiated. The paralysis crisis was resolved after the medication, and the patient was referred to the clinic for the etiologic diagnosis. During the investigation, Graves' disease was diagnosed with TSH <0.05 mUI/L (Normal range: 0.5-4.5 mUI/L), free T4 >6.0 ng/dL (Normal range: 0.6-1.5 ng/dL), and total T3=535 ng/dL (Normal range: 30-200 ng/dL). The ultrasound revealed diffuse enlargement of the thyroid gland and increased vascularization detected by Doppler. [1, 31] I scintigraphy revealed an uptake of 21% over 2 hours (normal range from 1 to 8%) and 50% over 24 hours (normal range from 3 to 23%). Methimazole and propranolol treatments were initiated followed by the definitive hyperthyroidism therapy with radioactive iodine.

The case above illustrates the importance of a proper diagnosis to determine the specific treatment. Many patients already exhibit signs of hyperthyroidism due to Graves' disease (goiter and exophthalmia) or thyrotoxicosis symptoms at the time of the paralysis crisis, but often the thyroid alteration is not recognized at the time and may be confused with hysteria or neuro-anxiety. Often, patients are erroneously classified as psychiatric and consequently treated with benzodiazepines.

The paralysis crises are transient and remit spontaneously, and their frequency, duration and intensity vary. [1] Because of this variability in the clinical presentation, the delayed diagnosis is not uncommon. Many patients report multiple visits to the emergency department with a sudden onset of muscle weakness of the limbs before the diagnosis.

Muscle weakness typically affects the proximal muscles of the lower limbs and is usually symmetric. [31] Some patients may present with tetraparesis or tetraplegia, which can be confused with Guillain-Barre syndrome, transverse myelitis, myasthenia gravis, or an acute spinal cord compression. However, in TPP, there is no urinary incontinence or intestinal dysfunction, nor is there a history of infection or trauma. [32] Although rare, there are reports of respiratory muscle paralysis that requires mechanical ventilation. [1, 33] It is important to distinguish TPP from other neuromuscular disorders that also presents with proximal muscle weakness inherent to thyrotoxic myopathy. In these other disease, the patients exhibit muscle atrophy and increased tendon reflexes, and the symptoms are proportional to the severity of the thyrotoxic state. [34]

TPP may be preceded by prodromal symptoms such as muscle pain, cramps, and/or stiffness of muscles of the affected limbs. [32] Frequently, the patients report that crises occur when they get up during the night or early in the morning after a day of intensive exercise and/or consumption of a large amount of food.

Sensitivity is preserved in the physical-neurological examination. However, as shown in Figure 3, the tendon reflexes are decreased or absent in the majority of the patients, [32] in contrast to the expected hyperreflexia in a thyrotoxic patient without paralysis. The duration of the crisis is variable, lasting up to 72 hours. [31] In a recently published study, the average duration of most cases was two to six hours. [2]

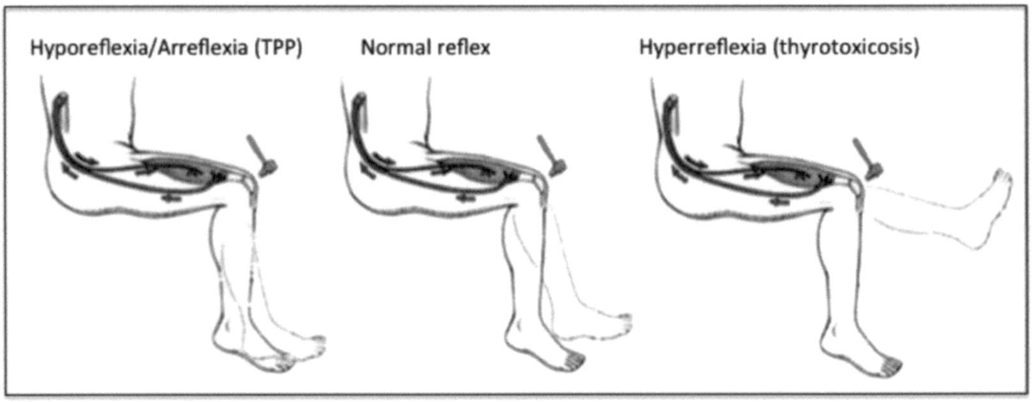

Figure 3. Patellar tendon reflex in patients with TPP, normal individuals, and individuals with thyrotoxicosis.

6. Laboratory and differential diagnosis

The confirmation of thyrotoxicosis, i.e., TSH suppressed in the presence of high levels of thyroid hormones (total and free T3 and T4), is essential for the definitive diagnosis of TPP. Hypokalemia is the primary laboratory alteration at the time of crisis. [9, 35] There are some reports of normokalemia, [36, 37] but we believe that these reports are due to errors during data collection, i.e., data collection in a late stage of the crisis after the serum concentrations of potassium have already recovered, [9] or due to improper storage of the samples, predisposing them to hemolysis. [2]

Hypokalemia results from the influx of ion into the intracellular compartment and does not indicate total depletion of the body potassium. [28] Calcium levels are normal, and creatine phosphokinase (CPK) might be elevated. [2] Some patients exhibit hypophosphatemia and *hypomagnesemia,* [9] both without need for replacement.

Other complementary exams, such as ultrasound, thyroid scintigraphy, and antibody measurements (anti-thyroglobulin, anti-peroxidase, and anti-TSH receptors (TRAb), may be necessary to define the etiology of hyperthyroidism. During the paralysis crisis, some patients exhibit a myopathic pattern on electromyography, which disappears in the remission period. [38] Muscle biopsy demonstrates nonspecific histological findings, and the study of the cerebrospinal fluid does not add any information to the diagnosis, both being dispensable during the investigation of TPP. [2]

We present a table 1 summarizing the major clues for differential diagnosis of acquired muscular disorders in young adults, including clinical and analytical features.

	Thyrotoxic hypokalemic periodic paralysis (TPP)	Familial hypokalemic periodic paralysis (FPP)	Guillain-Barré syndrome	Proximal myopathy
Thyrotoxicosis	Yes (symptoms can be very subtle)	No	No	Yes (duration rather than severity of the thyrotoxic state is proportional to muscle weakness)
Age of onset (years)	20-45 (95%)	Before 16 (80%)	All	All
Frequency	Rare	Rare	Rare	Common (67% of thyrotoxic patients)
Male to female ratio	30:1	3:1	1.5:1	More common among men
Muscle paralysis	Yes (sporadic recurrent acute paralysis)	Yes (sporadic recurrent acute paralysis)	Yes (weakness and paralysis with ascending progression)	No
Ethnicity most frequently affected	East Asian	White	Any	Any
Family history of paralysis	No	Yes	No	No
Precipitating factors	Heavy carbohydrate and/or salt meal, alcohol, exercise, stress	Heavy carbohydrate and/or salt meal, alcohol, exercise, dehydration	Usually preceded by an infection	No
Dysautonomia	No	No	Yes	No
Deep tendon reflexes	Usually absent or depressed	Usually absent or depressed	Absent or depressed	Normal and often hyperactive
Severe respiratory muscle weakness	Very rare	Rare	10-30% of patients	Very rare (in the acute thyrotoxic myopathy only)
Facial muscles weakness	No	No	Common (≥ 50%)	Very rare
Duration of muscle symptoms	30 min-6h	≥ 24h	Progressive over days to 4 weeks	Throughout thyrotoxic state
Potassium level during the muscle symptoms (mmol/L)	1.5-3.0	2.8-3.5	Normal	Normal

	Thyrotoxic hypokalemic periodic paralysis (TPP)	**Familial hypokalemic periodic paralysis (FPP)**	**Guillain-Barré syndrome**	**Proximal myopathy**
Cerebral spinal fluid	Normal	Normal	Albuminocytologic dissociation	Normal
Nerve conduction analysis	Not specific, not necessary	Not specific	Useful and helpful for diagnosis	Not specific, not necessary
Clinical course	Remission when euthyroidism is reached	Chronic myopathy	Recovery; residual deficit in up to 20%; death in some patients	Weakness of proximal muscles that remits when euthyroidism is reached
Genetic inheritance	Mutation in KCNJ18 gene in up to 33% of patients	Mutation in CACN1AS gene (80%) and SCN4A gene (15%)	None	None

(Adapted with permission from reference [2])

Table 1. Clues for differential diagnosis of acquired muscular disorders in young adults

7. Treatment and follow-up

The administration of oral and/or intravenous (IV) potassium is recommended during the paralysis crisis to accelerate the recovery and prevent a possible cardiac arrhythmia. [2] The oral use of potassium should be preferred, [39] but if a faster recovery is necessary, potassium may be slowly IV infused, usually over 2 hours. The main concern about potassium replacement is rebound hyperkalemia [40] because the potassium abnormality is not due to total potassium depletion but intracellular ion trapping. Therefore, monitoring the serum K levels during the treatment and suspending the infusion at the first sign of the muscular force recovery is recommended. [2]

Non-selective beta blockers, especially oral propranolol (80-240 mg/day), [2] may be useful in TPP treatment, especially when awaiting the FT4 and TSH results, by limiting the time of the crisis without inducing rebound hyperkalemia. [41, 42] These drugs block the adrenergic stimulation of the Na^+/K^+-ATPase pump activity, resulting in lower K influx to skeletal muscle.

Early treatment for the underlying cause of thyrotoxicosis is the most important procedure in patients with TPP. When euthyroidism is reached, the paralysis crises remits definitively. [34] Triggering factors such as high intake of carbohydrates, alcohol, and intense physical exercise should be avoided until the resolution of the *thyroid* disease. [43] In cases of thyrotoxicosis caused by excessive intake of thyroid hormones, the drug is suspended. In hyperthyroidism associated with Graves' disease, toxic multinodular goiter, or toxic adenoma, the definitive treatment with radioactive iodine or thyroidectomy should be established immediately. Anti-thyroid drugs (methimazole or propylthiouracil) should be prescribed as adjuvant while the patient waits for the definitive therapy.

Acknowledgements

The authors' work is supported by the Brazilian research funding agencies: CNPq (Conselho Nacional de Desenvolvimento Científico e Tecnológico), CAPES (Coordenação de Aperfeiçoamento de Pessoal de Nível Superior) and FAPESP (Fundação de Amparo à Pesquisa do Estado de São Paulo). A.L.R.R is an M.S. student from the CNPq.

Author details

Ana Luiza R. Rolim and Magnus R. Dias da Silva

Laboratory of Molecular and Translational Endocrinology, Department of Medicine, Escola Paulista de Medicina, Universidade Federal de São Paulo, São Paulo, SP, Brazil

References

[1] Silva MR, Chiamolera MI, Kasamatsu TS, Cerutti JM, Maciel RM. [Thyrotoxic hypokalemic periodic paralysis, an endocrine emergency: clinical and genetic features in 25 patients]. Arquivos brasileiros de endocrinologia e metabologia 2004;48:196-215.

[2] Maciel RM, Lindsey SC, Dias da Silva MR. Novel etiopathophysiological aspects of thyrotoxic periodic paralysis. Nat Rev Endocrinol 2011;7:657-67.

[3] Hay ID, McDougall IR. Letter: Thyrotoxic periodic paralysis in Britain. British medical journal 1975;4:761.

[4] Hackshaw KV, Coker E. Hypokalemic periodic paralysis in a hyperthyroid black woman. Journal of the National Medical Association 1988;80:1343-4.

[5] Lin SH. Thyrotoxic periodic paralysis. Mayo Clin Proc 2005;80:99-105.

[6] Rosenfeld M. Akute aufsteigende Lahmungen bei Morbus Basedow. Berl Klin Wochenschr 1902;39:538-40.

[7] Dunlap HF, Kepler EJ. A syndrome resembling familial periodic paralysis occurring in the course of exolphthalmic goiter. Endocrinology 1931;15:541-6.

[8] Pereira VG, Wajchenberg BL, Quintao ER. Periodic paralysis associated with hyperthyroidism. Study of the precipitating factors. Arquivos brasileiros de endocrinologia e metabologia 1968;17:55-67.

[9] Manoukian MA, Foote JA, Crapo LM. Clinical and metabolic features of thyrotoxic periodic paralysis in 24 episodes. Arch Intern Med 1999;159:601-6.

[10] Hsieh MJ, Lyu RK, Chang WN, et al. Hypokalemic thyrotoxic periodic paralysis: clinical characteristics and predictors of recurrent paralytic attacks. Eur J Neurol 2008;15:559-64.

[11] Ptacek LJ. Channel surfing. J Clin Endocrinol Metab 2002;87:4879-80.

[12] McFadzean AJ, Yeung R. Familial occurrence of thyrotoxic periodic paralysis. British medical journal 1969;1:760.

[13] Leung AK. Familial "hashitoxic' periodic paralysis. J R Soc Med 1985;78:638-40.

[14] Ober KP. Thyrotoxic periodic paralysis in the United States. Report of 7 cases and review of the literature. Medicine (Baltimore) 1992;71:109-20.

[15] Ryan DP, Ptácek LJ. Ion Channel Disorders. In: Rosenberg RN, DiMauro S, Paulson HL, Ptácek LJ, Nestler EJ, eds. The molecular and genetic basis of neurologic and psychiatric disease. Philadelphia: Lippincott Williams & Wilkins; 2007:550-68.

[16] Dias da Silva MR, Cerutti JM, Tengan CH, et al. Mutations linked to familial hypokalaemic periodic paralysis in the calcium channel alpha1 subunit gene (Cav1.1) are not associated with thyrotoxic hypokalaemic periodic paralysis. Clin Endocrinol (Oxf) 2002;56:367-75.

[17] Ng WY, Lui KF, Thai AC, Cheah JS. Absence of ion channels CACN1AS and SCN4A mutations in thyrotoxic hypokalemic periodic paralysis. Thyroid 2004;14:187-90.

[18] Abbott GW, Butler MH, Bendahhou S, Dalakas MC, Ptacek LJ, Goldstein SA. MiRP2 forms potassium channels in skeletal muscle with Kv3.4 and is associated with periodic paralysis. Cell 2001;104:217-31.

[19] Dias Da Silva MR, Cerutti JM, Arnaldi LA, Maciel RM. A mutation in the KCNE3 potassium channel gene is associated with susceptibility to thyrotoxic hypokalemic periodic paralysis. J Clin Endocrinol Metab 2002;87:4881-4.

[20] Sternberg D, Tabti N, Fournier E, Hainque B, Fontaine B. Lack of association of the potassium channel-associated peptide MiRP2-R83H variant with periodic paralysis. Neurology 2003;61:857-9.

[21] Plaster NM, Tawil R, Tristani-Firouzi M, et al. Mutations in Kir2.1 cause the developmental and episodic electrical phenotypes of Andersen's syndrome. Cell 2001;105:511-9.

[22] Ryan DP, Dias da Silva MR, Soong TW, et al. Mutations in potassium channel Kir2.6 cause susceptibility to thyrotoxic hypokalemic periodic paralysis. Cell 2010;140:88-98.

[23] Okihiro MM, Nordyke RA. Hypokalemic periodic paralysis. Experimental precipitation with sodium liothyronine. Jama 1966;198:949-51.

[24] Cohen-Lehman J, Charitou MM, Klein I. Tiratricol-induced periodic paralysis: a review of nutraceuticals affecting thyroid function. Endocrine practice : official journal of the American College of Endocrinology and the American Association of Clinical Endocrinologists 2011;17:610-5.

[25] Fontaine B, Fournier E, Sternberg D, Vicart S, Tabti N. Hypokalemic periodic paralysis: a model for a clinical and research approach to a rare disorder. Neurotherapeutics 2007;4:225-32.

[26] Plassart E, Elbaz A, Santos JV, et al. Genetic heterogeneity in hypokalemic periodic paralysis (hypoPP). Hum Genet 1994;94:551-6.

[27] Rolim ALR, Lindsey SC, Kunii IS, et al. Ion channelopathies in endocrinology: recent genetic findings and pathophysiological insights. Arquivos brasileiros de endocrinologia e metabologia 2010;54:755-63.

[28] Chan A, Shinde R, Chow CC, Cockram CS, Swaminathan R. In vivo and in vitro sodium pump activity in subjects with thyrotoxic periodic paralysis. BMJ 991;303:1096-9.

[29] Chan A, Shinde R, Chow CC, Cockram CS, Swaminathan R. Hyperinsulinaemia and Na+, K(+)-ATPase activity in thyrotoxic periodic paralysis. Clin Endocrinol (Oxf) 1994;41:213-6.

[30] Lin SH, Huang CL. Mechanism of thyrotoxic periodic paralysis. Journal of the American Society of Nephrology : JASN 2012;23:985-8.

[31] Magsino CH, Jr., Ryan AJ, Jr. Thyrotoxic periodic paralysis. Southern medical journal 2000;93:996-1003.

[32] Kung AW. Clinical review: Thyrotoxic periodic paralysis: a diagnostic challenge. J Clin Endocrinol Metab 2006;91:2490-5.

[33] Wu CZ, Wu YK, Lin JD, Kuo SW. Thyrotoxic periodic paralysis complicated by acute hypercapnic respiratory failure and ventricular tachycardia. Thyroid 2008;18:1321-4.

[34] Kung AW. Neuromuscular complications of thyrotoxicosis. Clin Endocrinol (Oxf) 2007;67:645-50.

[35] Shizume K, Shishiba Y, Sakuma M, Yamauchi H, Nakao K, Okinaka S. Studies on electrolyte metabolism in idiopathic and thyrotoxic periodic paralysis. I. Arteriovenous differences of electrolytes during induced paralysis. Metabolism: clinical and experimental 1966;15:138-44.

[36] Wu CC, Chau T, Chang CJ, Lin SH. An unrecognized cause of paralysis in ED: thyrotoxic normokalemic periodic paralysis. Am J Emerg Med 2003;21:71-3.

[37] Gonzalez-Trevino O, Rosas-Guzman J. Normokalemic thyrotoxic periodic paralysis: a new therapeutic strategy. Thyroid 1999;9:61-3.

[38] Puvanendran K, Cheah JS, Wong PK. Electromyographic (EMG) study in thyrotoxic periodic paralysis. Aust N Z J Med 1977;7:507-10.

[39] Chen DY, Schneider P, Zhang XS, He ZM, Chen TH. Fatality after Cardiac Arrest in Thyrotoxic Periodic Paralysis due to Profound Hypokalemia Resulting from Intravenous Glucose Administration and Inadequate Potassium Replacement. Thyroid 2012.

[40] Lu KC, Hsu YJ, Chiu JS, Hsu YD, Lin SH. Effects of potassium supplementation on the recovery of thyrotoxic periodic paralysis. Am J Emerg Med 2004;22:544-7.

[41] Lin SH, Lin YF. Propranolol rapidly reverses paralysis, hypokalemia, and hypophosphatemia in thyrotoxic periodic paralysis. Am J Kidney Dis 2001;37:620-3.

[42] Tassone H, Moulin A, Henderson SO. The pitfalls of potassium replacement in thyrotoxic periodic paralysis: a case report and review of the literature. The Journal of emergency medicine 2004;26:157-61.

[43] Cesur M, Bayram F, Temel MA, et al. Thyrotoxic hypokalaemic periodic paralysis in a Turkish population: three new case reports and analysis of the case series. Clin Endocrinol (Oxf) 2008;68:143-52.

Chapter 7

Hematopoiesis Dysfunction Associated with Abnormal Thyroid Hormones Production

Miłosz P. Kawa and Bogusław Machaliński

Additional information is available at the end of the chapter

http://dx.doi.org/10.5772/58531

1. Introduction

Thyroid hormones (THs), the only known iodine-containing compounds with biological activity, are important for normal development of human organism, affecting the function of virtually all systems [1]. The thyroid gland releases primarily thyroxine (T4), which is converted in peripheral tissues by the enzyme thyroxine 5′-deiodinase to the active TH form, 3,3', 5-triiodo-L-thyronine (T3) [1]. Thyroid hormone action is predominantly the result of T3 binding to high-affinity nuclear TH receptors (TRs) that have different tissue distribution and metabolic targets. TRs subsequently interact with specific DNA sequences, called thyroid hormone response elements (TREs), located in the regulatory region of different target genes [2]. Although both T3 and T4 enter the cells, only T3 is the ligand for TRs. When T3 binds to TR, specific co-factors are recruited and transmit signals to basal transcriptional machinery, thus inducing conformational changes of the chromatin, and making the selected genes accessible to the transcription process [3]. Accordingly, the transcription of the target genes is regulated by T3 and, in this way triiodothyronine exerts its biological effects through the chosen products of the transcription process. There are two thyroid hormone receptor genes, *TRα* and *TRβ*, located in humans on chromosomes 17 and 3, respectively. Although various TR isoforms have been reported, these isoforms can be categorized into TRα1, TRα2, TRβ1, which are widely distributed in the body, and a form with more limited expression, TRβ2 [4]. TRα1 and TRβ1 are the major products of *TRα* and *TRβ* genes, respectively. Alternative splicing of the 3'-most exon of TRα1 results in the generation of TRα2. Since the discovery of these TR isoforms, many studies have attempted to demonstrate their relative contribution to mediate thyroid hormone action in various tissues. However, a number of tissues that are well known targets of THs, is so far limited, and include the pituitary, bones, liver, skeletal and cardiac muscle, fat tissue and developing brain [1]. In addition to the variable expression of

TRs in different tissues, the role of TH can vary in particular tissues. Likewise, the numerous effects by a single hormone on so many distinct tissues is surprising and underscores the vital role of thyroid hormones in cellular function. Therefore, the interpretation of studies on action of biological TH/TRs axis is dependent on understanding the complex nature of thyroid hormone action. It was found that TRs are a multi-functional proteins: they act as transcriptional repressors in the absence of ligand and as transcriptional activators in the presence of T3 [5]. Of note, there are reports that TRα2 reveals an inhibitory action against other active TRs [6]. Importantly, the majority of thyroid hormone actions are thought to be mediated by nuclear receptors, although a wide range of nongenomic effects of TH at the cellular level have been recognized in the last decade [7]. Cellular uptake of iodothyronines and the nuclear TRs are not implicated in the nongenomic actions of thyroid hormones. These specific TH activities have been described to be present in the cell membrane, various organelles, the cytoskeleton, and in cytoplasm. Plasma membrane-initiated actions of TH begin at $\alpha v\beta 3$ receptor for integrin,which activates ERK1/2-dependant cascade of kinases and culminate in local membrane processes, like a modulation of ion transport systems or in complex intracellular events, such as cell proliferation [8].

The objective of this chapter is to provide a current overview of the impact of hyperthyroidism on physiological hematopoiesis in humans and experimental animals. The molecular mechanisms involved in thyroid-dependent regulation of hematopoietic cell growth and development, with insight on the effects of hyperthyroidism on hematopoietic stem cell proliferation, apoptosis and cell cycle have been described. Moreover, the potential direct role of thyroid hormones in regulating the development of main hematopoietic lineages, erythropoiesis and leukopoiesis, are discussed. Finally, a summary on hyperthyroidism and its correlation with thrombocytopoiesis and platelet counts in circulating blood is also given.

2. Hyperthyroidism and hematopoiesis

Thyroid hormones significantly affect the cell cycle, proliferation, apoptosis as well as differentiation and metabolism in different types of human cells throughout the entire life [9]. THs also play an important role in specific tissues during their growth and development. THs have been known to be important regulators of bone development and metabolism [10-12]. In this notion, thyroid hormones may also regulate a wide array of hematological parameters of peripheral blood due to their potential influence on cell functions of hematopoietic system. The association of thyroid disorders and abnormalities in hematological parameters is well known, however, evidence for a role of THs/TRs in hematopoiesis is unclear so far and mostly indirect. In 1881, Charcot showed for the first time that Graves' disease is associated with anemia. Two years later, Kocher observed a decreased number of red blood cells (RBCs) in the peripheral blood (PB) of patients after thyroidectomy. Likewise, direct and indirect effects of excessive or insufficient thyroid hormones on hematopoietic cell maturation and function, on the synthesis and action of hematogenous humoral factors, and on changes in established blood composition may play a role in the pathogenesis of abnormal functions of hematopoietic system that accompany different thyroid diseases. Moreover, various abnormalities in hematological status that occur in patients with thyroid diseases may range from subclinical laboratory abnormalities to clinically significant disorders that might strongly complicate the clinical course of particular thyroid disease. Indeed, erythrocytosis is fairly common in the course of hyperthyroidism [13-14], and importantly, all parameters involved in erythropoiesis return to normal, when an euthyroid state is obtained [15]. However, also anemia is present in 10 to 25 percent of these patients. With regard to white blood cells, elevated, normal, but also depressed, total leukocyte counts have been reported in hyperthyroid patients. Observing the specific types of leukocytes in circulating blood, only the slight decrease in the number of neutrophils and relative increase in the number of eosinophils and mononuclear cells have been recorded in hyperthyroid patients. Nevertheless, the hyperplasia of all myeloid lineages in the bone marrow has been described in several cases of hyperthyroidism [16]. Interestingly, treatment with thyroid hormones has been suggested to improve reconstitution of the immune system after hematopoietic stem cell transplantation [17]. Besides, the clinical relationship between thyroid diseases and the hemostatic system was first defined in 1913 by Kaliebe and coworkers [18]. At that time authors have reported an episode of central vein thrombosis in a thyrotoxic patient. Different overt thyroid dysfunctions may cause thrombosis or hemorrhage by affecting primary and secondary physiologic hemostasis as this system requires careful regulation, also hormonal, in order to work properly [19].

Altogether, according to recent knowledge, the relationship between thyroid diseases and hematopoiesis is more complex than assumed and there are several molecular and patient-based studies on this subject in the scientific literature. Nevertheless, appropriate and adequate studies of high quality are lacking. In most of the reported studies, there are important methodological limitations, such as lack of control groups, small number of cases, and heterogeneity in etiology of the diseases, the severity of thyroid dysfunction and the usage of different laboratory methods. We review here some of the major advances in this area by initially focusing on what is known about molecular mechanisms of TH action on hematopoietic cells, with the particular insight into hematopoietic stem and progenitor cells, and discuss the implications of TH functioning in specific hematopoietic lineages. Although there is a great body of evidence that TH affect early hematopoietic cells in the indirect manner, the recent studies of our group suggested that THs may play a direct role in the regulation of the growth and apoptosis of human early hematopoietic cells [20-21].

2.1. Thyroid hormone receptor expression in hematopoietic stem/progenitor cells

In order to prove that thyroid hormones can directly influence hematopoiesis it is necessary to investigate in the first line the presence of the thyroid hormone receptor in hematopoietic stem/progenitor cells (HSPC). The expression of different TRs has been documented in mature cells of mouse bone marrow (BM), particularly in stromal cells [22], as well as in rat BM cells [23]. Besides, expression of mRNA for *TRα1* receptor was reported in mononuclear cells isolated from human peripheral blood [17]. Recently, our group demonstrated for the first time that TH receptors (TRα1 and TRβ1) are expressed at mRNA and protein level in human $CD34^{+}$HSPCs that were derived from different sources such as bone marrow and peripheral blood [20]. Importantly, we also analyzed TRα1 and TRβ1 expression in HSPC circulating in human umbilical cord blood and we found that TR*α*1 was expressed in both mRNA and protein form, however, *TRβ1* gene had only the expression at the mRNA and not at the protein level [20]. The presence of different TRs in human early CD34$^+$hematopoietic cells is summarized in Figure 1.

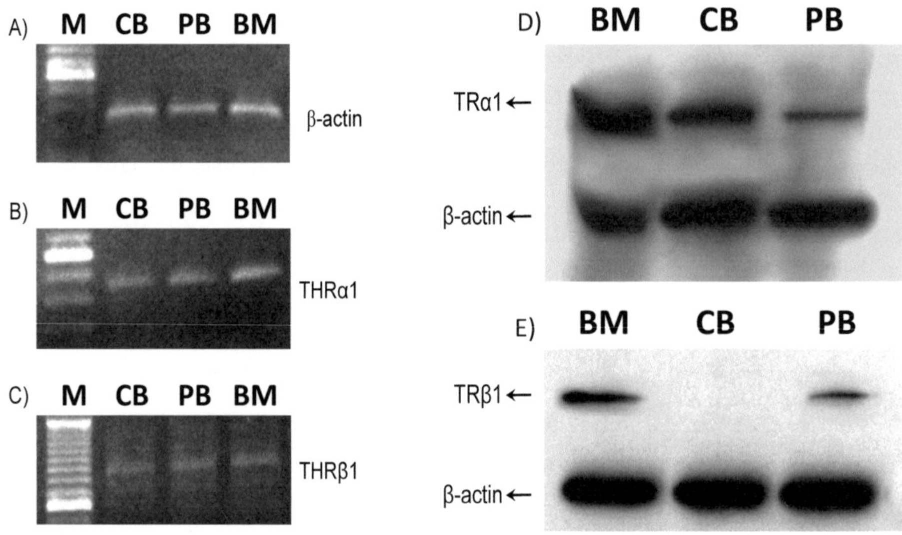

Figure 1. Analysis of TRα1 and TRβ1 expression at transcriptomic and translational level in human CD34$^+$-enriched hematopoietic stem/progenitor cells. Left panel: expression of mRNA for *β-actin* (A), *TRα1* (B) and *TRβ1* (C) in CD34$^+$human cells obtained from cord blood (CB), peripheral blood (PB), and bone marrow (BM). Right panel: expression of protein for TRα1 (D) and TRβ1 (E) in CD34$^+$human cells obtained from bone marrow (BM), cord blood (CB), and peripheral blood (PB). M-molecular marker of DNA weight. Modified from: [20].

Interestingly, we recently observed that the abnormal concentrations of thyroid hormones may influence the rate of expression of different TRs in hematopoietic cells. To investigate the molecular changes underlying the enhanced influence of THs on circulatory HSPCs, we analyzed the expression of *TRα-1* gene in CD34$^+$-enriched HSPCs isolated from the PB of healthy subjects. When HSPC population was subjected for period of 72 hours to triiodothyronine at concentration ten times higher than normal physiological concentration (equal to 3.7 pg/mL), which quite resemble the natural conditions of hyperthyroid state in human patients, the expression of mRNA for *TRα-1* gene was down-regulated in the majority of analyzed blood samples as shown in Figure 2 [21].

Furthermore, our group found that in patients with hyperthyroidism the levels of mRNA for *TRα-1* expressed by CD34$^+$-enriched HSPCs were significantly decreased by around 37% compared to HSPCs isolated from control healthy subjects (254.9 vs. 398.3, respectively; amount of the transcript given in arbitrary units; $P<0.01$) as determined by real-time PCR [21]. Additionally, the results indicating the direct influence of THs on TR expression were qualitatively corroborated by the immunocytofluorescence analysis of TR*α*-1 protein expression in PB-derived CD34$^+$-enriched HSPCs obtained from patients with overt thyroid dys-

http://dx.doi.org/10.5772/58531

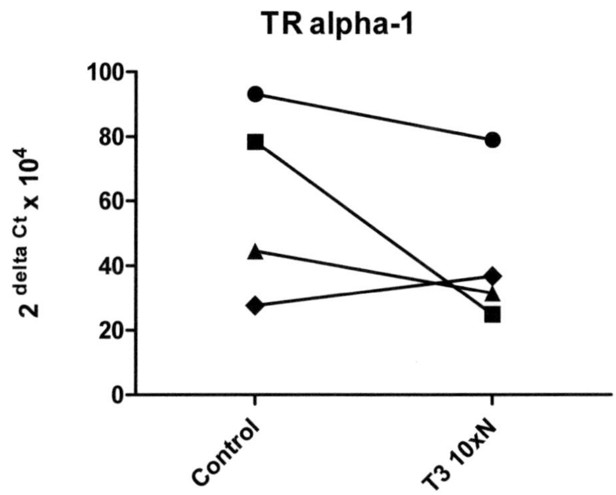

Figure 2. Expression of mRNA for *TRα-1* in human CD34⁺-enriched hematopoietic stem/progenitor cells incubated with increased concentration of T3. Gene expression of *TRα-1* was assessed by real-time RT-PCR in CD34⁺cells collected from healthy donors and incubated through 72 hours with serum saline (Control) or with ten times higher than normal concentration of T3 (T3 10xN). The amount of the transcript is expressed in the arbitrary units. Each line represents *TRα-1* expression in cells collected from particular subject [21].

function. Here, the fluorescence signal of cells from hyperthyroid patients was much weaker than signal of equal cell population from healthy donors. Interestingly, HSPCs from hypothyroid patients presented the most intense fluorescence signal in this analysis performed in the established and fixed conditions. The summary of data obtained from in vitro investigation using immunofluorescence to detect TRα-1 protein expression is presented in Figure 3.

Altogether, the above findings may indicate that T3 at high concentration might reduce the expression of TRα-1 in circulating CD34⁺-enriched HSPCs due to active trafficking of protein receptors and possible intense biodegradation after terminating its role in cell signaling. The process of shuttling of TR between cytoplasm and nucleus directly after TH stimulation was also observed [24]. Alternatively, a biologically controlled ligand-negative loop that form homeostatic mechanism regulating cell activity may prevent the possibility that more ligand binding to specific receptors could actively induce different cellular processes in TR-expressing cells. Therefore, the active reduction of mRNA expression or inhibition of TR protein production would result in prevention against cellular hyperactivity in the hyperthyroid state of the organism, also in the hematopoietic cells of patients with hyperthyroidism. Similar data were obtained by Meier–Heusler et al., who documented a decreased expression of TRβ-1 in mononuclear cells of peripheral blood from hyperthyroid patients and they noted that the levels of mRNA for TRβ-1 were about 40% lower than in euthyroid subjects [25]. Correspondingly, previous observations by Rao et al. suggested a significant trend towards a down-regulation of *TRα-1* mRNA levels in the other tissues under the hyperthyroid state, such as rat testes [26]. These data suggest that specific cellular TR expression is sensitive to the pathological conditions related to hyperthyroidism developed in the affected organism.

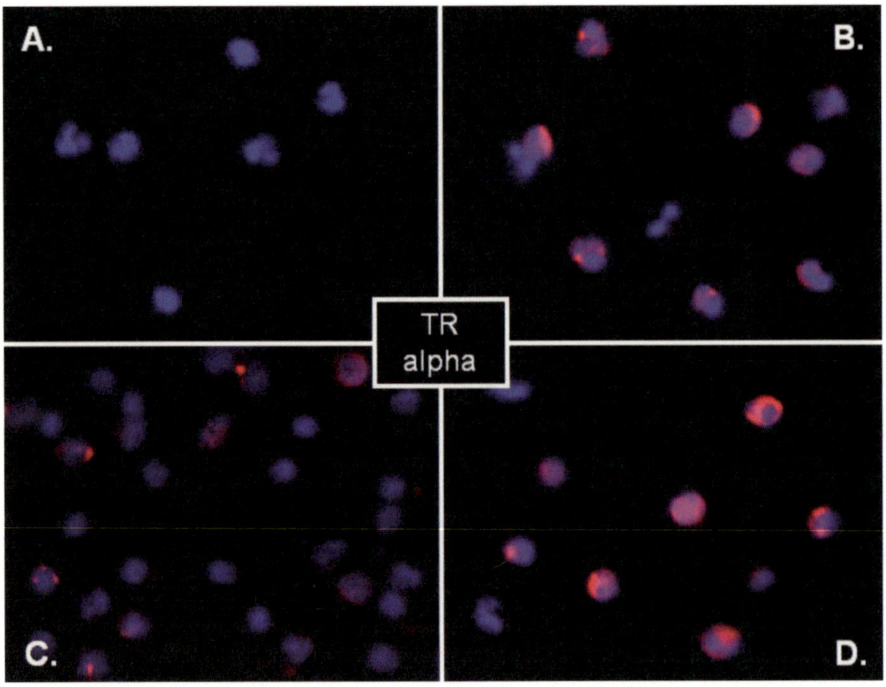

Figure 3. Immunocytofluorescence of TRα-1 protein in human CD34⁺-enriched hematopoietic stem/progenitor cells. CD34⁺cells from healthy donors (B), hyperthyroid patients (C), and hypothyroid patients (D) were stained with anti-TRα-1 antibody (pseudo-colored red). Cell nuclei (A-D) are visualized with DAPI (pseudo-colored blue) [21].

2.2. Hyperthyroidism and lineage-specific clonogenic growth of hematopoietic cells

The hematopoietic system is very sensitive to thyroid hormones and hyperthyroidism may induce significant alterations in growth of hematopoietic stem/progenitor cells, originally located in bone marrow as well as constantly circulating in peripheral blood, and thus significantly exposed to biologic activity of free THs. Unfortunately, our current knowledge concerning the influence of THs on clonogenicity of human HSPCs is very limited and mostly based on studies performed in animal models or human tissues cultured ex vivo. However, such studies, performed in part also by our group, expanded the understanding of the role of thyroid disorders in normal human hematopoiesis and could show a direct pathophysiological influence of T3 on this process.

2.2.1. *Erythropoiesis*

Erythropoiesis is the physiologic process in which red blood cells (RBCs) are produced. Hematopoietic development within the erythroid lineage requires a delicate balance between the opposing effects of proliferation-promoting factors that maintain the renewal capacity of immature erythroid progenitors and differentiation-inducing factors required for successful terminal maturation of erythroid progenitors into mature erythrocytes [27]. In vivo, both the renewal and maturation of human erythroid progenitors proceed in the bone marrow in

http://dx.doi.org/10.5772/58531

parallel. Although thyroid hormones are required for normal development and differentiation of many cell types, little is known about their role in physiologic erythropoiesis, especially in humans [4]. On one side, hyperthyroidism induced in experimental laboratory animals or in humans, generates increased RBC number and total RBC mass through stimulation of erythropoiesis [28-29], however, it has been postulated that this effect would be indirect and involves modulating function of biologically active substances important for erythropoiesis, such as kidney-derived erythropoietin (EPO) or other hematogenous humoral factors, which production by non-erythroid cells is also increased in hyperthyroid state [30-31]. Besides, there are evidences that THs may increase the concentration of 2,3-diphosphoglycerate in erythrocytes, which serves to enhance the delivery of oxygen to tissues, and thus affects steady-state levels of circulating EPO [32-33]. Interestingly, in vitro studies confirmed that both T4 and T3 stimulate EPO synthesis in the human liver cell line HepG2 and this stimulating effect could persist for 24 hours after the removal of THs from the cell culture [34]. However, in the established model of HSPCs cultures in vitro with standard amount of EPO performed for analysis of differential clonogenic growth of hematopoietic cells, we observed that proliferative potential of burst-forming units of erythrocytes (BFU-E) was increased only in the samples collected from the patients with hyperthyroidism and, in contrast, it was decreased in case of samples collected from the hypothyroid subjects [21]. Therefore, it seems that THs can induce signal transduction pathways implicated in proliferation of hematopoietic progenitors for erythroid lineage other than EPO-dependent mechanisms. Data from in the available literature corroborate our discovery indicating the direct role of THs in normal erythroid differentiation of human and animal origin [35-38]. For example, daily administration of thyroxine into mice stimulated the increase of indices significant for RBC production, such as packed red blood cell volume, total circulating RBC count and mass, and reticulocyte count [39]. Likewise, Malgor et al. have studied the TH role on modulation of erythropoiesis using the in vitro cultures of cells collected from bone marrow of normal rats in the absence of EPO [37]. They found that T3 produced a direct and significant stimulation of clonogenic growth of late colony-forming erythroid units (CFU-E) and a moderate increase of early erythroid burst-forming units (BFU-E) indicating an enhanced proliferative activity of committed erythroid progenitors in response to this hormone. In contrast, the addition of T3 to in vitro cultures of avian BM cells activates the TRα receptor in avian erythroblasts, blocks their self-renewal, and induces synchronous, terminal differentiation of erythroid lineage from hematopoietic progenitor cells [40]. Notwithstanding, Kendrick et al. recently verified the essential function of TRα in regulating erythropoiesis in mammals by characterizing the phenotype of TRα–/– mice deficient for TRα. These transgenic mice had significantly reduced numbers of erythroid progenitor cells in the fetal liver, decreased hematocrit in adult organism, and a diminished erythroid stress response to hemolytic anemia [41]. Similar results of direct TH influence on erythroid lineage growth were taken from observations of human erythropoiesis developed in vitro in established conditions. In pioneer studies of human BM-derived cells and THs action Golde et al. showed that THs do not shift the requirement for EPO in the course of human erythropoiesis, but both substances have synergistic effects in increasing the number of erythroid colonies growing in vitro [35]. These data were corroborated by Leberbauer et al., who recently demonstrated that terminal erythroid maturation in course of development of human erythroblasts obtained from umbilical cord blood is significantly improved by supplementation of T3 to the defined culture medium [42]. Likewise, we performed a quantitative molecular analysis of hematopoietic stem/progenitor cell proliferation based on the expression levels of mRNA for the *Cyclin D1* and *PCNA* genes, which are concerned to be important for the cell cycle regulation. We found in our study, the nearly 100% increase in expression of mRNA for both analyzed genes in PB-derived CD34⁺-enriched HSPCs collected from subjects with hyperthyroidism (Figure 4), thus indicating that THs significantly stimulates up-regulation of genes involved in the induction of hematopoietic cell proliferation [21].

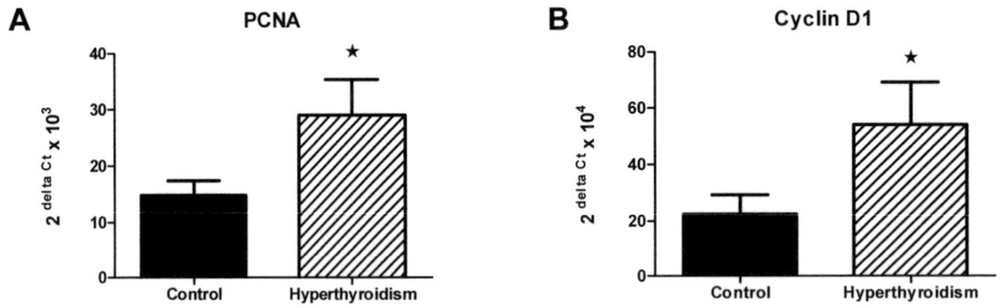

Figure 4. Expression of mRNA for *PCNA* and *Cyclin D1* in human $CD34^+$-enriched hematopoietic stem/progenitor cells collected from hyperthyroid patients. Gene expression of *PCNA* (panel A) and *Cyclin D1* (panel B) was assessed by real-time RT-PCR in $CD34^+$cells isolated from PB of patients with hyperthyroidism and healthy donors (Control). The mean amount of the selected gene transcript (± SD) is expressed in the arbitrary units. $P < 0.05$. [21]

These molecular data correlate strongly with increased potential of erythroid progenitor cell growth observed in our study performed on $CD34^+$-enriched HSPCs from PB of patients with thyroid dysfunction using in vitro proliferation assays [21]. Erythroid BFU-E colonies cultivated from $CD34^+$cells that were collected from circulating blood of patients with hyperthyroidism exhibited in average a 40% increase of their clonogenic growth compared to the healthy control group ($P<0.05$). Importantly, in the group of patients with hyperthyroidism comprised of 25 persons of whom 52% were patients with Graves' disease and 48% with toxic nodular goiter, we also observed a significant increase in the number of mature RBCs in the PB. Furthermore, RBCs from our cohort possessed increased mean corpuscular volume, but reduced mean corpuscular hemoglobin concentration and mean hemoglobin mass. These findings together might indicate that erythroid progenitors that are overproduced in BM of hyperthyroid patients under the abnormal T3 stimulation would generate mature RBCs circulating in excess in peripheral blood. However, cellular structure and composition of circulating RBCs was also affected. Of note, our study group presented the mild increase in free T3 concentration compared to healthy volunteers who served as control group (2.71±1.14 vs. 6.95±3.13 pg/mL of T3, respectively).

However, there is a few studies with contradictory results investigating the functional effect of thyroid abnormalities on the RBC counts in peripheral blood. Gianoukakis et al. have measured the RBCs in 87 hyperthyroid patients with Graves' disease and 19 healthy subjects. The average number of RBCs was found to be lower in the 36% of recruited hyperthyroid subjects compared to the healthy individuals. Nevertheless, in the group of selected patients with anemia, the mean EPO levels were significantly higher (P=0.004) than those of the non-anemic controls [43]. According to other authors, anemia is present in 10 to 25 percent of patients with hyperthyroidism [15, 44]. This finding may be the result of increased plasma volume, as reported effect of increased T3 concentration in humans [45] and animal model [39], but also the result of autoimmune processes leading to anemia in Graves' disease, such as pernicious anemia and autoimmune hemolytic anemia, which concurrently may develop [46]. In addition, decreased RBC survival and ineffective erythropoiesis in course of hyperthyroidism have been described [47-48]. Pancytopenia in the setting of hyperthyroidism has also been reported in the literature. Most cases of pancytopenia have been associated with Graves' disease and one case with toxic adenoma, and TH-related stem cell dysfunction has been suggested there as one possible mechanism among others [49-51]. Likewise, our group observed that heavily non-physiological concentrations of T3, such as ten times higher or fifty times higher than physiological concentration of free T3 significantly negatively influenced the in vitro growth of erythroid BFU-E colonies in proliferation assays derived from human $CD34^{+}$HSPCs circulating in peripheral blood. This effect was even more noticeable after prolonged exposure to increased non-physiological T3 amounts [20]. This may explain the abnormalities in RBC counts observed in some patients with hyperthyroidism, especially those with advanced and chronic disease. In contrast, the in vitro clonogenic potential of erythroid BFU-E progenitors was considerably increased in physiological concentration of free T3 as well as in mildly increased concentration of T3 such as five times higher than normal physiological one [21]. The mean numbers of the colonies of erythroid BFU-E obtained in our study are presented in Table 1.

Free T3 concentration		**N**	**5xN**	**10xN**	**50xN**
Parameter	**Incubation**	**%**	**%**	**%**	**%**
Growth of BFU-E from BM	24 hours	100.00	103.5 ± 30.7	85.6 ± 29.1	70.6 ± 54.4
	72 hours	100.00	108.9 ± 43.9	88.25 ± 46,9	49.2 ± 18.2*
Growth of BFU-E from PB	24 hours	100.00	114.0 ± 42.9*	104.0 ± 20.2	65.0 ± 12.2*
	72 hours	100.00	101.0 ± 50.3	63.0 ± 36.2	59.0 ± 13.9*
Growth of BFU-E from CB	24 hours	100.00	94.9 ± 32.2	88.8 ± 39.2	58.0 ± 31.9
	72 hours	100.00	90.5 ± 18.9	66.5 ± 11.6*	46.9 ± 14.5*

Table 1. Influence of T3 on clonogenicity of human BFU-E after 24-and 72-hour incubation with increasing free T3 concentrations. Cells (n=5) incubated with: N=physiological dose of T3 (3.7 pg/mL); 5×N=five times higher than N; 10×N=10 times higher than N; 50×N=50 times higher than N. Results are expressed as mean percentage (± SD) of the control value obtained with established physiological dose of T3 taken as 100%. $P < 0.05$ [20].

2.2.2. Leukopoiesis

Leukopoiesis is the process of white blood cells (WBCs) formation from hematopoietic stem cells placed in hematopoietic organs. Leukocytes are a heterogeneous group of blood cells that all have nuclei and include granulocytes (i.e. neutrophils, eosinophils, and basophils), monocytes, lymphocytes T and B, as well as natural killer cells. Leukopoiesis is stimulated by different cytokines, interleukins, colony-stimulating factors and several hormones. The body of information on the relationship between thyroid hormones and WBC biology is relatively large and describes contribution of thyroid hormones to the modulation of physiological leukocyte activities such as chemotaxis, phagocytosis, respiratory burst, cytolytic activity, and cytokine synthesis in monocytes/macrophages and different types of lymphocytes. Nevertheless, the data available are frequently difficult to interpret or even contradictory, when related to growth and proliferation of specific leukocyte types. This situation is even more complicated by the fact, that WBCs are able to produce several hormones or hormone-like molecules [52], and the expression of thyroid hormones has been reported in several WBCs, like monocytes, granulocytes, natural killer cells, mast cells, and lymphocytes [53-54]. It is also known that T3 is able to modulate functions of immune-related cells either via nuclear receptors that are responsible for genomic TH activities, and by interactions with other membrane receptors for THs that conduct non-genomic actions of THs [1].

In general, it was found that physiological concentrations of thyroid hormones positively correlates with the immune cell parameters/functions, such as cell counts and induction of different physiological activities of particular WBC populations. Few reports analyzing the in vitro actions of THs showed modifications in lymphocyte reactivity [55-56]. However, the direction and magnitude of these alterations might depend on the type and concentration of the TH encountered by the responding cells, and the species source of lymphoid cells. For example, it was found that THs within the normal physiological range may increase a mitogen-induced normal T lymphocytes proliferation through both the genomic and non-genomic mechanisms [57]. Furthermore, Hodkinson et al. measured plasma thyroid hormone levels in 93 late-middle aged healthy euthyroid subjects, and calculated the mean T3/T4 ratio, and next used these numbers to distinguish between low-and high-thyroid hormones concentration, but still within the normal physiological range, and found a significant positive association between thyroid hormones concentration and natural killer T-cell percentage and monocytes count [58]. In addition, in the same study there was also a significant inverse association of THs levels with the expression of early lymphocyte apoptosis markers [58]. Recently, it has been proposed that thyroid hormones are significant for leukopoesis as highly involved in maintaining immune system homeostasis in response to environmental changes or stress-mediated immunosuppression [59]. Further evidences from studies on mammals indicate that thyroid hormones have important immunomodulatory effects. Likewise, T3 enhances phytohaemagglutinin stimulation of human lymphocytes [60]. Concurrently, El-Shaikh et al. have shown that the daily subcutaneous supplementation of T4 in BALB/c mice for one month induces an increase in the total number of peripheral blood leukocytes, as well as augments cellularity of thymus and spleen parenchyma, and peripheral lymph nodes [61]. In general, developed hyperthyroid state induces the increase in the immune system functions related to the antibody production, immune cell migration, and reactive oxygen species production, whereas it decreases the proinflammatory markers expression, the antioxidant enzymes production, and their cellular activity [62]. Notwithstanding, in other in vivo study performed in rats, the induction of hyperthyroidism did not affect the ratio of helper to suppressor T lymphocytes in the examined immune system [63].

Due to the contrasting results revealed in some previous reports, it is quite difficult to establish a clear correlation between hyperthyroidism and immune functions [62]. These discrepancies may be largely attributed to differences in the duration of disease, age and gender of animal and human subjects and hyperthyroidism origin, or even the treatment mode given to the patients with thyroid disease. Especially, previous studies on human different WBC population counts and function during hypo-and hyperthyroid states produced conflicting results. Indeed, a significant decrease in the lymphocyte and increase in monocyte count were observed in patients with autoimmune thyroiditis [64], however, similar changes in the number of lymphocytes were also observed in autoimmune hyperthyroidism [65]. Thus, it is supposed that the changes in number of lymphocytes in different thyroid autoimmune dysfunctions are due to the autoimmune process alone, and not due to the direct influence of thyroid hormones specifically on lymphopoiesis. Possibly, the elevated number of lymphocytes in autoimmune-related thyroid disorders may demonstrate a nonspecific activation of the immune system as it is found in some other autoimmune-derived diseases in humans [66-67]. Our own results performed in the selected group of patients with hyperthyroidism showed a tendency to decrease the general WBC number in circulating peripheral blood. Thus, we were mostly interested in biology of hematopoietic stem and progenitor cells of myelomonocytic lineage from these subjects, as appeared that this lineage may be clearly independent from autoimmune responses developed in this patient group and might be affected by abnormal THs concentration. It appears from the available literature that the relationship between thyroid hormones and myelopoiesis has been studied mainly based on hematopoietic cells collected from peripheral blood of healthy subjects. Unfortunately, the current knowledge concerning the influence of THs on clonogenicity of progenitors for granulocytes and monocytes that grown as colony forming units of granulocytes and monocytes (CFU-GM) is very limited. There are only few reports on the influence of physiological T3 concentration on clonogenic potential of human CFU-GM cells. For example, Notario et al. observed that both thyroid hormones, T3 and T4, are able to enhance the colony growth of CFU-GM obtained from normal PB, and interestingly, the response is more evident for T4 than T3 [68]. Moreover, the second report of this group revealed that there is a synergistic effect of THs and different hematopoietic growth factors, like G-CSF, GM-CSF, and IL-3, which are substantial for proliferation of progenitors for myelomonocytic lineage [69]. In contrast, Ponassi et al. reported an abnormal granulopoiesis in nearly 50 percent of patients with untreated Graves' disease, based on the pharmacological test with mobilization of the marrow granulocyte reserve by hydrocortisone [70]. However, no data on clonogenic potential of hematopoietic progenitor cells in the presence of different nonphysiological concentrations of thyroid hormones were reported in either of these studies. Therefore, our group recently analyzed the in vitro growth of myeloid CFU-GM colonies derived from human $CD34^{+}$HSPCs in proliferation assays with growing non-physiological concentrations of free T3. We observed that clonogenic potential of CFU-GM colonies from $CD34^{+}$HSPCs of healthy subjects was considerably increased in concentration of T3 only moderately higher (5x) than the physiological T3 concentration [20]. In contrast, the much higher non-physiological concentrations of T3, such as ten times higher or fifty times higher than physiological T3 concentration significantly negatively influenced the growth of myeloid CFU-GM colonies derived from CD34⁺HSPCs collected from peripheral blood as well as umbilical cord blood. This effect was even more significant in case of myeloid CFU-GM colonies derived from CD34⁺HSPCs harvested from the bone marrow of healthy donors [20]. In addition, we noticed an enhanced negative effects of non-physiological concentrations of T3 in the case of prolonged in vitro exposure to the triiodothyronine (72-hour-period). The mean numbers of the colonies of myeloid CFU-GM obtained in our study are presented in Table 2.

Free T3 concentration		**N**	**5xN**	**10xN**	**50xN**
Parameter	**Incubation**	**%**	**%**	**%**	**%**
Growth of CFU-GM from BM	24 hours	100.00	77.8 ± 19.6*	72.6 ± 18.7*	50.1 ± 8.7
	72 hours	100.00	91.0 ± 36.7	97.2 ± 47,7	49.2 ± 18.2*
Growth of CFU-GM from PB	24 hours	100.00	154.0 ± 18.7*	101.0 ± 14.5	90.0 ± 35.8*
	72 hours	100.00	292.0 ± 26.6*	205.0 ± 17.5*	141.0 ± 29.4*
Growth of CFU-GM from CB	24 hours	100.00	106.3 ± 28.4	92.7 ± 11.6	93.8 ± 35.7
	72 hours	100.00	96.1 ± 16.2	65.1 ± 9.9	55.9 ± 7.5

Table 2. Influence of T3 on clonogenicity of human CFU-GM after 24-and 72-hour incubation with increasing free T3 concentrations. Cells (*n*=5) incubated with: N=physiological dose of T3 (3.7 pg/mL); 5×N=five times higher than N; 10×N=10 times higher than N; 50×N=50 times higher than N. Results are expressed as mean percentage (± SD) of the control value obtained with established physiological dose of T3 taken as 100%. $P < 0.05$ [20].

The abovementioned results clearly correlated with clonogenic potential of CD34⁺-enriched HSPCs collected from subjects with diagnosed thyroid dysfunction [21]. In our clinical study, we examined the clonogenicity of CD34⁺HSPCs harvested from PB of hyperthyroid patients using the in vitro proliferation assays, and we found that the number of CD34⁺-expanded CFU-GM colonies was significantly lower in this group than that observed in healthy euthyroid subjects (66 vs. 100% respectively; $P < 0.05$).

One of the possible explanations for the diminished clonogenic growth of CFU-GM derived from hyperthyroid patients might be the TH-dependent cell death induced in circulating and BM residual HSPCs. Cell death has been broadly classified into two categories, necrosis and apoptosis. Of note, there is ongoing debate as to the mutually exclusive nature of these two categories of cell death, and it seems possible that there are many intermediate subcategories. However, necrotic cell death is always a pathological event occurring in response to strong cell/tissue injury or environmental insult. In contrast, apoptosis is an energy-requiring process that often involves altered expression of key cell proliferation and death-inducing genes. It is known that THs, like many other hormones acting through nuclear receptors, are important regulators of cellular proliferation and apoptosis [71-72]. At the cellular level, both T3 and T4 induce apoptosis in different cell types, like rat pituitary cell lines [73-74], rat cardiomyocytes [75], and human breast cancer cells [76], when exposed to THs in vitro or in vivo. It was observed that in HeLa cervix cancer cell line T3 induces caspase activity, which plays a key role in the execution of apoptosis [77]. In contrast, the physiological concentrations of both T3 and T4 inhibited apoptosis in rat brain-derived endothelial cells in vitro through alterations in the mRNA levels of apoptosis-related genes, such as *BCL-2* and *BAD* [78]. T4 was able to inhibit the resveratrol-induced apoptosis in glioma cells in vitro through nongenomic mechanisms, employing integrin receptor and ERK-mediated cascade [79]. Alike, previously mentioned Hodkinson et al. observed that under normal physiological conditions T3 reduced incidence of lymphocyte apoptosis in healthy older individuals [58]. Similarly, Barreiro Arcos et al. observed, that TH treatment augments the mitogen-induced proliferation of normal T lymphocytes [80]. Altogether, TH-mediated effects on cellular apoptosis depend on the type and developmental or pathophysiological state of the selected cells and tissues. Importantly, there are many compounds and circumstances that can induce cell apoptosis. It is known that a particular agent may produce apoptosis in a given cell or tissue, but may not in another, or in a given cell at one period of the cell cycle, but not at another. Whether a cell responds to such an agent by induction of programmed cell death, it must therefore depend on the specific array of interactive molecular regulatory systems active in that cell at that time [81]. In case of cells related to hematopoietic system, the pro-apoptotic actions of THs were defined in normal and tumor-derived lymphocytes. In this notion, Mihara et al. demonstrated that T lymphoma cells from the human Jurkat cell line, cultured in vitro for 2 weeks with addition of T3 and T4, showed their enhanced apoptosis [82]. This group also showed that T lymphocytes from healthy volunteers cultured with T3, but not T4, for five days exhibited an increase in the percent of spontaneous apoptosis, thus indicating that long-term exposure to T3 induces accelerated lymphocyte apoptosis in vitro [82]. Indeed, Mihara and coworkers found also significantly higher percentage of apoptotic T lymphocytes in vivo from patients with chronic Graves' disease than from healthy subjects [82]. Moreover, Gandrillon et al. determined that THs increased apoptosis rate in early erythrocytic progenitor cells [83], and similar effect was observed by Hara et al. in hematopoietic HL-60 cells of promyeloleukemic lineage [84]. To put the light on the possible pathophysiological mechanisms of such decreased proliferative potential of $CD34^+$HSPCs in high non-physiological T3 concentrations reported by our group, we analyzed the process of apoptosis in HSPCs collected from different compartments of human hematopoietic system, such as bone marrow, peripheral blood or umbilical cord blood [20]. In our study, we performed the analysis of potential influence of T3 on the apoptosis induction in human $CD34^+$-enriched hematopoietic progenitor cells collected from the above hematopoietic cell sources of healthy subjects. Importantly, we analyzed the apoptosis in these cells employing three different molecular techniques as, according to specialists in this field, it is crucial for reliable detection of this phenomenon to confirm it by applying at least three distinct laboratory methods. For this reason, we used the flow cytometry-based detection of annexin-V, TUNEL technique detecting apoptosis-related abnormalities in cell genetic material, and finally, analysis of the expression level of pro-apoptotic *Bax* and both anti-apoptotic *Bcl-xL* and *Bcl-2* genes in the $CD34^+$HSPCs that were incubated with different non-physiological T3 concentrations (5×N; 10×N; and 50×N; where N is equal to established physiological

T3 dose) for period of 24 or 72 hours. We found that after 24 hours all three used non-physiological T3 concentrations markedly induced the apoptosis in analyzes hematopoietic progenitors, however the percentage of apoptotic CD34⁺HSPCs was significantly higher in samples collected from PB, CB and BM incubated with the highest dose [20]. Similar results were obtained for longer incubation through 72-hour-period. It was especially clearly noticeable in the detailed analysis of the apoptosis detected by TUNEL technique presented in Table 3. Correspondingly, when analyzing the mRNA expression for genes crucial for apoptosis in human early hematopoietic $CD34^+$cells after incubation with the fixed increasing T3 concentrations, we observed an augmented expression of pro-apoptotic *BAX* gene and decreased expression of the anti-apoptotic genes: *BCL-xL* and *BCL-2* in these cells under exposure to T3 amount 50 times higher than the established physiological T3 concentration [20].

Free T3 concentration		**N**	**5xN**	**10xN**	**50xN**
Parameter	**Time**	**%**	**%**	**%**	**%**
Apoptotic $CD34^+$ HSPCs from BM	24 hours	100.00	144.5 ± 39.4*	94.3 ± 33.9	87.4 ± 47.6
	72 hours	100.00	179.0 ± 25.5*	107.3 ± 9,6	119.1 ± 11.0*
Apoptotic $CD34^+$ HSPCs from PB	24 hours	100.00	115.1 ± 20.5	166.6 ± 31.7*	98.8 ± 20.4
	72 hours	100.00	105.3 ± 36.5	122.5 ± 17.8*	125.1 ± 16.1*
Apoptotic $CD34^+$ HSPCs from CB	24 hours	100.00	105.3 ± 36.5	122.5 ± 47.8	105.1 ± 26.1
	72 hours	100.00	167.8 ± 6.9*	177.4 ± 34.6*	213.6 ± 32.0*

Table 3. Percentage of apoptotic cells detected with the established TUNEL method after 24-and 72-hour incubation of human $CD34^+$cells with increasing free T3 concentrations. Cells (n=5) incubated with: N=physiological dose of T3 (3.7 pg/mL); 5×N=five times higher than N; 10×N=10 times higher than N; 50×N=50 times higher than N. Results are expressed as mean percentage (± SD) of the control value obtained with established physiological dose of T3 taken as 100%. $P < 0.05$ [20].

Our group was also interested to assess the influence of THs on apoptosis rate in PB-derived $CD34^+$HSPCs circulating in peripheral blood of the patients with hyperthyroidism [21]. For this analysis, we used combined annexin-V and propidium iodate staining of hematopoietic cells detected by flow cytometry. This method especially provides the chance to assess apoptosis in two distinct stages, the early and late phase of apoptosis. In fact, we observed a significant increase in the percentage of cells undergoing the late, executive phase of apoptosis in the group of patients with hyperthyroidism compared to euthyroid control subjects (1823.43 ± 1334.15 vs. 100% of the control population, respectively; $P<0.05$). The results are displayed in Figure 5. However, there were no differences between analyzed groups in percentage of $CD34^+$cells undergoing the early stage of apoptosis (103.1 ± 74.16 vs. 100% of the control population, respectively).

Concurrently, expression of mRNA for *BCL-2* and *BCL-xL* genes was assessed by real-time RT-PCR in $CD34^+$cells isolated from PB of patients with hyperthyroidism and healthy controls.

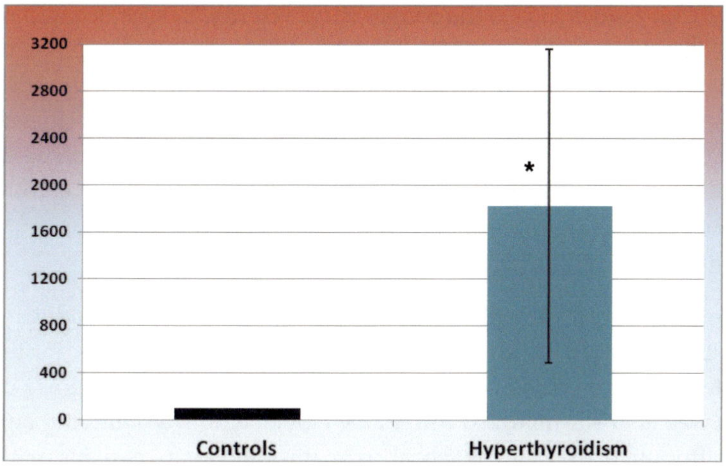

Figure 5. Percentage of human CD34⁺-enriched hematopoietic stem/progenitor cells in the late apoptotic stage collected from hyperthyroid patients. Apoptosis in hematopoietic progenitor cells collected from patients with hyperthyroidism and healthy subjects (Controls) was scored by cytometric detection of annexin-V and propidium iodate. Results are expressed as mean percentage (± SD) in relation to control values considered as 100%. *P<0.05 vs. controls. [21]

We found that both examined anti-apoptotic genes, *BCL-2* and *BCL-xL*, were significantly down-regulated compared to healthy volunteers (40% and 67% vs. 100% respectively; P<0.05). In the same manner the expression of *BAX* gene of pro-apoptotic activity was analyzed. Interestingly, this gene was also significantly down-regulated compared to control subjects (36% vs. 100% respectively; P<0.05). The above data strongly correlate with the previously observed tendency to decrease the clonogenic potential of $CD34^+$hematopoietic stem/progenitor cells of myeloid lineage of hyperthyroid subjects and may indicate that THs at higher concentrations negatively modulate the expression of genes important for hematopoietic cell survival, such as anti-apoptotic *BCL-2* and *BCL-xL* genes. On the other side, the parallel decrease of expression level of pro-apoptotic *BAX* gene might be related with significant augmentation of late, executive phase of apoptosis in circulating $CD34^+$cells due to the chronic exposure to elevated concentrations of T3 found in hyperthyroid patients (Fig. 5). Indeed, *BAX* is expressed at high levels during the period when programmed cell death is activated by intracellular or extracellular stimuli, and down-regulation of the gene expression occurs thereafter, when signal transduction pathways triggered the performance of apoptotic protein cascade inside the cell [21].

2.2.3. Thrombocytopoiesis

Thrombocytopoiesis is the process of thrombocyte generation from the cytoplasm of megakaryocytes located in bone marrow hematopoietic niche. Megakaryocyte maturation comes to completion with the release of thrombocytes, known as platelets, into the bloodstream and each day an adult produces about 100 billion platelets. They are necessary for normal blood clotting. Megakaryocytes normally account for 1 out of 10.000 bone marrow cells but their number can increase or decrease in the course of certain diseases, thus resulting in abnormal megakaryocyte function and abnormal platelet quantity or function, and this influences hemostatic system in peripheral blood [85]. In the specialized microenvironment of the bone marrow the megakaryocyte development and subsequent platelets production is regulated through a complex crosstalk between many cell types and cytokines. Especially, thrombopoietin was identified as the major regulator of platelet production, however, other biologically active substances, such as hormones, may play an important role in the regulation of megakaryocyte growth and proliferation [86].

Exactly, one century ago appeared the first report of Kaliebe et al. indicating the clinical relationship between thyroid disease and the dysfunction in hemostatic system. In 1913 the authors have described an episode of central vein thrombosis in a thyrotoxic patient and this medical report was later summarized in 1927 by Doyle, who was studying a possible association between thyrotoxicosis and cerebral vein thrombosis in patients with neurological symptoms [87]. Likewise, various diseases of hemostatic system, ranging from hemostasis disorders, and rarely life-threatening hemorrhages to hypercoagulability and thrombotic events, could be observed in parallel to thyroid gland dysfunctions. However, some contradictory results regarding hemostatic system functions have been obtained in clinical studies of patients with thyroid disorders.

Several published reports have shown a hypercoagulable state in patients with hyperthyroidism [19, 88]. For certain, patients with hyperthyroidism showed a tendency toward thromboembolic process (8–40%), including major emboli at cerebral vasculature, which accounts for nearly 18% of all deaths associated with thyrotoxicosis [89]. Another systematic analysis also supports an increased risk of venous thrombotic complications, including cerebral venous thrombosis, deep vein thrombosis and pulmonary embolism in patients with hyperthyroidism [90]. Hypercoagulability state that is observed in hyperthyroidism is produced by various coagulation factor (e.g. clotting factors and their inhibitors) abnormalities that occur in patients with hyperthyroidism and are not directly related to thrombocytes and thrombocytopoiesis. Researchers hypothesized that THs may affect the synthesis of many proteins originating from the liver and endothelium by altering the specific gene expression. Indeed, collected data have specified that hyperthyroidism, regardless of its etiology, influences endothelial function by up-regulating the expression levels of vascular adhesion molecules and endothelium-derived proteins important for fibrinolysis, such as tissue-type plasminogen activator and plasminogen activator inhibitor-1 [91]. On the other hand, it is known that there is a general increase of metabolism in hyperthyroid state, which may affect cell components of the peripheral blood and bone marrow. Likewise, it was found that the life-span of platelets is shortened in patients with hyperthyroidism resulting in thrombocytopenia [92]. Moreover, the same group observed that the platelet count increased upon reduction of the concentration of circulating thyroid hormones [92]. Similar data were obtained by Kurata et al., who showed that the platelets count are low and their lifespan shorter in almost one-half of 214 studied patients with Graves' disease [93]. Notwithstanding, thrombocytopenia in patients with hyperthyroidism may have several causes, such as autoimmunity against thromobocytes [94-95] in parallel to nonspecific thyroid antibodies binding to platelets that augment their non-specific degradation or due to thrombocyte clearance from plasma by the enhanced phagocytic activity of the reticuloendothelial system [96]. Finally, detected relative low platelet quantities could be due to increased circulating blood volume observed in patients with hyperthyroidism, as in case of other hematologic parameters of blood. Of note, patients with hyperthyroidism had significantly higher risks of having co-morbidities such as hypertension, hyperlipidemia, and diabetes that might affect the survival of platelets and their bone marrow progenitors. Although the pathomechanism is still not well known, altered glucose and lipid metabolism has been often reported in patients with hyperthyroidism [97]. Altogether, the above-mentioned studies have indicated that hyperthyroidism is associated with either increased blood coagulability and endothelial cell dysfunction based on examining the incidence of venous thrombosis, or with thrombocytopenia and decreased life-span of platelets, however, only few scientists attempted to explore the bone marrow-related mechanisms of abnormal functions of hemostatic system among patients with hyperthyroidism. Even the recent development of efficient megakaryocyte cultures in vitro that produce functional platelets has provided the means to study the biology of megakaryopoesis in abnormal pathophysiological conditions, such as hyperthyroid state, the number of reports covering this field is very scanty. In one attempt, to check whether non-physiological THs concentration may directly affect platelet production, it was necessary to determine the quantity of reticulated platelets (RP) circulating in peripheral blood. RP represent young cells recently released from the bone marrow, and according to some reports, their number in peripheral blood reflects thrombopoietic activity [98]. Indeed, Stiegler et al. confirmed that hyperthyroidism was associated with an increased marrow thrombocytopoiesis resulting in elevated RP counts. Moreover this finding was corroborated by observation that RP increase in course of hyperthyroidism was reversible upon achievement of euthyroid state [99]. Furthermore, to confirm the clinical reports indicating that excessive THs exert depressive effects on platelets production, Sullivan et al. used a mouse model to investigate the effects of the hyperthyroid state on thrombocytopoiesis in vivo by administration of T4 into normal healthy mice. They observed that daily thyroxine administration significantly decreased total circulating platelet count and platelet mass due to decreased platelet production. This mechanism was confirmed using the most sensitive methods of assessing platelet production, i.e. percentage of S-35 incorporation into platelets and determination of megakaryocyte size and number [39]. Likewise, Sullivan and coworkers observed that percentage of S-35 incorporation into platelets was reduced and megakaryocyte size and number in bone marrow were considerably decreased [39]. These are only a few available evidences that hyperthyroidism plays a direct role in the fine regulation of thrombocytopoiesis in vivo.

3. Conclusion

In recent years there have been published several studies indicating that the thyroid dysfunction could have important implications in human hematopoiesis, and thus might affect various hematological parameters of circulating blood. This chapter demonstrates that hyperthyroid state might be responsible for profound disturbances in functions of the hematopoietic system due to the fact that THs modulate hematopoietic cell production in the bone marrow. The hyperthyroidism-related symptoms in peripheral blood comprise increased plasma volume, anemia (10-25%), leukopenia (10%), neutropenia, lymphopenia, thrombocytopenia, decreased MCV, and reduced RBC survival, as well as general pancytopenia. Of note, erythrocytosis, lymphocytosis and increased counts of monocytes are also fairly common. Potential molecular mechanisms of reported hematologic symptoms has been explained in part in this paper. Importantly, increased thyroid hormone concentrations influence the mechanisms of the development of hematological abnormalities through both genomic and non-genomic actions. As a result, in patients with different thyroid endocrinopathies, overt hyperthyroidism should be also considered as a possible cause of clinically detectable abnormalities in peripheral blood of these patients. Novel pathophysiological insights into the mechanisms of thyroid hormone actions in the hematopoietic system may help to improve the understanding of the interactions between THs and human hematopoiesis and offer a potential for the future development of novel therapeutic interventions in thyroid diseases.

Author details

Miłosz P. Kawa* and Bogusław Machaliński

*Address all correspondence to: kawamilosz@gmail.com

Department of General Pathology, Pomeranian Medical University in Szczecin, Szczecin, Poland

References

[1] Yen PM. Physiological and molecular basis of thyroid hormone action. Physiol Rev. 2001;81(3):1097-142

[2] Murata Y. Multiple isoforms of thyroid hormone receptor: an analysis of their relative contribution in mediating thyroid hormone action. Nagoya J Med Sci. 1998;61(3-4):103-15.

[3] Horwitz KB, Jackson TA, Bain DL, Richer JK, Takimoto GS, Tung L. Nuclear receptor coactivators and corepressors. Mol Endocrinol. 1996;10(10):1167-77.

[4] Lazar MA. Thyroid hormone receptors: Multiple forms, multiple posibilities. Endocr. Rev. 1993;14:184-193.

[5] Wu Y, Koenig RJ. Gene regulation by thyroid hormone. Trends Endocrinol Metab. 2000;11(6):207-11.

[6] Koenig RJ, Lazar MA, Hodin RA, Brent GA, Larsen PR, Chin WW, Moore DD. Inhibition of thyroid hormone action by a non-hormone binding c-erbA protein generated by alternative mRNA splicing. Nature. 1989;337(6208):659-61.

[7] Davis PJ, Leonard JL, Davis FB. Mechanisms of nongenomic actions of thyroid hormone. Front Neuroendocrinol. 2008;29(2):211-8.

[8] Cheng SY, Leonard JL, Davis PJ. Molecular aspects of thyroid hormone actions. Endocr Rev 2010;31:139-170.

[9] Pascual A, Aranda A. Thyroid hormone receptors, cell growth and differentiation. Biochim Biophys Acta. 2013;1830:3908-16.

[10] Allain TJ, McGregor AM. Thyroid hormones and bone. J Endocrinol. 1993;139(1): 9-18.

[11] Varga F, Rumpler M, Zoehrer R, Turecek C, Spitzer S, Thaler R, Paschalis EP, Klaushofer K. T3 affects expression of collagen I and collagen cross-linking in bone cell cultures. Biochem Biophys Res Commun. 2010;402(2):180-5.

[12] Gorka J, Taylor-Gjevre RM, Arnason T. Metabolic and clinical consequences of hyperthyroidism on bone density. Int J Endocrinol. 2013;2013:638727

[13] Fein HG, Rivlin RS. Anemia in thyroid diseases. Med Clin North Am. 1975;59(5): 1133-45.

[14] Corrocher R, Querena M, Stanzial AM, De Sandre G Microcytosis in hyperthyroidism: haematological profile in thyroid disorders. Haematologica. 1981;66:779–786.

[15] Perlman JA, Sternthal PM. Effect of 131I on the anemia of hyperthyroidism. J Chronic Dis. 1983;36(5):405-12.

[16] Axelrod AR, Bergman L. The bone marrow in hyperthyroidism and hypothyroidism. Blood 1951, 6, 436–453.

[17] Omazic B, Näsman-Björk I, Johansson J, Hentschke P, Mattsson J, Permert J, Lundkvist I. Altered expression of receptors for thyroid hormone and insulin-like growth factor-I during reconstitution after allogeneic hematopoietic stem cell transplantation. Bone Marrow Transplant. 2001;27(11):1163-71.

[18] Squizzato A, Gerdes VE, Brandjes DP, Büller HR, Stam J. Thyroid diseases and cerebrovascular disease. Stroke. 2005;36(10):2302-10.

[19] Squizzato A, Romualdi E, Büller HR, Gerdes VE.J Clinical review: Thyroid dysfunction and effects on coagulation and fibrinolysis: a systematic review. Clin Endocrinol Metab. 2007;92(7):2415-20.

[20] Grymuła K, Paczkowska E, Dziedziejko V, Baśkiewicz-Masiuk M, Kawa M, Baumert B, Celewicz Z, Gawrych E, Machaliński B. The influence of 3,3',5-triiodo-L-thyronine on human haematopoiesis. Cell Prolif. 2007;40(3):302-15.

[21] Kawa MP, Grymula K, Paczkowska E, Baskiewicz-Masiuk M, Dabkowska E, Koziolek M, Tarnowski M, Kłos P, Dziedziejko V, Kucia M, Syrenicz A, Machalinski B. Clinical relevance of thyroid dysfunction in human haematopoiesis: biochemical and molecular studies. Eur J Endocrinol. 2010;162(2):295-305.

[22] Gruber R, Czerwenka K, Wolf F, Ho GM, Willheim M, Peterlik M Expresion of the vitamin D receptor, of estrogen and thyroid hormone receptor alfa-and beta-isoforms, and of the androgen receptor in cultures of native mouse bone marrow and stromal/osteoblastic cells. Bone. 1999;24:465–473.

[23] Milne M, Kang MI, Cardona G, Quail JM, Braverman LE, Chin WW, Baran DT Expression of multiple thyroid hormone receptor isoforms in rat femoral and vertebral bone marrow and in bone marrow osteogenic cultures. J. Cell. Biochem. 1999;74:684–693.

[24] Davis PJ, Davis FB, Lin HY. Promotion by thyroid hormone of cytoplasm-to-nucleus shuttling of thyroid hormone receptors. Steroids. 2008;73(9-10):1013-7.

[25] Meier-Heusler S, Pernin A, Liang H, Goumaz MO, Burger AG, Meier CA. Quantitation of beta 1 triiodothyronine receptor mRNA in human tissues by competitive reverse transcription polymerase chain reaction. J Endocrinol Invest. 1995;18(10):767-73

[26] Rao JN, Liang JY, Chakraborti P, Feng P. Effect of thyroid hormone on the development and gene expression of hormone receptors in rat testes in vivo. J Endocrinol Invest. 2003;26(5):435-43.

[27] Bauer A, Gandrillon O, Samarut J, Beug H. Nuclear receptors in hematopoietic development: cooperation with growth factor receptors in regulation of proliferation and differentiation. In: Zon L, ed. Hematopoiesis: A Developmental Approach. Oxford, UK: Oxford University Press; 2001; 268-290.

[28] Shalet M, Coe D, Reissmann KR. Mechanism of erythropoietic action of thyroid hormone. Proc Soc Exp Biol Med. 1966;123(2):443-6.

[29] Ford HC, Carter JM. The haematology of hyperthyroidism: abnormalities of erythrocytes, leucocytes, thrombocytes and haemostasis. Postgrad Med J. 1988;64(756): 735-42.

[30] Dainiak N, Sutter D, Kreczko S 1-triiodothyronine augments erythropoietic growth factor release from peripheral blood and bone marrow leukocytes. Blood. 1986;68:1289–1297.

[31] Fandrey J, Pagel H, Frede S, Wolff M, Jelkmann W. Thyroid hormones enhance hypoxia-induced erythropoietin production in vitro. Exp Hematol. 1994;22(3):272-7.

[32] González-Cinca N, Pérez de la Ossa P, Carreras J, Climent F. Effects of thyroid hormone and hypoxia on 2,3-bisphosphoglycerate, bisphosphoglycerate synthase and phosphoglycerate mutase in rabbit erythroblasts and reticulocytes in vivo. Horm Res. 2004;62(4):191-6.

[33] Tokay A, Raymondjean M, Aliciguzel Y. The effect of thyroid hormones on erythrocyte 2,3-diphosphoglycerate. The Endocrinologist 2006;16:57–60.

[34] Brenner B, Fandrey J, Jelkmann W. Serum immunoreactive erythropoietin in hyper- and hypothyroidism: clinical observations related to cell culture studies. Eur J Haematol. 1994;53(1):6-10.

[35] Golde DW, Bersch N, Chopra IJ, Cline MJ. Thyroid hormones stimulate erythropoiesis in vitro. Br. J. Haematol. 1977;37:173–177.

[36] Schroeder C, Gibson L, Zenke M, Beug H. Modulation of normal erythroid differentiation by the endogenous thyroid hormone and retinoic acid receptors: a possible target for v-erbA oncogene action. Oncogene 1992;7:217–227.

[37] Malgor LA, Valsecia ME, Verges EG, de Markowsky EE. Enhancement of erythroid colony growth by triiodothyronine in cell cultures from bone marrow of normal and anemic rats with chronic renal failure. Acta Physiol Pharmacol Ther Latinoam. 1995;45(2):79-86.

[38] Perrin MC, Blanchet JP, Mouchiroud G. Modulation of human and mouse erythropoiesis by thyroid hormone and retinoic acid: evidence for specific effects at different steps of the erythroid pathway. Hematol. Cell Ther. 1997;39:19–26.

[39] Sullivan PS, McDonald TP. Thyroxine suppresses thrombocytopoiesis and stimulates erythropoiesis in mice. Proc Soc Exp Biol Med. 1992;201(3):271-7.

[40] Bauer A, Mikulits W, Lagger G, Stengl G, Brosch G, Beug H. The thyroid hormone receptor functions as a ligand-operated developmental switch between proliferation and differentiation of erythroid progenitors. EMBO J. 1998;17(15):4291-303.

[41] Kendrick TS, Payne CJ, Epis MR, Schneider JR, Leedman PJ, Klinken SP, Ingley E. Erythroid defects in TRalpha-/-mice. Blood. 2008;111(6):3245-8.

[42] Leberbauer C, Boulmé F, Unfried G, Huber J, Beug H, Müllner EW. Different steroids co-regulate long-term expansion versus terminal differentiation in primary human erythroid progenitors. Blood. 2005;105(1):85-94.

[43] Gianoukakis AG, Leigh MJ, Richards P, Christenson PD, Hakimian A, Fu P, Niihara Y, Smith TJ. Characterization of the anaemia associated with Graves' disease. Clin Endocrinol (Oxf). 2009;70(5):781-7.

[44] Nightingale S, Vitek PJ, Himsworth RL. The haematology of hyperthyroidism. Q J Med. 1978;47(185):35-47.

[45] Muldowney FP, Crooks J, Wayne EJ. The total red cell mass in thyrotoxicosis and myxoedema. Clin Sci (Lond). 1957;16(2):309-14.

[46] Boelaert K, Newby PR, Simmonds MJ, Holder RL, Carr-Smith JD, Heward JM, Manji N, Allahabadia A, Armitage M, Chatterjee KV, Lazarus JH, Pearce SH, Vaidya B,

Gough SC, Franklyn JA. Prevalence and relative risk of other autoimmune diseases in subjects with autoimmune thyroid disease. Am J Med. 2010;123(2):183.e1-9.

[47] McClellan JE, Donegan C., Thorup OA, Leavell BS. Survival time of the erythrocyte in myxedema and hyperthyroidism. J Lab Clin Med. 1958;51(1):91-6.

[48] Donati RM, Warnecke MA, Gallagher NI. Ferrokinetics in hyperthyroidism. Ann Intern Med. 1965;63(6):945-50.

[49] Duquenne M, Lakomsky D, Humbert JC, Hadjadj S, Weryha G, Leclère J. Pancytopenia resolved by the treatment of hyperthyroidism. Presse Med. 1995;24(17):807-10.

[50] Shaw B, Mehta AB. Pancytopenia responding to treatment of hyperthyroidism: a clinical case and review of the literature. Clin Lab Haematol. 2002;24(6):385-7.

[51] Lima CS, Zantut Wittmann DE, Castro V, Tambascia MA, Lorand-Metze I, Saad ST, Costa FF. Pancytopenia in untreated patients with Graves' disease. Thyroid. 2006;16(4):403-9.

[52] Haddad JJ, Saadé NE, Safieh-Garabedian B. Cytokines and neuro-immune-endocrine interactions: a role for the hypothalamic-pituitary-adrenal revolving axis. J Neuroimmunol. 2002;133(1-2):1-19.

[53] Pállinger E, Csaba G.; A hormone map of human immune cells showing the presence of adrenocorticotropic hormone, triiodothyronine and endorphin in immunophenotyped white blood cells. Immunology. 2008;123(4):584-9.

[54] Csaba G, Pállinger E. Thyrotropic hormone (TSH) regulation of triiodothyronine (T(3)) concentration in immune cells. Inflamm Res. 2009;58(3):151-4.

[55] Balázs C, Leövey A, Szabó M, Bakó G. Stimulating effect of triiodothyronine on cell-mediated immunity. Eur J Clin Pharmacol. 1980;17(1):19-23.

[56] Ong ML, Malkin DG, Malkin A. Alteration of lymphocyte reactivities by thyroid hormones. Int J Immunopharmacol. 1986;8(7):755-62.

[57] Barreiro Arcos ML, Sterle HA, Paulazo MA, Valli E, Klecha AJ, Isse B, Pellizas CG, Farias RN, Cremaschi GA. Cooperative nongenomic and genomic actions on thyroid hormone mediated-modulation of T cell proliferation involve up-regulation of thyroid hormone receptor and inducible nitric oxide synthase expression. J Cell Physiol. 2011;226(12):3208-18.

[58] Hodkinson CF, Simpson EE, Beattie JH, O'Connor JM, Campbell DJ, Strain JJ, Wallace JM. Preliminary evidence of immune function modulation by thyroid hormones in healthy men and women aged 55-70 years. J Endocrinol. 2009;202(1):55-63.

[59] Dorshkind K, Horseman ND. The roles of prolactin, growth hormone, insulin-like growth factor-I, and thyroid hormones in lymphocyte development and function: insights from genetic models of hormone and hormone receptor deficiency. Endocr Rev. 2000;21(3):292-312.

[60] Bloehr H, Bregengaard C, Povlsen JV. Triiodothyronine stimulates growth of peripheral blood mononuclear cells in serum-free cultures in uremic patients. Am J Nephrol. 1992;12(3):148-54.

[61] El-Shaikh KA, Gabry MS, Othman GA. Recovery of age-dependent immunological deterioration in old mice by thyroxine treatment. J Anim Physiol Anim Nutr (Berl). 2006;90(5-6):244-54.

[62] De Vito P, Incerpi S, Pedersen JZ, Luly P, Davis FB, Davis PJ. Thyroid hormones as modulators of immune activities at the cellular level. Thyroid. 2011;21(8):879-90.

[63] Pacini F, Nakamura H, DeGroot LJ. Effect of hypo-and hyperthyroidism on the balance between helper and suppressor T cells in rats. Acta Endocrinol (Copenh). 1983;103(4):528-34.

[64] Christ-Crain M, Meier C, Huber P, Zulewski H, Staub JJ, Müller B. Effect of restoration of euthyroidism on peripheral blood cells and erythropoietin in women with subclinical hypothyroidism. Hormones (Athens). 2003;2(4):237-42.

[65] Porter L, Mandel SJ. The Blood in Thyrotoxicosis. In: Brawerman LE, Utiger RD, eds. Werner & Ingbar's The Thyroid, Philadelphia: Lippincott Williams, Wilkins; 2000; 627-630.

[66] Garcia-Suarez J, Prieto A, Reyes E, Arribalzaga K, Perez-Machado MA, Lopez-Rubio M, Manzano L, Alvarez-Mon M. Persistent lymphocytosis of natural killer cells in autoimmune thrombocytopenic purpura (ATP) patients after splenectomy. Br J Haematol. 1995;89(3):653-5.

[67] Grossi A, Nozzoli C, Gheri R, Santini V, Marrani C, Zoccolante A, Ferrini PR. Pure red cell aplasia in autoimmune polyglandular syndrome with T lymphocytosis. Haematologica. 1998;83(11):1043-5.

[68] Notario A, Torriani A, Bravi M, Broglia M, Borghi G, Guerra G. The influence of thyroid hormones on colony growth of peripheral CFU-GM from normal and leukemic subjects. Tumori. 1988;74(5):507-12.

[69] Notario A, Mazzucchelli I, Fossati L, Baldi A, Rolandi ML. Qalqili A. International Journal of Immunopathology and Pharmacology 1997;10:133-138.

[70] Ponassi A, Morra L, Caristo G, Parodi GB, Biassoni P, Sacchetti C. Disorders of granulopoiesis in patients with untreated Graves' disease. Acta Haematol. 1983;70(1): 19-23.

[71] Kucharova S, Farkas R. Hormone nuclear receptors and their ligands: role in programmed cell death (review). Endocr Regul. 2002;36(1):37-60.

[72] Alisi A, Demori I, Spagnuolo S, Pierantozzi E, Fugassa E, Leoni S. Thyroid status affects rat liver regeneration after partial hepatectomy by regulating cell cycle and apoptosis. Cell Physiol Biochem. 2005;15(1-4):69-76.

[73] Yehuda-Shnaidman E, Kalderon B, Bar-Tana J. Modulation of mitochondrial transition pore components by thyroid hormone. Endocrinology. 2005;146(5):2462-72.

[74] Chiloeches A, Sánchez-Pacheco A, Gil-Araujo B, Aranda A, Lasa M. Thyroid hormone-mediated activation of the ERK/dual specificity phosphatase 1 pathway augments the apoptosis of GH4C1 cells by down-regulating nuclear factor-kappaB activity. Mol Endocrinol. 2008;22(11):2466-80.

[75] Wang YY, Jiao B, Guo WG, Che HL, Yu ZB. Excessive thyroxine enhances susceptibility to apoptosis and decreases contractility of cardiomyocytes. Mol Cell Endocrinol. 2010;320(1-2):67-75.

[76] Sar P, Peter R, Rath B, Das Mohapatra A, Mishra SK. 3, 3'5 Triiodo L thyronine induces apoptosis in human breast cancer MCF-7 cells, repressing SMP30 expression through negative thyroid response elements. PLoS One. 2011;6(6):e20861.

[77] Yamada-Okabe T, Satoh Y, Yamada-Okabe H. Thyroid hormone induces the expression of 4-1BB and activation of caspases in a thyroid hormone receptor-dependent manner. Eur J Biochem. 2003;270(14):3064-73

[78] Zhang L, Cooper-Kuhn CM, Nannmark U, Blomgren K, Kuhn HG. Stimulatory effects of thyroid hormone on brain angiogenesis in vivo and in vitro. J Cereb Blood Flow Metab. 2010;30(2):323-35.

[79] Lin HY, Tang HY, Keating T, Wu YH, Shih A, Hammond D, Sun M, Hercbergs A, Davis FB, Davis PJ. Resveratrol is pro-apoptotic and thyroid hormone is anti-apoptotic in glioma cells: both actions are integrin and ERK mediated. Carcinogenesis. 2008;29(1):62-9.

[80] Barreiro Arcos ML, Gorelik G, Klecha A, Genaro AM, Cremaschi GA. Thyroid hormones increase inducible nitric oxide synthase gene expression downstream from PKC-zeta in murine tumor T lymphocytes. Am J Physiol Cell Physiol. 2006;291(2):C327-36.

[81] Medh RD, Thompson EB. Hormonal regulation of physiological cell turnover and apoptosis. Cell Tissue Res. 2000;301(1):101-24.

[82] Mihara S, Suzuki N, Wakisaka S, Suzuki S, Sekita N, Yamamoto S, Saito N, Hoshino T, Sakane T. Effects of thyroid hormones on apoptotic cell death of human lymphocytes. J Clin Endocrinol Metab. 1999;84(4):1378-85.

[83] Gandrillon O, Ferrand N, Michaille JJ, Roze L, Zile MH, Samarut J. C-erbA alpha/T3R and RARs control commitment of hematopoietic self-renewing progenitor cells to apoptosis or differentiation and are antagonized by the v-erbA oncogene. Oncogene 1994;9,749–758

[84] Hara M, Suzuki S, Mori J, Yamashita K, Kumagai M, Sakuma T, Kakizawa T, Takeda T, Miyamoto T, Ichikawa K, Hashizume K. Thyroid hormone regulation of apoptosis induced by retinoic acid in promyeloluekemic HL-60 cells: studies with retinoic acid

receptor–specific and retinoid X receptor–specific ligands. Thyroid 2000;10,1023–1034.

[85] Branehög I, Ridell B, Swolin B, Weinfeld A. Megakaryocyte quantifications in relation to thrombokinetics in primary thrombocythaemia and allied diseases. Scand J Haematol. 1975;15(5):321-32.

[86] Kaushansky K. Historical review: megakaryopoiesis and thrombopoiesis. Blood. 2008;111(3):981-6.

[87] Doyle JB. Obstruction of the longitudinal sinus. Arch Neurol Psychiatry. 1927;29,374–382.

[88] Marongiu F, Cauli C, Mariotti S. Thyroid, hemostasis and thrombosis. J Endocrinol Invest. 2004;27(11):1065-71.

[89] Hofbauer LC, Heufelder AE. Coagulation disorders in thyroid diseases. Eur J Endocrinol. 1997;136(1):1-7.

[90] Franchini M, Lippi G, Targher G. Hyperthyroidism and venous thrombosis: a casual or causal association? A systematic literature review. Clin Appl Thromb Hemost. 2011;17(4):387-92.

[91] Burggraaf J, Lalezari S, Emeis JJ, Vischer UM, de Meyer PH, Pijl H, Cohen AF. Endothelial function in patients with hyperthyroidism before and after treatment with propranolol and thiamazol. Thyroid. 2001;11(2):153-60.

[92] Panzer S, Haubenstock A, Minar E. Platelets in hyperthyroidism: studies on platelet counts, mean platelet volume, 111-indium-labeled platelet kinetics, and platelet-associated immunoglobulins G and M. J Clin Endocrinol Metab. 1990;70(2):491-6.

[93] Kurata Y, Nishioeda Y, Tsubakio T, Kitani T. Thrombocytopenia in Graves' disease: effect of T3 on platelet kinetics. Acta Haematol. 1980;63(4):185-90.

[94] Bizzaro N. Familial association of autoimmune thrombocytopenia and hyperthyroidism. Am J Hematol. 1992;39(4):294-8

[95] Cordiano I, Betterle C, Spadaccino CA, Soini B, Girolami A, Fabris F. Autoimmune thrombocytopenia (AITP) and thyroid autoimmune disease (TAD): overlapping syndromes? Clin Exp Immunol. 1998;113(3):373-8.

[96] Adrouny A, Sandler RM, Carmel R. Variable presentation of thrombocytopenia in Graves' disease. Arch Intern Med. 1982;142(8):1460-4.

[97] Dimitriadis G, Mitrou P, Lambadiari V, Boutati E, Maratou E, Koukkou E, Tzanela M, Thalassinos N, Raptis SA. J Clin Endocrinol Metab. Glucose and lipid fluxes in the adipose tissue after meal ingestion in hyperthyroidism. 2006;91(3):1112-8.

[98] Ault KA, Knowles C. In vivo biotinylation demonstrates that reticulated platelets are the youngest platelets in circulation. Exp Hematol. 1995;23(9):996-1001.

[99] Stiegler G, Stohlawetz P, Brugger S, Jilma B, Vierhapper H, Höcker P, Panzer S. Elevated numbers of reticulated platelets in hyperthyroidism: direct evidence for an increase of thrombopoiesis. Br J Haematol. 1998 Jun;101(4):656-8.

Chapter 8

Surgical Management of Hyperthyroidism

Z. Al Hilli, C. Cheung, E.W. McDermott and
R.S. Prichard

Additional information is available at the end of the chapter

http://dx.doi.org/10.5772/57499

1. Introduction

Hyperthyroidism is a syndrome characterised by the signs and symptoms of hyper-metabolism and excess sympathetic nervous system activity. It has an overall prevalence of 27 per 1000 women and 2.3 per 1000 men within the United Kingdom [1]. Hyperthyroidism occurs as a result of either the excess synthesis or secretion of thyroid hormones by the thyroid gland itself. It must be distinguished from thyrotoxicosis, in which excess thyroid hormone may come from other sources, such as excess thyroid hormone ingestion, struma ovarii and functional metastatic thyroid carcinoma[2,3].

Patients present with a variety of symptoms and clinical findings on physical examination. It is important for clinicians to remember that these may be more subtle in the elderly population who may present with fatigue or weakness, a condition known as apathetic hyperthyroidism, or with predominantly cardiovascular signs such as atrial fibrillation, ischaemic heart disease and congestive cardiac failure [4,5]. The routine use of serum thyrotropin (TSH) as a screening investigation may allow earlier identification and treatment of the disease [6,7]. Radiological imaging with iodine-123 uptake scanning and thyroid scintigraphy may aid in the identification of the underlying cause [6].

The management of hyperthyroidism is based on three treatment modalities, namely anti-thyroid medication, radioactive iodine ablation or surgery. Patient, physician and geographically preferences may dictate the choice of therapy. Given the overall healthcare costs of hyperthyroidism, surgical intervention performed with minimal morbidity in high volume centres may offer the highest chance of success with the lowest chance of recurrence [8].

The aim of this chapter is to discuss the role of surgical intervention in hyperthyroidism. Firstly, to examine the evidence supporting surgical intervention in the management of Graves' disease and that of toxic nodular goitres including toxic multi-nodular goitre and solitary toxic nodule. Secondly, and perhaps more controversially, the evidence for the extent of surgical intervention in hyperthyroidism will be discussed focusing specifically on the evidence for total compared with subtotal thyroidectomy.

2. Surgical anatomy

The thyroid gland is derived from the median thyroid diverticulum at the floor of the pharynx. The thyroglossal duct extends from the foramen caecum at the base of the tongue to the isthmus and is derived from the stalk of the diverticulum, which is later obliterated, with the distal portion forming the pyramidal lobe of the thyroid. The ultimobranchial bodies that arise from the fourth pharyngeal pouch become related to the lateral aspect of the gland and constitute the para-follicular and C cells, which produce calcitonin [9,10,11].

The thyroid gland consists of two lobes connected by an isthmus that is situated antero-lateral to the trachea and cricothyroid muscle. The gland itself has a bi-lobed shape and weighs 15 – 25g often depending on age and sex. Superiorly, the pyramidal extension (lobe) of the gland may be found on the anterior surface of the cricothyroid. Laterally, the tubercles of Zucker-kandl, which arise from median anlage and ultimobranchial fusion, may form significant protrusions of thyroid tissue within the tracheo-esophageal groove. Inferior to the thyroid lie the thyrothymic rests. These occur in up to 50% of individuals and are classified according to their connection to the thyroid [12).

The blood supply to the thyroid is derived from two main arteries; the superior thyroid artery, which is a branch of the external carotid artery, and the inferior thyroid artery, which is a branch of the thyrocervical trunk that itself is a branch of the subclavian artery. The main venous drainage is through the middle thyroid vein directly into the internal jugular vein. Other venous drainage includes the paired superior thyroid veins and a plexus of veins draining the inferior poles of the gland. The lymphatic drainage is to local lymph nodes situated in the central neck compartment and subsequently to cervical nodes [10,11].

The recurrent laryngeal nerve (RLN) and the external branch of the superior laryngeal nerve (EBSLN) are closely related to the thyroid gland and can be vulnerable to damage during thyroid surgery. An intimate knowledge of their anatomy in the neck is crucial to safe thyroid surgery. The recurrent laryngeal nerve (RLN) originates from the vagus (X Cranial nerve) nerve. The right RLN branches from the vagus as it crosses the subclavian artery and loops around it, while the left nerve arises at the level of the arch of aorta and loops under it. Both nerves lie and ascend in the tracheo-oesophageal groove, where they pass deep to the postero-medial surface of the thyroid lobes [10,11]. The angle of the nerve relative to the trachea is usually more oblique on the right. The nerve subsequently enters the larynx by passing behind the inferior constrictors, supplying all the intrinsic muscles of the larynx except the cricothy-roid and sensation to the mucosa below the vocal cords [10,11]. The right RLN may have a non-recurring course (0.3%) and derive directly from the vagus, approaching the cricothyroid directly without travelling in the tracheo-esophageal groove. This occurs as a consequence of a displaced right subclavian arterial takeoff from the aortic arch and may be identified preoperatively if cross-sectional imaging is performed. Both left and right RLNs may give multiple branches to the oesophagus and trachea. The RLN may bifurcate prior to insertion into the cricothyroid, with the majority of the motor fibres being carried in the anterior portion of the nerve [9,10,11].

The superior laryngeal nerve (SLN) also emanates from the vagus and travels deep and medial to the carotid arteries where it then divides into an internal and external branch above the superior horn of hyoid [all books Grays]. The internal branch travels in relation to the superior laryngeal vessels and supplies the mucosa to the level of the vocal cords. The external branch supplies the cricothyroid muscle and lies deep to superior thyroid artery [10], where it can be particularly vulnerable to damage. In an attempt to minimise trauma to the EBSLN numerous classifications have been proposed, the most widely adopted being that devised by Cernea et al [13,14]. Type 1 EBSLN is where the EBSLN crosses the superior thyroid artery (STA) greater than 1cm above the upper pole of the thyroid. It is the commonest (40 – 62%) type and suggests that the nerve may not be significantly at risk. In type 2a and b, the EBSLN crosses the artery less than 1 cm above the upper pole and may therefore be at risk during dissection [13,14]. Kierner et al proposed that these be further divided into type 3 EBSLN where the nerve crosses the STA under the cover of the thyroid gland and type 4 is where the EBSLN had descended dorsal to the artery and only crosses the branches of the STA immediately above the upper pole of the thyroid [14].

The paired inferior and superior parathyroid glands are derived from the third and fourth pharyngeal pouches respectively and are closely related to the thyroid in position. The majority of individuals (85%) will have four glands while approximately 13% will have five glands and an even smaller proportion will have greater than this. The superior gland is found in over 90% of cases within 1cm of the junction of the inferior thyroid artery and the recurrent laryngeal nerve on the posterior aspect of the middle third of the thyroid gland. The inferior parathyroid glands, in conjunction with the thymus, have a longer migration path and their location is therefore more variable. The majority will be found on the anterior or postero-lateral aspect of the thyroid lobe or within the thyrothymic tract and are typically symmetrical in location [9,10,11].

3. Hyperthyroidism

Hyperthyroidism, a disorder of the thyroid gland, arises as a result of either excess hormone synthesis or secretion [2,3]. It has a population prevalence of 2% for women and 0.2% for men [1]. It is common with the incidence of new cases in the UK per year among women being reported at 3 per 1000 [6]. The mean age of diagnosis is 48 years with an increasing incidence with age [6,15]. Grave's disease, being the most common cause of hyperthyroidism, accounts for 60-80% of all cases [16]. Other causes include hyperthyroidism resulting from a toxic nodular goitre (single or multiple nodule) and these constitute the remaining 5-15% of all causes. [16].

Hyperthyroidism must be distinguished from thyrotoxicosis, which is defined as the excess of circulating thyroid hormones in the bloodstream [17]. Causes for thyrotoxicosis vary and include excess thyroid hormone ingestion, struma ovarii and functional metastatic thyroid carcinoma [18]. These will not be discussed further in this chapter

4. Clinical features

Hyperthyroidism has a multi-system effect on the body, giving rise to a range of classic signs and symptoms which are caused by increased catabolism [19]. Patients present with nervousness, fatigue, palpitations, heat intolerance, polyphagia and weight loss [6,9]. It is important to note that the elderly may present with a different range of symptoms and exhibit more subtle signs [20]. Weight loss and anorexia are common symptoms in older patients and may be mistaken for the presence of a neoplastic process which can lead to over investigation [21].

As a result of the increased basal metabolic rate patients often present with a persisting tachycardia. This occurs characteristically during sleep and may be associated with palpitations [22]. In the elderly and in those with pre-morbid cardiac disease, cardiac arrhythmias may develop on this background [22]. Atrial fibrillation is the commonest arrhythmia and is present in up to 20% of patients [18]. Interestingly, up to 15% of new onset atrial fibrillation in the elderly population is due to hyperthyroidism [23]. This may be resistant to medical treatment and resolves only when the underlying hyperthyroidism itself is treated [24]. Cardiovascular mortality is increased in hypertoxic states primarily as a result of ischaemic heart disease and congestive heart failure [25,26].

Increasing dyspnoea may occur in hyperthyroid patients, limiting exercise tolerance. This is thought to be due to a reduction in respiratory muscle mass and strength with a corresponding reduction in the vital capacity [18]. Bone turnover is also increased in the thyrotoxic state due to the direct stimulation of osteoclasts and osteoblasts to increase bone resorption [27,28]. Low TSH levels, of themselves, have also been implicated in the dysregulation of bone turnover [29]. Longstanding thyrotoxicosis can lead to increase bone loss and subsequent osteoporosis. Thyrotoxic patients can be emotionally labile and restless. Other less common complaints include poor concentration and changes in personality[3]. Overt psychosis, although rare may occur [7].

5. Diagnosis

5.1. Biochemical

Serum thyrotropin (TSH) is the most commonly used screening test to diagnose hyperthyroidism with levels being low or undetectable [2]. TSH levels are measured using immunoradiometric and chemiluminescent methods which have a high sensitivity (100%) and specificity (99.1%) [30,31]. When an abnormally low TSH is detected, free Thyroxine (T4) and free Triiodothyronine (T3) levels are measured to determine the degree of hyperthyroidism. Indirect assays measure the free T4 and T3 level while sensitive and specific radioimmunoassays are used to measure total T4 and T3 levels [7]. The presence of a low TSH with normal T4 and T3 level is defined as sub-clinical hyperthyroidism [32]. Atrial fibrillation, other cardiac arrhythmias and cardiovascular mortality are all associated with prolonged sub-clinical hyperthyroidism, especially in the elderly [33,34]. The identification of a normal T4 but a high free T3 is known as T3 Thyrotoxicosis and may be an early manifestation of Grave's disease [3,35].

The measurement of auto antibodies, thyroglobulin, thyroxine peroxidase (TPO) and TSH receptor (TSHR) antibodies, may help in elucidating the underlying aetiology [6]. More than 90% of patients with Graves' disease have increased levels of circulating TSHR antibodies and in the setting of thyrotoxicosis it can confirm the diagnosis [3]. Similarly, TPO antibodies are also present in approximately 75% of patients with Graves' disease [2].

5.2. Radiological imaging

Radionuclide scanning and radioactive iodine uptake assesses the activity within the thyroid gland and may be used as an adjunct to biochemical analysis to identify the underlying aetiology of hyperthyroidism. Lesions are classified into three main categories: hot, whereby there is hyper-accumulation of radiotracer; warm, where there is increased uptake with suppression of background thyroidal tissue; or cold where the thyroid nodule is non-functioning [36]. Warm and hot nodules represent an increase in thyroid tissue turnover and may therefore suggest a benign toxic cause (Figure 1). Cold nodules, on the other hand are concerning for malignancy and should proceed to an ultrasound and FNAC [36,37]. Typically in Graves' disease, thyroid tissue is diffusely hyper-active with increased radio-tracer throughout the gland. In toxic nodular goitres, the radioactive iodine is focally concentrated in the nodules with suppression of the background tissue giving patchy uptake [38].

Early radionuclide scans were performed using radioactive iodine. This had been subsequently replaced by technetium (Tc-99m) pertechnetate. This has been shown to mimic the behaviour and uptake of iodine within the thyroid gland but involves a much lower dose of radioactivity and is cheaper [39].

Thyroid ultrasound has a limited role in patients with hyperthyroidism. It has been recommended to assess thyroid nodules, palpable thyroid abnormalities, nodular goitres and lesions found incidentally by other imaging modalities [37]. However, in the presence of a low TSH and a discrete hot nodule fine needle aspiration cytology should be avoided. Suspicious nodules on ultrasound or cold nodules should be subjected to a FNAC to allow for a cytological diagnosis to be made pre-operatively [37,38].

Chest radiography, CT and MRI scans can help in surgical planning for patients with compressive or obstructive symptoms although it is rarely used. CT scanning may allow assessment of size and extent of the goitre, including the presence of a retro-sternal component but predominantly aids in pre-operative assessment of the airway (narrowing and displacement) and the need for an awake fiber-optic intubation (Figure 1). When undertaking cross-sectional imaging, contrast should be avoided due to the high iodine content, which may acutely worsen or induce symptoms of hyperthyroidism [40].

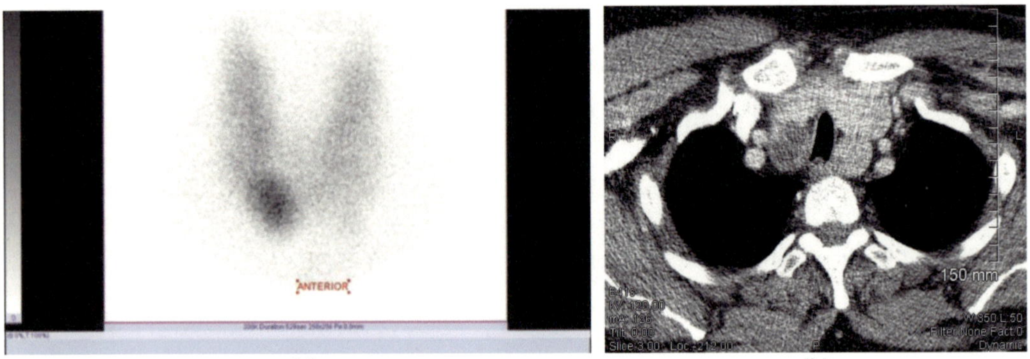

(a) (b)

Figure 1. (a) Solitary nodule (b) Retrosternal extension of a large multinodular goitre

6. Aetiology of hyperthyroidism

6.1. Graves' disease

Graves' disease is an autoimmune disorder with a familial predisposition first described by Robert James Grave in 1835 [41]. Overall the incidence of the disease is approximately 100-200 cases per 100,000 per year with a marked female predominance and accounts for approximately 60–80% of all causes of hyperthyroidism [1,16]. A strong family history among affected patients suggests a genetic predisposition however the incidence in monozygotic twins is approximately 20% suggesting that penetrance is not 100% and other environmental causes may play a role in pathogenesis [3,42]. It is typically associated with other autoimmune conditions such as rheumatoid arthritis, SLE, Sjogrens, Type 1 Diabetes Mellitus and pernicious anaemia [43]. Graves' disease is also closely associated with myasthenia gravis occurring in 3-5% of patients [18].

Graves' disease classically consists of a triad of hyperthyroidism with diffuse goitre, ophthalmopathy and pretibial myxoedema [44]. Each of these may run an independent course. The clinical presentation includes signs and symptoms of thyrotoxicosis, a symmetrically enlarged non tender goitre often with a palpable thrill or audible bruit [5]. However, it may also present with a variable degree of extra-thyroidal manifestations such as ophthalmopathy, pretibial myxoedema and acropachy [6]. Ophthalmopathy, proptoisis, extra-ocular muscle involvement and rarely optic nerve compression, are thought to arise as a result of an immune response to antigens within the retro-orbital tissues that are shared with the thyroid leading to oedema and glycosaminoglycan deposition and fibrosis of the retro-orbital tissues [45,46].

The diagnosis of Graves' disease is made by establishing the presence of hyperthyroidism, the presence of TSH auto-antibodies and diffuse increased symmetrical uptake on radio-iodine scanning [47].

Treatment options include anti-thyroid medication, radioactive iodine ablation or surgical intervention. The aim of treatment is to achieve a euthyroid state and in the presence of ophthalmopathy to ensure overall stability. The ultimate decision regarding optimal management is tailored to an individual patient.

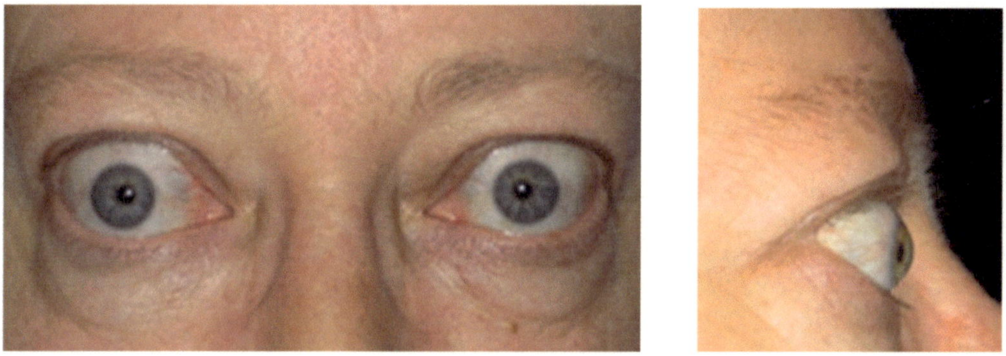

Figure 2. Graves opthalmopathy

6.2. Toxic nodular goitre

Toxic nodular disease, resulting from either multiple or single adenomatous nodules was first described as a separate entity to Graves' disease in 1913 by Henry Plummer [48]. Toxic nodular goitre includes two distinct entities, toxic multi-nodular goitre and a solitary toxic nodule, also known as Plummers' Disease. Both are characterised by abnormal thyroid function independent of TSH regulation. Together, they account for the second commonest cause of hyperthyroidism but there are differences in their pathogenesis and treatment and therefore will be considered separately.

Toxic Multi-nodular Goitre

Toxic multinodular goitre is defined as a thyroid gland with two or more autonomously functioning nodules [49]. It's incidence ranges from 5% of all hyperthyroid cases in iodine replete areas to 50% in iodine deficient areas and typically presents in older females [19]. Many aetiological factors are involved in the pathogenesis of toxic multi-nodular goitre including the functional heterogeneity of the thyroid follicles, the effects of growth factors and goitrogens, the presence or absence of iodine and genetic abnormalities. Concurrent autoimmune diseases are uncommon [50].

Patients present with less severe symptoms of hyperthyroidism and the onset may be more insidious [51]. Typically they have compressive symptoms from an enlarging multi-nodular goitre with retro-sternal extension [3]. The diagnosis is confirmed with a combination of biochemistry and radio-iodine scanning. Nuclear medicine scanning may show a heterogenous gland with mixed areas of hyper and hypo-activity [3,32]. Thyroid auto-antibodies are negative. [32].

The treatment of multinodular goitres is aimed at eradication of all autonomously functioning thyroid tissue. Given the concurrent compressive symptoms surgery may provide the most definitive treatment. Recurrence of disease is more common with either medical anti-thyroid medication or radio-iodine ablation [6,32].

Solitary Toxic Nodule

A solitary toxic nodule is an autonomously hyper-functioning nodule present within an otherwise normal thyroid gland. Approximately 50% of solitary nodules are truly solitary, while typically it presents as part of a nodular gland constituting a dominant nodule [52]. The prevalence of palpable nodules in a population ages 30-59 years can be up to 4.2% [53].

Patients present with a neck lump, visible or palpable. Appropriate investigation of a solitary nodule is crucial as the risk of malignancy is higher than in the presence of a multi-nodular goitre [37]. The incidence of malignancy in truly solitary nodules is 5-15%, but this figure would increase for solid or cold nodules to more than 25% [37]. Surgery remains the treatment of choice for these patients although they may be observed if asymptomatic.

Treatment Options

The management of hyperthyroidism is based on three different treatment modalities, namely anti-thyroid medication, radioactive iodine ablation or surgery. Patient, physician and geographical preferences will dictate the choice of therapy. The overall aim of treatment is to provide symptom relief, achieve a euthyroid state and to prevent recurrence. Given the overall healthcare costs of hyperthyroidism, surgical intervention performed with minimal morbidity in high volume centres may offer the highest chance of success with the lowest chance of recurrence [8]. However, a prospective study by Torring et al examining such outcome measures as patient satisfaction, time to euthyroidism and rates of sick leave demonstrated equivalence between all three treatment modalities [54].

6.3. Anti thyroid drugs

Anti-thyroid medication is used to render patients euthyroid to either induce long-term remission or as preparation for definitive treatment with radioactive ablation or surgery [2]. The main thioamide agents used are Carbimazole, Methamimazole and Propylthiouracil (PTU). By inhibiting thyroxine peroxidase and interfering with both the organification of iodide and the coupling of iodo-thyryronines a reduction in hormone synthesis is achieved [6,55]. Initial doses of medication are usually high and a euthyroid state can be achieved after 8-12 weeks of treatment whereupon doses can be titrated downwards to a maintenance dose [2]. PTU is preferred in pregnancy as at it less likely to cross the placenta due to protein binding [56,57]. Treatment may be discontinued after one year if sustained remission is achieved with the patient being euthyroid and TSH-R antibodies undetectable [19]. Remission can be variable with reported relapse rates of between 50% to 60% [19]. Factors influencing relapse include smoking, compliance with medication, the presence of a large goitres and the elevated TSH-R antibodies at end of treatment [58]. Side effects range from mild symptoms of urticaria, fever and rash to more serious neutropenia, hepatotoxicity and vascultitis [55,59,60]. Agranulocytocis occurs in approximately 0.1-0.5% of treated patients and the rate of development of hypothyroidism is 0.6% per annum [61,62]..

6.4. Radio-iodine ablation

Radio-iodine (RAI) can be used as first line treatment or for patients who have either failed medical management or present with recurrent disease following a sub-total thyroidectomy. Within the USA RAI is the first line treatment for patients with Graves' disease [55]. Iodine-131 is taken up by the thyroid cells causing local apopotosis and subsequent fibrosis of the gland thereby reducing the overall functional thyroid mass [22]. RAI is most suitable for patients with a small goitre in the absence of ophthalomopathy. A wide variety of dosages (200–600MBq) can be used [22]. The dosage however depends on the size and activity of the gland, associated failure rates with low doses and the increased rate of hypothyroidism when higher doses are utilised [19,63]. Absolute contra-indications include pregnancy, breastfeeding and coexisting differentiated thyroid cancer [55]. RAI is usually avoided in patients with severe ophthalmopathy as in approximately 15% of patient symptoms may worsen following treatment [64,65]. It may be used cautiously in patients with stable eye disease in combination with high dose glucocorticoids. [65].

Anti-thyroid agents are given for four to six weeks prior to radio-ablation in an attempt to render patients euthyroid and thus prevent the development of a thyrotoxic crisis during initial treatment [2]. These are discontinued two to three days prior to treatment to ensure functional thyroid tissue which is required to take up iodine [2,66]. The majority of patients (75%) require only a single dose of radio-iodine [67]. The effects of the RAI are not immediate and continue for months following treatment. Symptomatic improvement can take up to two months. Immediate complications include thyroid gland tenderness [32]. Long-term complications include the development of hypothyroidism in approximately 60% of patients at 1 year, and therefore regular long-term surveillance is warranted with T4 replacement as necessary [68].

6.5. Surgery

Surgery provides high cure rates in hyperthyroidism with minimal morbidity in high volume centres It gives almost immediate relief of the compressive symptoms of large goitres, achieves euthyroidism rapidly and consistently, and avoids the long term risks of radioactive iodine and anti-thyroid medications [69]. Surgical intervention is warranted where the disease has proved refractory to medical management, including both anti-thyroid medication and radioactive iodine. Other indications for surgery include large goitres with compressive symptoms, where RAI is contra-indicated including pregnancy (usually performed in the 2nd trimester) and severe ophthalomopathy, desire for pregnancy soon after treatment, suspicion or presence of underlying thyroid malignancy, for children and patient preference [5]

Historically thyroid surgery was rarely performed for indications other than cancer until the last quarter of the twentieth century [70]. The high peri-operative and post-operative morbidity and mortality made the procedure untenable and indeed in 1850 it was banned by the French Academy of Medicine [71]. However improvements in anti-sepsis, anaesthesia and the introduction of anti-thyroid medication to render patients euthyroid pre-operatively revolutionised thyroid surgery. It is now well established as an acceptable and efficacious form of treatment and the controversy focuses on the extent of intervention; sub-total versus total thyroidectomy.

Currently, total thyroidectomy is regarded as the surgical procedure of choice for Graves' disease, multi-nodular toxic and non toxic nodules [70,72-74]. A study by Efermidou et al reviewing 932 cases of total thyroidectomy for benign thyroid disease showed that surgery is safe and is associated with minimal morbidity. Patients achieved immediate and permanent cure with no risk of disease recurrent or repeated surgery [75]. This was supported by Ballentone et al who demonstrated in over 500 patietns a postoperative rates of haemorrhage of 1.5%, a permanent RLN palsy of 0.4% and a permanent rate of hypocalcaemia of 3.4%[76]. There was no recurrences noted during ther follow-up of 44 months (Ballintone). Another study by Pappalardo et al randomised 141 patients into receiving a total thyroidectomy or subtotal thyroidectomy and patients were followed up for a median of 14.5 months. The rate of goitre recurrence in the subtotal thyroidectomy group was higher at 14% [77].

Finally, a meta-analysis which included 1402 patients from 5 continents demonstrated higher relapse rates with anti-thyroid drugs than radioactive iodine (52.7% vs 15%) and with anti-thyroid drugs than surgery (52.7% vs 10%). In addition, examination of 31 scohort studies which included 5136 patinets found an adverse effect rate of 13% in patients treated with anti-thyroid drugs [78].

It is now widely accepted that high surgical volume in specialised units provides better patient outcome. A systematic review published in the British Journal of Surgery in 2007 examined 1075 studies and found that high volume surgeons had better outcomes in 75% of the studies and that specialised surgeons had significantly better outcomes than general surgeons in 91% of the studies [79]. The association between volume and outcome has also been demonstrated in thyroid surgery. Boudourakis et al performed a cross sectional analyses of a number of surgeries deemed to have demonstrated a volume-outcome relationship. There was a significant increased in number of procedures performed by high volume surgeons during the study period (23% for thyroidectomies). Unadjusted mortality and length of stay was significantly lower for high-volume surgeons compared with low-volume surgeons [80]. In a study by Pieracci et al, substernal thyroidectomy was compared with cervical thyroidectomy, with the main aim of assessing outcomes (all volume type hospitals were included). Increasing hospital volume predicted a decreased likelihood of overall complications, post-operative bleeding, blood transfusion, respiratory failure, mortality and length of stay [81].

7. Extent of surgery

7.1. Graves

Historically, a subtotal thyroidectomy was the procedure of choice in Graves' disease, minimizing the complications of surgery with potential cure of the disease. However, a randomized trial comparing anti-thyroid drugs, radioiodine treatment, and surgery in Graves' disease found all are equally effective in normalizing serum thyroid hormone concentrations within six weeks and over 95% of the patients were satisfied with their therapy [54].

The type of surgery in Graves' disease remains controversial. A total thyroidectomy ensures complete cure of symptoms but is obviously associated with surgical hypothyroidism and the need for lifelong thyroxine treatment. Conversely, subtotal thyroidectomy, given that a proportion of thyroid tissue is left in-situ is associated with a higher likelihood of recurrence and may still be associated with hypothyroidism. In a randomized trial of subtotal versus total thyroidectomy for Graves' disease involving 191 patients followed over five years, recurrent hyperthyroidism occurred in 4.7% of patients after subtotal versus 0% after total thyroidectomy, while transient hypoparathyroidism was seen in 6.8% and 12.6% respectively, and permanent hypoparathyroidism in 0% and 0.5% respectively confirming the advantages of total thyroidectomy without adversely affecting morbidity [82]. A meta-analysis published by Palit et al demonstrated in 35 studies with over 7241 patients that the rates of RLN injury and permanent hypo-parathyroidism were similar between subtotal and total thyroidectomy. More importantly they also demonstrated an 8% recurrence risk in those patients who had a subtotal thyroidectomy versus none in the total thyroidectomy group [83]. A further randomised trial published in the same year added weight to the call for total thyroidectomy as it failed to demonstrate a significant difference in the complication rates between a total or subtotal thyroidectomy [84]. Therefore total thyroidecomy should be considered the gold standard surgical intervention in Graves' disease.

7.2. Toxic multinodular goitre

Surgical resection remains the treatment of choice especially in the presence of a large goitre and compressive symptoms where surgery gives prompt relief [85]. The extent of surgical intervention and the comparative results of performing a near total or total thyroidectomy have been topical in the last decade. Attempts to perform more minimal surgery have been proposed to minimise the complications, such as RLN damage and permanent hypoparathyroidism, of thyroid surgery but are typically associated with higher rates of recurrence and an increased requirement for re-operative surgery. Stenmuller et al showed that a lobectomy plus a contralateral subtotal resection (known as the Dunhill procedure) and bilateral subtotal resection resulted in a low overall incidence of permanent hypoparathyroidism and RLN injury [86]. Rayes et al perfomed a prospective randomised study on 200 patients and concluded both can be performed with similar complication rates [87]. Remnant size was found to determine recurrence rates. Barczynski et al compared total thyroidectomy, Dunhill procedure and bilateral subtotal resection in 570 patients. Recurrence rates were 0.5% 4.7% and 11.6% respectively with recurrence highest in bilateral subtotal resection. However this study also shows that although recurrence rates differ, reoperation rates for these recurrences are comparable showing that not all of these recurrences may be clinically significant and require further surgery [88]. Several other papers have also supported the role for total thyroidectomy for multinodular goitre showing that it completely eradicates the disease process, lowers the local recurrence rate, allows for avoiding the substantial risk of reoperative surgery, and involves only a minimal risk of morbidity [89,90-91].

7.3. Toxic solitary nodule

For patients with a solitary toxic adenoma without evidence of nodules in the contralateral lobe, a thyroid lobectomy is adequate. For patients with toxic adenoma and a coexisting nonfunctioning nodule in the contralateral lobe, total thyroidectomy may be warranted especially if there is any suspicion regarding thyroid malignancy. The main advantages of surgery include immediate resolution of hyperthyroidsim symptoms, relief from compressive symptoms, avoidance of radiation exposure to normal tissue and confirmation of diagnosis in rare cases of suspected carcinoma [40]. The reported incidence of hypothyroidism is low (14% with surgery compared with 22% with radioiodine treatment [40].

8. Preparation for surgery

Historically the mortality and morbidity associated with thyroid surgery was extremely high, not only from intra-operative complications but from post-operative hormonal dysregulation [92,93]. Meticulous pre-operative preparation of hyperthyroid patients has reduced this to less that 1% in high volume centres [92,94].

8.1. Anti-thyroid drugs

The aim of preoperative preparation as previously discussed is to render patients as close as possible to being clinically and biochemically euthyroid [22]. Antithyroid drugs interfere with the incorporation of iodine into tyrosine residues and prevent the coupling of iodotyrosines into iodothyronines [55]. Anti thyroid agents such as Carbimazole and Propythiouracil are prescribed to achieve a euthyroid state [93,95]. The last dose should be given the day prior to surgery [22].

8.2. Beta-blockers

Many manifestations of hyperthyroidism relate to the cardiovascular system and to the sensitisation of the B-adrenergic receptors to catecholamines in patients who are thyrotoxic. Pre-operative treatment with a beta-blocker such as propranolol controls adrenergic effects [93]. It has also been shown to reduce the peripheral conversion of T4 to T3 [96]. Beta-blockers are used in combination with antithyroid drugs and play an important role in pre-operative patient preparation [97]. It is crucial to note that this drug should not be omitted on the morning of surgery and must be continued for at least 5 days postoperatively [22]. Beta-blockers are contraindicated in asthmatics, where a cardio-selective B-blocker may be considered [3].

8.3. Iodine treatment

The use of iodines in the pre-operative management of Graves disease was first documented in 1923 and its introduction saw a significant reduction in the mortality associated with thyroid surgery [98]. Iodines are now routinely used in the peri-operative management of hyperthyroid patients [93]. It is prescribed in the form of oral Lugol's iodine (drops) at a dose of 24mg divided over three doses administered 7–10 days pre-operatively to reduce the vascularity of the gland [93]. It has been postulated that organic iodide such as Lugol's solution usage can decrease the vascularity of the thyroid gland pre-operatively by inhibiting vascular endothelial growth factor A expression in thyroid follicles [99]. A randomised control trial by Erbil et al using colour flow Doppler ultrasonography, immunohistochemical and western blot analysis to compare thyroid vascularity with or without preoperative Lugol's solution in 36 patients. It showed a decrease in rate of blood flow to thyroid, thyroid vascularity and intra-operative blood loss in the preoperative Lugol solution treatment group. They concluded that preoperative Lugols treatment reduces intraoperative bleeding which in turn improves the safety profile of the procedure [100].

Large doses of iodine act by producing a transient remission of hormone synthesis by 'stunning' the thyroid gland an effect known as the Wolff-Chaikoff effect. It is a phenomenon where higher than normal doses of iodine inhibit organification of thyroid hormone resulting in a decrease in hormone synthesis and release [101]. Onset of action begins 24 hours post administration peaking at approximately 10 days [102]. This can be seen as an auto-regulatory system in dealing with supra-physiologic levels of iodine [93]. In normal euthyroid subjects thyroid synthesis normalises due to down-regulation of the sodium iodine symporter known as the escape phenomenon [103].

However, in hyperthyroid patients the escape phenomenon does not occur and Jod-Basedow phenomenon occurs instead [93]. The Jod Basedow effect occurs due to dysregulation of iodine in hyperthyroid patients where excess iodine stimulates more hormone production by acting as the substrate [104]. It can result in a temporary hyperthyroidism, worsening of existing hyperthyroidism or rarely a permanent rise in thyroid hormone [93]. Therefore iodines should be used cautiously and for a limited time period in conjunction with anit-thryoid medication in the pre-operative period.

9. Surgical intervention

9.1. Anaesthesia

The majority of thyroid surgery is performed under general anaesthetic without neuromuscular blockade using an endotracheal cuffed tube to allow for intra-operative neuromonitoring. Local anasethic is given pre-operatively along the incision to ensure minimal post-operative discomfort. In selective patients with small thyroid nodules and favourable anatomy local anaesthetic has been documented as being utilised. Local anesthetic techniques require the use of cervical block anesthesia. The disadvantage of this is risk of bilateral paralysis of the recurrent laryngeal nerve resulting from blockade with the local anaeasthetic, with consequent difficulty in breathing postoperatively [105].

9.2. Intra-operative nerve monitoring

The primary complication of thyroid surgery is damage to either the recurrent laryngeal nerve or the external branch of the superior laryngeal nerve. Routine visual identification of the RLN decreases the incidence of injury and is standard practice (Figure 3). However, a recent survey of members of the American Association of Endocrine Surgeons found that 63% of respondents do not use neuromonitoring, 14% of surgeons used it routinely and 23% were selective users [106]. Non-users were in practice longer, reported a lower case volume, were less familiar with the technology and had limited access to the equipment [106].

The main role for intra-operative monitoring is to identify the RLN nerve, to aid in safe dissection once it is identified and for prognostication of neural function postoperatively [107]. The two main components of monitoring are stimulation of the RLN and assessment of the vocal cord response to stimulation. Several techniques have been described and are in routine use. The most common method is the use of a laryngeal surface electrode which is applied to the surface of the endotracheal tube in a proximal location to the vocal cord [108,109]. An attached probe is used to deliver the low voltage electric current. During thyroid resection an auditory signal or visual EMG signal can be used to provide information about the presence and course of the RLN.

A systematic review of the literature demonstrated that neuromonitoring of the RLN during thyroid surgery reduced RLN injury compared with routine nerve identification [110]. Other studies comparing intra-operative nerve monitoring have demonstrated a benefit for its use although a statistically significant difference between the groups could not be identified [111, 112]. A randomized trial of 1000 patients showed a decrease in transient but not permanent RLN paresis compared to visualization alone [113]. In addition, there are studies which show low sensitivity and positive predictive value of intra-operative neuromonitoring for predicting nerve injury [114]. Despite this evidence, monitoring, when used appropriately, has been shown to be feasible, safe and reproducible and should be considered for all cases. It must be noted that neuromonitoring does not replace adequate intra-operative visualization and meticulous surgical technique.

10. Surgical procedures in hyperthyroidism

10.1. Dunhill and Holtz procedures

Hartely and Dunhill described the procedure of subtotal thyroidectomy where a total thyroid lobectomy is performed on one side and a small remnant is left in situ (weighing approximately 4 grams) on the contralateral side [5]. However it has been consistently difficult to assess the residual remnant thyroid size and it may vary between 2–12 gms. The surgery is performed through a collar incision placed halfway between the sternal notch and the thyroid cartilage.

http://dx.doi.org/10.5772/57499

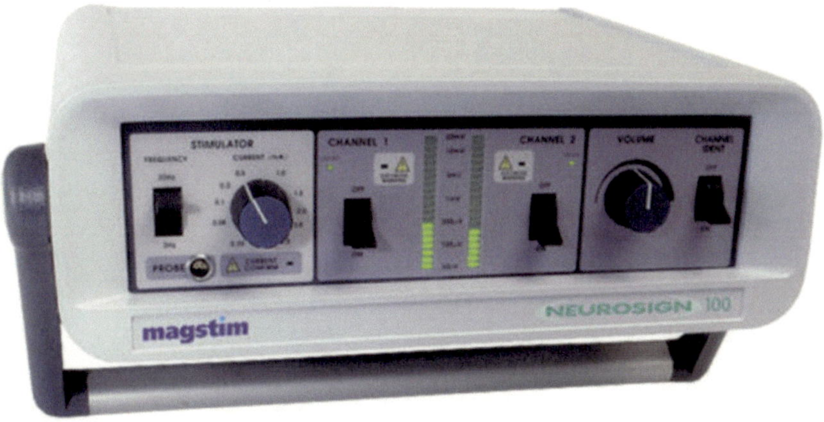

Figure 3. Nerve stimulator used for intra-operative recurrent laryngeal nerve monitoring

As the thyroid gland is approached, the middle thyroid vein is identified and ligated. The entire lobe and isthmus are excised on the diseased side. On the contralateral side, the superior pole is freed by dividing the superior vessels and the remaining thyroid lobe is approached from a postero-lateral plane through the thyroid tissue leaving a posterior remnant. This keeps the dissection plane away from the parathyroid glands and the recurrent laryngeal nerve on this sub-total operative side [115].

The Enderlen Holtz procedure involves performing a subtotal bilateral thyroidectomy. The procedure is similar to the Dunhill procedure and involves mobilisation of the thyroid gland supero-laterally. In this case remnant tissue of 2 grams or more are left on both sides. Disadvantages of both these procedures, as previously discussed include the high risk of recurrence as well as an increased rate of complications (RLN damage and permanent hypoparathyroidism) associated with re-operative surgery [115].

10.2. Total thyroidectomy

The patient is positioned supine on the operating table in a slight reverse Trendelenburg position. A gel pad or sand bag is placed transversely under the shoulders and the neck is extended and placed in a head ring. This allows the thyroid gland to become more prominent and applies tension to the skin, platysma, and strap muscles aiding in dissection. In a total thyroidectomy complete excision of the gland, including the pyramidal lobe is performed [22,105].

A curved incision is made midway between the suprastenal notch and the thyroid cartilage. The incision is deepened through the skin, subcutaneous tissue and platysma. Skin flaps are then raised upwards to the thyroid notch and downwards to the suprasternal notch. The deep cervical fascia is then divided in the midline down and in-between the strap muscles to the plane of the thyroid gland. The strap muscles are then retracted laterally and mobilised off the

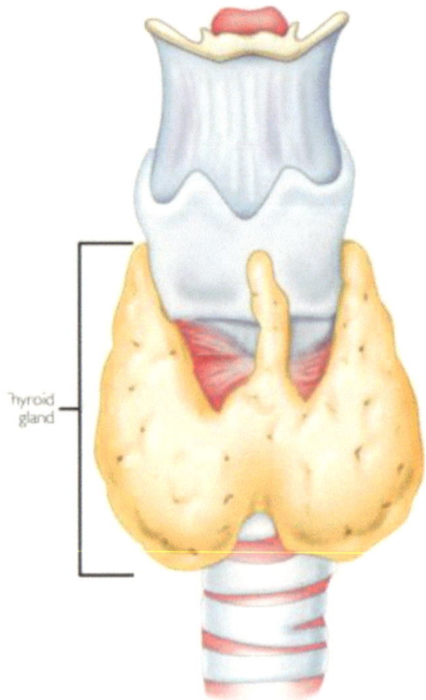

Figure 4. Thryoid gland and pyramidal lobe [116]

thyroid gland using an advanced surgical sealing instrument, such as the Ligasure vessel sealing device (Covidien) [22,105].

The middle thyroid vein is encountered laterally, and this drains directly into the internal jugular vein. This is ligated and divided. The plane between the medial pole of the upper lobe and the cricothyroid muscle is subsequently developed, ensuring close proximity to the thyroid in order to avoid trauma or injury to the external branch of the superior laryngeal nerve. The branches of the superior thyroid artery are then ligated and divided, allowing downward delivery of the upper pole. Capsular dissection is then performed and this invovles commencing the lateral component of the dissection high on the surface of the thyroid gland, diviging only the tertiary branches of the inferior thyroid artery and progressing posteriorly. In this process, the vascular supply of the parathyroid glands is often well preserved [22,105,117].

The recurrent laryngeal nerve is identified in its course in the tracheo-esophageal groove. This is first identified and sought below the level of the inferior thyroid artery, where it passes obliquely upwards and forwards. The tubercle of Zuckerkandl serves as a useful landmark in the identification of the RLN. Situated on posterolateral aspect of the gland in the tracheo-esphageal groove in proximity of the cricothryoid membrane it is a constant landmark for RLN identification which is aided by further mobilisation of the thyroid. The nerve is followed upwards until it passes into the larynx under the inferior border of the inferior constrictor behind the inferior cornu of the thyroid cartilage. In cases where the right nerve is difficult to

http://dx.doi.org/10.5772/57499

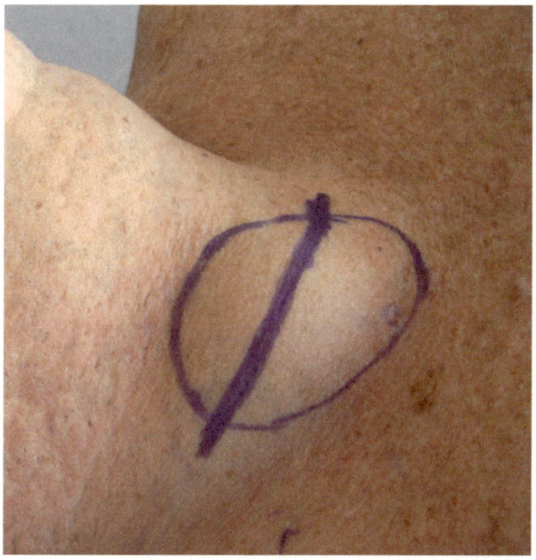

Figure 5. Marking of incision

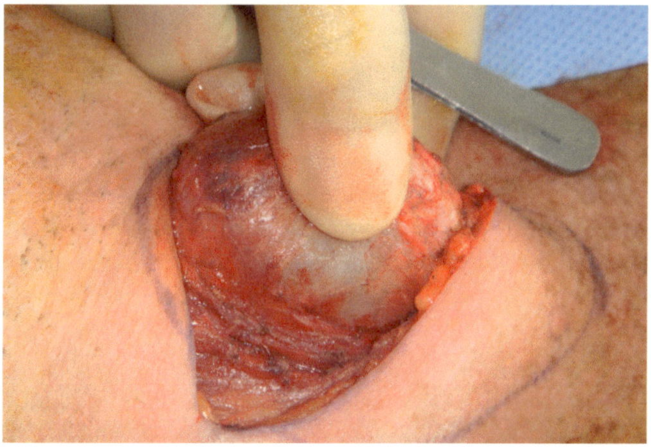

Figure 6. Mobilisation of the thyroid

identify one must consider an anomalous (non-recurrent) nerve, which is pesent in 1 percent of patients. A non-recurrent RLN passes behind the carotid sheath and curves medially, forwards and upwards and can be mistaken for the inferior thyroid artery. It is important to be careful with diathermy and newer advanced sealing devices as heat conduction may damage the RLN, the blood supply to the parathyroid's or to the delicate areas within the larynx [22,105,117].

The parathyroid glands must be identified in all cases. This is done by careful inspection of the common locations and by utilising capsular dissection they can be peeled away from the thyroid gland itself. Care is taken not to damage the branches of the inferior thyroid artery which supply the parathyroid glands. If a parathyroid gland is accidentally excised or devascularised inadvertantly then it should be fragmented into small pieces and autotransplanted immediately within the sternocleidomastoid muscle [22,105,117].

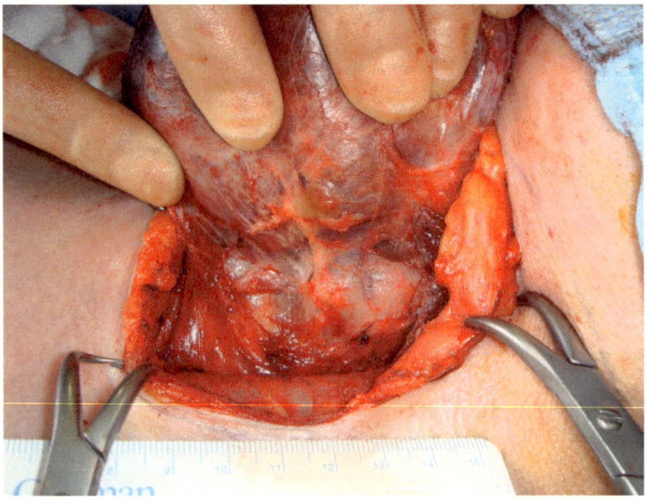

Figure 7. Postero-lateral aspect of the thyroid

The pretacheal and cercval fascia are closed using interrupted sutures. Routine drain placement after thyroid surgery is not necessary. A meta-analysis of 11 randomized clinical trials showed no significant difference in the incidence of hematoma or seroma between routine drainage and no drainage [118]. If the thyroid is very large with a significant retrosternal component or the dissection is extensive,a closed-suction drain can be placed to prevent a serous fluid collection [118]. This can be removed safely when the drain output is serous and decreasing in volume.

10.3. Thyroid lobectomy

Thyroid lobectomy is predominantly the treatment of choice in the management of solitary toxic nodules because it not only removes the stimulus of excess thyroid production, but it also allows definitive histological assessment of the nodule.

The details of the procedure, patient positing and exposure are similar to that of a total thyroidectomy, as described above. In a thyroid lobectomy, the isthmus is transected using a haemostatic device such as the harmonic scalpel or Ligasure [22,105,116].

10.4. Subtotal thyroidectomy

The thyroid gland is exposed in a similar manner to a total thyroidectomy. The middle thyroid vein is encountered upon retractionof the strap muscles and is ligated and divided. The superior poles of the thyroid are then ligated taking care to avoid the EBSLN [22,105,116]. The inferior thyroid artery is identified and ligated lateral to the recurrent laryngeal nerve. The procedure then entails dividing across each lobe of the thyroid from the lateral edge towards the trachea, leaving intact a posterior capsule with the attached remnant of the thyroid. For ease of closure the thicker remnant of the gland is left laterally and incised more on the medial aspect. This allows the folding over of the remnant laterally to medially, allowing the capsular edges to be sutured together using a Vicryl suture. As a general guide the remnant strip is often recommended to be 3cm x 1cm on each side. This operation is rarely used in modern surgical practice [22,105,116].

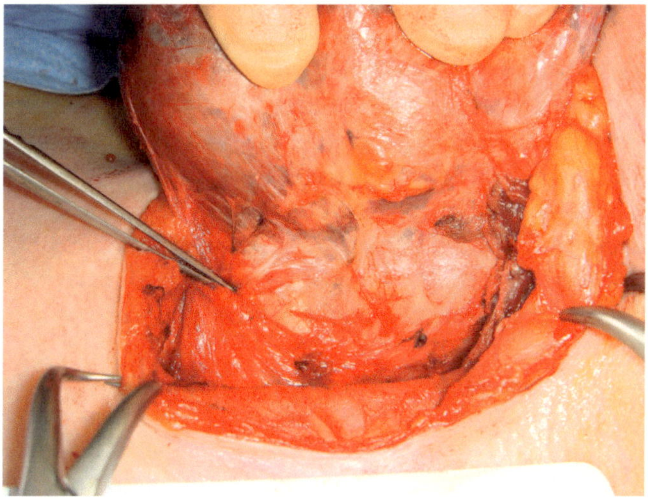

Figure 8. Identification of recurrent laryngeal nerve

10.5. Surgery in recurrent thyroid disease

Re-operative thyroid surgery is technically challenging due to the formation of adhesions and scar tissue, and is associated with increased rates of recurrent laryngeal nerve injury and hypoparathyroidism [119,120,121]. Operative intervention for recurrence accounts for anywhere between 5–12% of all thyroidectomies performed [122,123]. However, the last twenty years have seen a shift away from conservative primary operations such as bilateral subtotal thyroidectomy and this should begin to be mirrored by declining recurrence rates [124].

The risks associated with reoperation should be carefully examined and balanced with the options of medical management or observation [119,120,121]. The extent of the disease should be assessed in addition to the location and possible complications such as nerve injury and excision of the parathyroid glands [124].

The operation of choice in all cases of recurrent nodular goiter should be a completion total thyroidectomy. The surgical approach is dependent on the extent of the initial operation and the size and location of the recurrent goitre. Re-operation following a subtotal or total thyroidectomy is hazardous and requires a methodical and standardized operative approach [124]. The key is the initial identification of anatomical landmarks outside the original operative field.

The dissection must commence laterally by mobilization of the sternocleidomastoid muscle to expose the carotid sheath. The carotid sheath may however be displaced medially and lie abutting both fibrous tissue and the thyroid remnant. Dissection continues until the lateral aspect of the gland in encountered. It is important to ensure that the nerve is not encased within the strap muscles prior to their division. Identification of standard landmarks is vital. Therefore the esophagus posteriorly and the trachea anteriorly should be identified next. This helps to narrow down the location of the recurrent laryngeal nerve, which should be lying within the trachea-oesophageal groove. Protection of the recurrent laryngeal nerve is best achieved by identifying it in virgin territory. Dissection should thus begin low down in the trachea-esophageal groove, if necessary as low as the thoracic inlet, where the nerve can be safely identified in an undisturbed, non-operated field. Once the nerve has been identified, its course is traced through to the insertion into the cricothyroid muscle. The recurrent laryngeal nerve should not be sought at the fibrosed upper pole, as the risk of subsequent damage is extremely high. Mobilization of the thyroid is by capsular dissection. Sub-sternal recurrent goitre may increase the difficulty of surgical management and may be associated with a significantly higher rate of recurrent laryngeal nerve damage as it exits the thoracic inlet. A sternal split is rarely required. However, where there is excessive local bleeding or where removal of the gland is prevented by excessive fibrosis a partial sternal split provides adequate access [124].

10.6. Retrosternal thyroid extension

Given the embryological descent of the thyroid most extension of the thyroid gland is into the anterior and superior mediastinum. In the majority of cases the retrosternal component of the thyroid gland can be delivered into the neck with gentle traction upwards given the position the patient on the operation table [105]. In the small number of cases where the thyroid extends behind the trachea and enters into the posterior mediastinum, there is a risk of injury to major vessels and structures within the chest and a median sternotomy in conjunction with the cardio-thoracic surgeons should be performed [105].

10.7. Postoperative care

Post operative patients are monitored closely for complications. Typically, thyroid surgery is performed as a 23 hour surgical stay but increasingly in smaller cases there has been a move to day case surgery. Patients are observed for exclusion of a post-operative haematoma and subsequent airway compromise as well as for signs and symptoms of hypocalcemia in the immediate post-operative period. Close monitoring of calcium levels especially in symptomatic patients is crucial. Clinical tests of hypocalcaemic, including Chvostek's sign (tapping of facial nerve causing facial muscles to twitch) and Trousseu's sign (finger and wrist spasm on insufflation of a sphygnomanomator cuff around arm), may be present [125]. Studies have shown that oral calcium and vitamin D supplementation has been found to decrease the development of hypocalcaemic symptoms. However, a randomized trial that included 143 patients undergoing a total thyroidectomy, showed that patients with a PTH level >10 pg/mL obtained on post-operative day one could be safely discharged without routine calcium supplementation [126]. Calcium levels need to be followed up as hypercalcaemia may occur.

http://dx.doi.org/10.5772/57499

In addition short term courses are usually sufficient and supplementation may be discontinued once levels are normalised.

It is recommended that thyroid hormone is started on the first post-operative day in patients who have undergone a total thyroidectomy. Serum TSH and free T4 are tested 6 weeks postoperatively and the dose of oral thyroxine adjusted accordingly. Anti-thyroid medications are stopped following surgery and beta-blockers may be weaned.

11. Complications of surgery

The most important complications of thyroid surgery include recurrent laryngeal nerve injury, external superior laryngeal nerve injury, hypoparathyroidism, laryngeal oedema, bleeding, hypothyroidism/hyperthyroidism, wound infection and keloid scarring. Morbidity from thyroid surgery is minimised with meticulous anatomical dissection and operating in a bloodless field.

11.1. Airway obstruction

This complication, although rare, remains life-threatening. This can be due to sub-glottic and laryngeal oedema caused by venous and lymphatic obstruction, post-operative haematoma formation or bilateral recurrent laryngeal nerve damage. The identification of early signs of airway obstruction are crucial. It is recognised by a distressed patient and the presence of increasing stridor. Immediate suture removal and exploration of the wound is warranted. If no haematoma is demonstrated then one may proceed with conservative treatment with humidified oxygen and the administration of intravenous glucocorticoids. Anaesthetic input is recommended as intubation may be necessary to secure the patient's airway [22].

11.2. Haemorrhage

Haemostasis is paramount in thyroid surgery. Bleeding from the thyroid arteries and veins or the thyroid remnant can lead to the development of a haematoma deep to the strap muscles. A haematoma requires immediate decompression by opening all the layers of the wound and return to the operating room to control the underlying bleeding. The airway must be secured and sometimes a definitive airway is required although intubation for 24 hours with use of glucocorticoids and subsequent trial of extubation may save the patient a tracheostomy [22].

11.3. Nerve damage

Recurrent laryngeal nerve injury is rare and has been reported to occur 0.3-3% of cases permanently [127]. The incidence is increased in recurrent thyroid surgery and total thyroidectomy compared with thyroid lobectomy. The nerve can be typically injured or divided during ligation of the inferior thyroid artery or as it enters the larynx at the ligament of Berry. Mobilisation of large goitres can also stretch the nerve and make it more vulnerable to damage [10]. Paresis or partial damage of RLN, which is more common than complete transection, results in the vocal cord on the affected side adopting a midline adducted position [10]. Transient paresis of the RLN can occur with rates of 1.8% at one month and 0.5% at 3 months for first time operations suggesting improvement with time [22]. Symptoms of unilateral RLN damage include hoarseness, inability to speak loudly, fatiguable of the voice and an increased risk of aspiration [128]. In bilateral RLN damage both cords adopt a midline position and symptoms include total loss of voice, stridor and airway compromise requiring tracheostomy [10]. Measures to reduce RLN injury include pre-operative laryngoscopy to assess vocal cord function, direct identification of RLN and use of vocal cord stimulator intra-operatively.

The external branch of the superior laryngeal nerves lies close to the superior thyroid artery and can be damaged as the vessels are ligated and divided. Damage to the SLN causes the inability of the cricothyroid to tighten the vocal cords resulting in a weakness in phonation and a change in pitch of the voice [10]. These findings are more subtle than damage to the RLN and may be overlooked unless patients are specifically asked regarding symptoms [10]. Measures to avoid SLN injury include individually ligating the arterial branches close to the thyroid gland and identifying the nerve where possible [22].

11.4. Hyperthyroidism / Hypothyroidism

Hypothyroidism occurs with total thyroidecomy. In thyroid lobectomy, the incidence of hypothyroidism can be as high as 50% although the rate quoted is predominantly less than this, typically 20% [129]. Port-operative monitoring and follow-up of thyroid function is therefore needed. Hyperthyroidism, on the other hand, represents failure of the operation or the presence of thyroid remnants left in situ at the time of the operation. This occurs in around 5% of patients. The three common site of embryological recurrence or persistence of nodular goitre are within the pyramidal lobe, within thyroid rests in the thyrothymic tract or within posterior remnants associated with the tubercle of Zuckerkandl (Figure 9).

11.5. Parathyroid insufficiency and hypocalcaemia

Inadvertent damage or removal of a parathyroid gland can result in either temporary or permanent hypoparathyroidism post operatively. Careful identification of the parathyroid glands and their preservation are crucial in order to avoid this complication as discussed above. A study by Thomusch et al demonstrated transient hypoparathyroidism in 7.3% of patients and permanent parathyroid dysfunction in 1.5% of patients [130]. Ionised calcium and PTH levels should be measured immediately postoperatively, before discharge and at outpatient review. Thomusch et al demonstrated a correlation between long term hypoparathyroidism and the extent of initial surgery [130]. Further work within this group demonstrated other significant factors for the development of hypoparathyroidism which included patient gender, hospital operative volume, and Graves' disease [131].

The symptomatic outcome of hypoparathyroidism if either temporary or permanent hypocalcemia [132]. Symptoms of hypocalcemia include paresthesia (especially circumorally and in digits), cramps, carpopedal spasm, tetany and convulsions. Treatment is with calcium supplementation orally or intravenously depending on degree of hypocalcemia and the

http://dx.doi.org/10.5772/57499

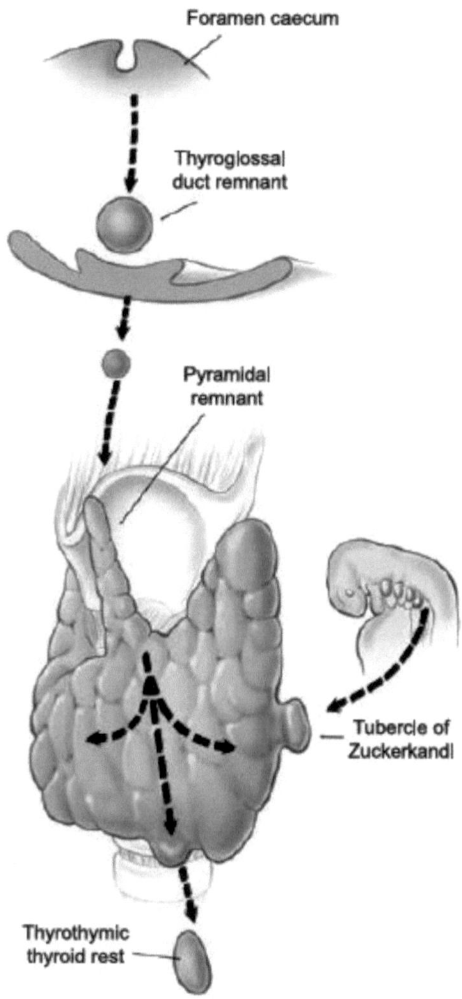

Figure 9. Embryological development of the thyroid gland [118]

presence of symptoms. Oral Vitamin D replacement can also be required. If calcium levels fail to increase the serum magnesium should be assessed and replaced as required [132].

Surgeons should be aware of the possibility of thyrotoxic patients developing Hungry bone syndrome post-operatively. As previously mentioned the presence of hyperthyroidism increases bone turnover [133,134] Therefore similar to its pathogenesis in parathyroid bone disease, removal of the excess thyroid hormone stimulation post thyroidectomy causes an imbalance in bone formation-resorption leading to an increase uptake of calcium, phosphate and magnesium in the osteoporotic bones [135,136] This leads to profound hypocalcemia, hypophosphatemia and hypomagnesemia. Treatment is with careful monitoring and electrolyte replacement [136].

11.6. Thyroid storm

This life-threatening condition is rarely seen post-operatively and is an acute exacerbation of thyroitoxicosis with an associated adrenergic response [137]. It accounts for less than 1–2% of all hospital admissions with hyperthyroidism but the mortality remains high at approximately 20–30% [138,139]. It typically occurs in patients who do not have an underlying diagnosis of hyperthyroidism. The crisis has an abrupt onset and is almost always evoked by a precipitating factor, such as infection, trauma, thyroidal surgery or radioactive iodine [3,16]. It is usually documented in patients undergoing thyroid surgery without adequate pre-operative preparation or where the diagnosis of thyrotoxicosis was not established [22]. Hormones released as a result of thyroid gland manipulation result in acute post-operative thyrotoxicosis[140]. Patients in crisis present with fever, abdominal pain, vomiting, diarrhoea, psychosis, altered mental state and coma. Signs include tachycardia, hypertension or hypotension, hyperpyrexia, atrial fibrillation and signs of congestive heart failure [141]. Treatment is aimed at reducing thyroid hormone secretion, supportive treatment and treatment of any underlying cause. It includes immediate fluid resuscitation, cooling with ice packs, supplemental oxygen, intravenous dextrose, diuretics and digoxin [22]. Specific treatments include intravenous beta blockers, propylthiouracil, potassium iodide and high dose steroids. Ensuring adequate and meticulous pre-operative preparation of patients should prevent this situation.

11.7. Tracheomalacia

Tracheomalacia represents a rare entity that is not completely understood. This condition is postulated to occur secondary to longstanding extrinsic tracheal compression with subsequent loss of tracheal cartilage rigidity, culminating in dynamic airway collapse in excess of 50% of diameter [142]. The typical manifestation of post-operative tracheomalacia is acute respiratory distress following extubation not explained by any other cause. This necessitates prompt re-intubation or a tracheostomy and the addition of high doses of glucocorticoids. A number of series failed to show cases of tracheomalacia [143,144], while a small number has been reported in others [145]. It has been postulated that this entity has been mistaken for unrecognised bilateral vocal cord paralysis [146]. Tracheomalacia is treated with intubation, tracheotomy, mesh repair of the posterior tracheal wall, trachelopexy and grafting.

12. Conclusion

Hyperthyroidism occurs as a result of an increase in thyroid hormone synthesis and secretion by the thyroid gland. This most commonly manifests as Graves' disease, multi-nodular goitre or a solitary toxic nodule. The management of hyperthyroidism is based on three treatment modalities, namely anti-thyroid medication, radioactive iodine ablation or surgery. Surgery increasingly plays an important role in the management of benign thyroid disease and has evolved into a cost-effective treatment with minimal associated morbidity and mortality. Total thyroidectomy is the surgery of choice in Graves' disease, while a total thyroidectomy or thyroid lobectomy are utilised in patients with toxic nodular goitres and this choice is dictated by the disease site and extent. Although thyroid surgery can be associated with significant complications, in high volume operative centres surgery provides effective long-lasting resolution of hyperthyroidism and therefore should be considered an integral component of treatment rather than the last resort of clinicians

Author details

Z. Al Hilli, C. Cheung, E.W. McDermott and R.S. Prichard

Department of Endocrine Surgery, St Vincent's University Hospital, Dublin, Ireland

References

[1] Turnbridge WM, Evered DC, Hall R, Appleton D, Brewis M, Clark F, et al. (2012) The spectrum of thyroid disease in a community: the Whickham survey. Clin Endocrinol (Oxf) 1977;7:481-93

[2] Franklyn JA, Boelaert K. Thyrotoxicosis. Lancet. 2012 Mar 24;379(9821):1155-66

[3] Cooper DS. Hyperthyroidism. Lancet. 2003 Aug 9;362(9382):459-68

[4] Lahey FA. Nonactivated (apathetic) type of hyperthyroidism. N Engl J Med 1931; 204: 747–48.

[5] Alsanea O, Clark OH. Treatment of Graves' disease: the advantages of surgery. Endocrinol Metab Clin North Am. 2000 Jun;29(2):321-37

[6] Little JW. Thyroid disorders. Part I: hyperthyroidism. Oral Surg Oral Med Oral Pathol Oral Radiol Endod. 2006 Mar;101(3):276-84

[7] Jameson JL, Weetman AP. Disorders of the thyroid gland: thyrotoxicosis.In: Kasper DL, Braunwald E, Fauci AS, Hauser SL, Longo DL, Jameson JL, et al., editors. Harrison's principles of internal medicine. 16th ed. New York: McGraw-Hill; 2005. p. 2113-2117, Chapter 320

[8] Pieracci FM, Fahey TJ 3rd. Effect of hospital volume of thyroidectomies on outcomes following substernal thyroidectomy. World J Surg. 2008 May;32(5):740-6

[9] Jameson JL, Weetman AP. Disorders of the thyroid gland: anatomy and development. In: Kasper DL, Braunwald E, Fauci AS, Hauser SL, Longo DL, Jameson JL, et al., editors. Harrison's principles of internal medicine. 16th ed. New York: McGraw-Hill; 2005. p. 2105, Chapter 320

[10] Harold Ellis (2002) The Thyroid Gland in Clinical Anatomy Tenth Edition Blackwell p284-285

[11] Drake RL, Vogl W, Mitchell AWM (2005) Head and Neck In Gray's Anatomy for medical students. Elsevier Churchill Livingstone p916-918

[12] McMullen TPW, Delbridge LW Thyroid Embryology, Anatomy, and Physiology: A Review for the Surgeon In Hubbard J, Inabnet WB,Lo CY(editors), Endocrine Surgery, Principles and Practice, Springer London 2009 p3-16

[13] Cernea CR, Ferraz AR, Nishio S, Dutra A Jr, Hojaij FC, dos Santos LR. Surgical anatomy of the external branch of the superior laryngeal nerve. Head Neck. 1992 Sep-Oct; 14(5):380-3

[14] Kierner AC, Aigner M, Burian M. The external branch of the superior laryngeal nerve: its topographical anatomy as related to surgery of the neck. Arch Otolaryngol Head Neck Surg. 1998 Mar;124(3):301-3

[15] Levy EG. Thyroid disease in the elderly. Med Clin North Am. 1991 Jan;75(1):151-67

[16] Weetman AP. Graves' disease. N Engl J Med. 2000 Oct 26;343(17):1236-48

[17] O'Hanlon KM, Baustian GH, Toth DW, In: Hyperthyroidism. contributors: First Consult [database on the internet]. St. Louis: Elsevier, Inc.; c2006 [cited 2006 Aug 10]. Available from: http://www.firstconsult.com/fc_home/members/?urn=com.firstconsult/1/101

[18] Davies TF, Larsen PR. Thyrotoxicosis In Larsen PR, Kronenberg HM, Melmed D, Polonsky KS editors. Willams Textbook of Endocrinology 10thed Philadelphia W.B. Saunders:2003 p374-414

[19] Reid JR, Wheeler SF. Hyperthyroidism: diagnosis and treatment. Am Fam Physician. 2005 15;72(4):623-30

[20] Knudson PB. Hyperthyroidism in adults: variable clinical presentations and approaches to diagnosis. J Am Board Fam Pract 1995;8:109-13

[21] Ronnov-Jessen V, Kirkegaard C. Hyperthyroidism: a disease of old age? BMJ 1973;1: 41–43.

[22] Krukowski ZH (2008) The Thyroid and Parathyroid glands. In: Williams N, Bulstrode CJK, O'Connell PR Bailey and Love's Short Practice of Surgery 25th edition. Hodder Arnold p772-800

[23] Cobler JL, Williams ME, Greenland P. Thyrotoxicosis in institutionalized elderly patients with atrial fibrillation. Arch Intern Med1984; 144: 1758–60

[24] Shimizu T, Koide S, Noh JY, Sugino K, Ito K, Nakazawa H. Hyperthyroidism and the management of atrial fibrillation. Thyroid 2002; 12: 489–93

[25] Franklyn JA, Sheppard MC, Maisonneuve P. Thyroid function and mortality in patients treated for hyperthyroidism. JAMA. 2005 Jul 6;294(1):71-80

[26] Siu CW, Zhang XH, Yung C, Kung AW, Lau CP, Tse HF. Hemodynamic changes in hyperthyroidism-related pulmonary hypertension: a prospective echocardiographic study. J Clin Endocrinol Metab. 2007 May;92(5):1736-42

[27] Barsal G, Taneli F, Atay A, Hekimsoy Z, Erciyas F. Serum osteocalcin levels in hyperthyroidism before and after antithyroid therapy. Tohoku J Exp Med. 2004 Jul;203(3): 183-8

[28] Britto JM, Fenton AJ, Holloway WR, Nicholson GC. Osteoblasts mediate thyroid hormone stimulation of osteoclastic bone resorption. Endocrinology. 1994 Jan;134(1): 169-76

[29] Galliford TM, Murphy E, Williams AJ, Bassett JH, Williams GR. Effects of thyroid status on bone metabolism: a primary role for thyroid stimulating hormone or thyroid hormone? Minerva Endocrinol. 2005 Dec;30(4):237-46

[30] Wang, X, et.al. Development of a Highly Sensitive and Selective Microplate Chemiluminescence Enzyme Immunoassay for the Determination of Free Thyroxine in Human Serum. Int. J. Biol. Sci. 2007; 3(5):274-280

[31] Villalta D. et.al. Analytical and diagnostic accuracy of "second generation" assays for thyrotropin receptor antibodies with radioactive and chemiluminescent tracers. J Clin Pathol. 2004; 57:378-382

[32] Sharma M, Aronow WS, Patel L, Gandhi K, Desai H. Hyperthyroidism. Med Sci Monit. 2011 ;17(4): 85-91.

[33] Auer J, Scheibner P, Mische T, Langsteger W, Eber O, Eber B. Subclinical hyperthyroidism as a risk factor for atrial fibrillation. Am Heart J. 2001 Nov;142(5):838-42.

[34] Haentjens P, Van Meerhaeghe A, Poppe K, Velkeniers B. Subclinical thyroid dysfunction and mortality: an estimate of relative and absolute excess all-cause mortality based on time-to-event data from cohort studies. Eur J Endocrinol. 2008 Sep;159(3): 329-41

[35] Horace K. Ivy, MD; Heinz W. Wahner, MD; Colum A. Gorman, MB, BCh"Triiodothyronine (T3) Toxicosis"Its Role in Graves' Disease Arch Intern Med. 1971;128(4): 529-534.

[36] Grossman ET, Yousmen DM. Extramucosal Diseases of the Head and Neck In Neuroradiology. Second Edition: Mosby: 2003. p 697-750

[37] American Thyroid Association (ATA) Guidelines Taskforce on Thyroid Nodules and Differentiated Thyroid Cancer, Cooper DS, Doherty GM, Haugen BR, Kloos RT, Lee SL, Mandel SJ, Mazzaferri EL, McIver B, Pacini F, Schlumberger M, Sherman SI, Steward DL, Tuttle RM. Revised American Thyroid Association management guidelines for patients with thyroid nodules and differentiated thyroid cancer. Thyroid. 2009 Nov;19(11):1167-214.

[38] Randolph GW. Surgery of the Thyroid and Parathyroid Glands. Second Edition: Elsevier: 2013

[39] Lee JC, Harris AM, Khafagi FA. Thyroid scans. Aust Fam Physician. 2012 Aug;41(8): 584-6.

[40] McHenry CR, Lo CY. The Surgical Management of Hyperthyroidism. In Randolph GW. Surgery of the Thyroid and Parathyroid Glands. Second Edition: Elsevier: 2013p 85-94

[41] Graves RJ. Clinical lectures delivered during the sessions 1834–5 and 1836–7. In: Dunglison's American Medical Library. Philadelphia: Adam Waldie; 1838. p.134–6.

[42] Brand OJ, Gough SC. Genetics of thyroid autoimmunity and the role of the TSHR. Mol Cell Endocrinol. 2010 Jun 30;322(1-2):135-43

[43] Boelaert K, Newby PR, Simmonds MJ, Holder RL, Carr-Smith JD, Heward JM, Manji N, Allahabadia A, Armitage M, Chatterjee KV, Lazarus JH, Pearce SH, Vaidya B, Gough SC, Franklyn JA. Prevalence and relative risk of other autoimmune diseases in subjects with autoimmune thyroid disease. Am J Med. 2010 Feb;123(2):183.e1-9

[44] Maitra A, Abbas AK. Thyroid Gland In:Robbin's and Cotran Pathologic Basis of Disease, Kumar, Abbas, Fausto 7th edition. Elsevier Saunders p1164-1183

[45] Burch HB, Wartofsky L. Graves' ophthalmopathy: current concepts regarding pathogenesis and management. Endocr Rev. 1993 Dec;14(6):747-93

[46] Bartalena L, Pinchera A, Marcocci C. Management of Graves' ophthalmopathy: reality and perspectives. Endocr Rev. 2000 Apr;21(2):168-99

[47] Schott M, Hermsen D, Broecker-Preuss M, Casati M, Mas JC, Eckstein A, Gassner D, Golla R, Graeber C, van Helden J, Inomata K, Jarausch J, Kratzsch J, Miyazaki N, Moreno MA, Murakami T, Roth HJ, Stock W, Noh JY, Scherbaum WA, Mann K. Clinical value of the first automated TSH receptor autoantibody assay for the diagnosis of Graves' disease (GD): an international multicentre trial. Clin Endocrinol (Oxf). 2009 Oct;71(4):566-73.

[48] Hamburger JI. The autonomously functioning thyroid nodule: Goetsch's disease. Endocr Rev. 1987 Nov;8(4):439-47

[49] Siegel RD, Lee SL. Toxic nodular goiter: toxic adenoma and toxic multinodular goiter. Endocrinol Metab Clin North Am 1998; 27:151–68

[50] Baliga R R 250 cases in Clinical Medicine 4th edition. Saunders Elesevier Case 140 Multinodular Goitre: p524-527

[51] Corvilain B, Dumont JF, Vassart G. Toxic adenoma and toxic multinodular goiter. In: Werner SC, Ingbar SH, Braverman LE, Utiger RD, eds. Werner & Ingbar's the thyroid: a fundamental and clinical text. 8th ed. Philadelphia: Lippincott Williams & Wilkins, 2000:564-72.

[52] Hegedus L: Clinical practice. The thyroid nodule. N Engl J Med 2004, 351:1764-1771

[53] Vander JB, Gaston EA, Dawber TR. The significance of non toxic thyroid nodules: final report of a 15 year study of the incidence of thyroid malignancy. Ann Intern Med 1968; 69: 537-540

[54] Törring O, Tallstedt L, Wallin G, Lundell G, Ljunggren JG, Taube A, Säaf M, Hamberger B. Graves' hyperthyroidism: treatment with antithyroid drugs, surgery, or radioiodine--a prospective, randomized study. Thyroid Study Group. J Clin Endocrinol Metab. 1996 Aug;81(8):2986-93

[55] Poshyachinda M Management of Hyperthyroidism in Therapeutic applications of radiopharmaceuticals, Proceedings of an international seminar held in Hyderabad, India, 18–22 January 1999 International Atomic Energy Agency 2001. P39-46 available online at http://www-pub.iaea.org/MTCD/publications/PDF/te_1228_prn.pdf

[56] Wartofsky L, Treatment options for hyperthyroidism, Hosp. Prac. 31(1996 Sep 15) 69–83

[57] Bender JM, Dworkin JM., "Therapy of hyperthyroidism", Nuclear Medicine, Vol II (Henkin, R., et al., Eds.), Mosby-Year Book, St Louis (1996) p 1549–1556.

[58] Nedrebo BG, Holm PI, Uhlving S, Sorheim JI, Skeie S, Eide GE, Husebye ES, Lien EA, Aanderud S. Predictors of outcome and comparison of different drug regimens for the prevention of relapse in patients with Graves' disease. Eur J Endocrinol. 2002 Nov;147(5):583-9

[59] Woeber KA. Methimazole-induced hepatotoxicity. Endocr Pract. 2002 May-Jun;8(3): 222-

[60] Noh JY, Asari T, Hamada N, Makino F, Ishikawa N, Abe Y, Ito K, Ito K. Frequency of appearance of myeloperoxidase-antineutrophil cytoplasmic antibody (MPO-ANCA) in Graves' disease patients treated with propylthiouracil and the relationship between MPO-ANCA and clinical manifestations. Clin Endocrinol (Oxf). 2001 May; 54(5):651-4

[61] Cooper DS. Antithyroid drugs. N Engl J Med. 2005 Mar 3;352(9):905-17

[62] Lamberg BA, Salmi J, Wägar G, Mäkinen T. Spontaneous hypothyroidism after antithyroid treatment of hyperthyroid Graves' disease. J Endocrinol Invest. 1981 Oct-Dec;4(4):399-402

[63] Harper MB, Mayeaux EJ Jr. Thyroid disease. In: Taylor RB. Family medicine:principles and practice. 6th ed. New York: Springer, 2003:1042-52

[64] Ginsberg J. Diagnosis and management of Graves' disease. CMAJ. 2003 Mar 4;168(5): 575-85

[65] Bartalena L, Marcocci C, Bogazzi F, Manetti L, Tanda ML, Dell'Unto E, Bruno-Bossio G, Nardi M, Bartolomei MP, Lepri A, Rossi G, Martino E, Pinchera A. Relation be-

tween therapy for hyperthyroidism and the course of Graves' ophthalmopathy. N Engl J Med. 1998 Jan 8;338(2):73-8.

[66] Bonnema SJ, Bennedbaek FN, Veje A, Marving J, Hegedüs L. Continuous methimazole therapy and its effect on the cure rate of hyperthyroidism using radioactive iodine: an evaluation by a randomized trial. J Clin Endocrinol Metab. 2006 Aug;91(8): 2946-51

[67] Poshyahinda M, Boonvisut S, Buacum V, Onthuam Y. "Analysis of I–131 treatment for Graves' disease with long term follow-up", the Third Asia and Oceania Congress of Nuclear Medicine (Abstract), Seoul (1984) 112

[68] Kendall-Taylor P, Keir MJ, Ross WM. Ablative radioiodine therapy for hyperthyroidism: long term follow up study. Br Med J (Clin Res Ed). 1984 Aug 11;289(6441):361-3

[69] Boger MS, Perrier ND. Advantages and disadvantages of surgical therapy and optimal extent of thyroidectomy for the treatment of hyperthyroidism. Surg Clin North Am. 2004 Jun;84(3):849-74

[70] Gough IR, Wilkinson D. Total thyroidectomy for management of thyroid disease. World J Surg 2000; 24:962-965

[71] Bliss R, Gauger PG, Delbridge L. Surgeon's approach to the thyroid gland: Surgical anatomy and the importance of technique. World J S 2000: 24: 891-897

[72] Bron LP, O'Brien CJ. Total thyroidectomy for clinically benign disease of the thyroid gland. Br J Surg 2004;91:569-574

[73] Friguglietti CU, Lin CS, Kulesar MA. Total thyroidectomy for benign thyroid disease. Laryngoscopy 2003; 113: 1820-1826

[74] Rios A, Rodriguez JM, Balsalbore MD et al. Results of surgery for toxic multinodular goiter. Surg Today 2005;35:901-906

[75] Efremidou EI, Papageorgiou MS, Liratzopoulos N, Manolas KJ. The efficacy and safety of total thyroidectomy in the management of benign thyroid disease: a review of 932 cases. Can J Surg. 2009 Feb;52(1):39-44

[76] Ballentone R, Lombardi CO, BOssola M, Boscherini M, De Crea C, Alesina P, Traini E, Princi P, Raffaelli M. Total thyroidectomy for the management for benign thyroid disease: review of 526 cases. World J Surgery 2002; 26(12): 1468-1471

[77] Pappalardo G, Guadalaxara A, Frattaroli FM, Illomei G, Falaschi P. Total compared with subtotal thyroidectomy in benign nodular disease: personal series and review of published reports. Eur J Surg. 1998 Jul;164(7):501-6

[78] Sundaresh V, Brito JP, Wang Z, Prokop LJ, Stan MN, Murad MH, Bahn RS. Comparative Effectiveness of Therapies for Graves' Hyperthyroidism: A Systematic Review and Network Meta-analysis. J Clin Endocrinol Metab. 2013 Jul 3

[79] Coudhury MM, Dagash H, Pierro A. A systematic review of the impact of volume of surgery and specialization on patient outcome. Br J Surg 2007: 94(2): 145-161

[80] Boudourakis LD, Want TS, Roman SA, Desei R, Sosa JA. Evolution of the surgeon-volume, patient-outcome relationship. Ann Surg 2009; 250(1): 159-165

[81] Pieracci FM, Fahey TJ 3rd. Effect of hospital volume of thyroidectomies on outcomes following substernal thyroidectomy. World J Surg 2008; 32(5): 740-746

[82] Barczyński M, Konturek A, Hubalewska-Dydejczyk A, Gołkowski F, Nowak W Randomized clinical trial of bilateral subtotal thyroidectomy versus total thyroidectomy for Graves' disease with a 5-year follow-up. Br J Surg. 2012 Apr;99(4):515-22

[83] Palit TK, Miller CC 3rd, Miltenburg DM. The efficacy of thyroidectomy for Graves' disease: A meta-analysis. J Surg Res. 2000 May 15;90(2):161-5

[84] Witte J, Goretzki PE, Dotzenrath C, Simon D, Felis P, Neubauer M, Röher HD Surgery for Graves' disease: total versus subtotal thyroidectomy-results of a prospective randomized trial. World J Surg. 2000 Nov;24(11):1303-11

[85] Erickson D, Gharib H, Li H, van Heerden JA. Treatment of patients with toxic multinodular goiter. Thyroid 1998; 8: 277–82

[86] Steinmüller T, Ulrich F, Rayes N, Lang M, Seehofer D, Tullius SG, Jonas S, Neuhaus P:Surgical procedures and risk factors in therapy of benign multinodular goiter. A statistical comparison of the incidence of complications. Chirurg. 2001 Dec;72(12): 1453-7

[87] Rayes N, Steinmüller T, Schröder S, Klötzler A, Bertram H, Denecke T, Neuhaus P, Seehofer D.Bilateral subtotal thyroidectomy versus hemithyroidectomy plus subtotal resection (Dunhill procedure) for benign goiter: long-term results of a prospective, randomized study. World J Surg. 2013 Jan;37(1):84-90

[88] Barczynski M, Konturek A, Hubalewski-Dydejczyk A et al (2010) Five-year follow up of a randomized clinical trial of total thyroidectomy versus Dunhill operation versus bilateral subtotal thyroidectomy for multinodular nontoxic goiter. World J Surg 34:1203–1213

[89] Wheeler MH (1998) Total thyroidectomy for benign thyroid disease. Lancet 351:1526–1527

[90] Agarwal G, Aggarwal V (2008) Is total thyroidectomy the surgical procedure of choice for benign multinodular goiter? An evidence-based review. World J Surg 32:1313–1324

[91] Delbridge L (2008) Symposium on evidence-based endocrine surgery (2): benign thyroid disease. World J Surg 32:1235–1236

[92] Mayo CH, Mayo CW. Pre-iodine and post-iodine days: a review of 37,228 cases of goiter at the Mayo Clinic. Western J Surg 1935;9:477–820

[93] Langley RW, Burch HB. Perioperative management of the thyrotoxic patient. Endocrinol Metab Clin North Am. 2003 Jun;32(2):519-34

[94] Lahey FH. The decisions for surgery and the management of the patient with hypertension. Surg Clin N Am 1933;13:731–4

[95] Wool MS. Hyperthyroidism. In: Cady C, Rossi RL, editors. Surgery of the thyroid and parathyroid glands. 3rd edition. Philadelphia: WB Saunders; 1991. p. 121–30

[96] Cooper DS, Daniels GH, Ladenson PW, Ridgway EC. Hyperthyroxinemia in patients treated with high-dose propranolol. Am J Med 1982;73:867–71

[97] Farling PA. Thyroid disease. Br J Anaesth. 2000 Jul;85(1):15-28

[98] Plummer HS. Results of administering iodine to patients having exophthalmic goiter. JAMA 1923;80:155–6.

[99] Yamada E, Yamazaki K, Takano K, Obara T, Sato K 2006 Iodide inhibits vascular endothelial growth factor-A expression in cultured human thyroid follicles: a microarray search for effects of thyrotropin and iodide on angiogenesis factors. Thyroid 16:545–554

[100] Erbil Y, Ozluk Y, Giriş M, Salmaslioglu A, Issever H, Barbaros U, Kapran Y, Ozarmağan S, Tezelman S. Effect of lugol solution on thyroid gland blood flow and microvessel density in the patients with Graves' disease. J Clin Endocrinol Metab. 2007 Jun;92(6):2182-9

[101] Wartofsky L, Ransil BJ, Ingbar SH. Inhibition by iodine of the release of thyroxine from the thyroid glands of patients with thyrotoxicosis. J Clin Invest 1970;49:78–86.

[102] Wolff J, Chaikoff IL, Goldberg RC, Meier JR. The temporary nature of the inhibitory action of excess iodide on organic iodine synthesis in the normal thyroid. Endocrinology 1949;45:504–13

[103] Eng PH, Cardona GR, Fang SL, Previti M, Alex S, Carrasco N, Chin WW, Braverman LE. Escape from the acute Wolff-Chaikoff effect is associated with a decrease in thyroid sodium/iodide symporter messenger ribonucleic acid and protein. Endocrinology. 1999 Aug;140(8):3404-10

[104] Vagenakis AF, Braverman LE. Adverse effects of iodides on thyroid function. Med Clin N Am 1975;59:1075–88

[105] Kirk RM. General Surgical Operations. Fifth Edition: Chirchill Livingstone: 2006

[106] Sturgeon C, Sturgeon T, Angelos P Neuromonitoring in thyroid surgery: attitudes, usage patterns, and predictors of use among endocrine surgeons World J Surg. 2009;33(3):417

[107] Randolph GW, Dralle H, International Intraoperative Monitoring Study Group, Abdullah H, Barczynski M, Bellantone R, Brauckhoff M, Carnaille B, Cherenko S, Chiang FY, Dionigi G, Finck C, Hartl D, Kamani D, Lorenz K, Miccolli P, Mihai R,

Miyauchi A, Orloff L, Perrier N, Poveda MD, Romanchishen A, Serpell J, Sitges-Serra A, Sloan T, Van Slycke S, Snyder S, Takami H, Volpi E, Woodson G Electrophysiologic recurrent laryngeal nerve monitoring during thyroid and parathyroid surgery: international standards guideline statement. Laryngoscope. 2011 Jan;121 Suppl 1:S1-16

[108] Dralle H, Sekulla C, Haerting J, Timmermann W, Neumann HJ, Kruse E, Grond S, Mühlig HP, Richter C, Voss J, Thomusch O, Lippert H, Gastinger I, Brauckhoff M, Gimm O. Risk factors of paralysis and functional outcome after recurrent laryngeal nerve monitoring in thyroid surgery. Surgery. 2004;136(6):131

[109] Angelos P Recurrent laryngeal nerve monitoring: state of the art, ethical and legal issues. Surg Clin North Am. 2009;89(5):1157

[110] Dralle H, Sekulla C, Lorenz K, Brauckhoff M, Machens A; German IONM Study Group. Intraoperative monitoring of the recurrent laryngeal nerve in thyroid surgery. World J Surg. 2008 Jul;32(7):1358-66. doi: 10.1007/s00268-008-9483-2. Review.

[111] Atallah I, Dupret A, Carpentier AS, Weingertner AS, Volkmar PP, Rodier JF. Role of intraoperative neuromonitoring of the recurrent laryngeal nerve in high-risk thyroid surgery. J Otolaryngol Head Neck Surg. 2009 Dec;38(6):613-8

[112] Chan WF, Lang BH, Lo CY. The role of intraoperative neuromonitoring of recurrent laryngeal nerve during thyroidectomy: a comparative study on 1000 nerves at risk. Surgery. 2006 Dec;140(6):866-72; discussion 872-3

[113] Barczyński M, Konturek A, Cichoń S. Randomized clinical trial of visualization versus neuromonitoring of recurrent laryngeal nerves during thyroidectomy. Br J Surg. 2009 Mar;96(3):240-6

[114] Chan WF, Lo CY. Pitfalls of intraoperative neuromonitoring for predicting postoperative recurrent laryngeal nerve function during thyroidectomy. World J Surg. 2006 May;30(5):806-12

[115] Clark OH, Caron NR. Chapter 34: Fine needle aspiration biopsy of the thyroid, Thyroid lobectomy and sub-total and total thyroidectomy. In Josef E. Fischer, Kirby I. Bland, Mark P. Callery: Mastery of Surgery, Volume 1, Lippincott Williams & Wilkins, p398-411

[116] Mosby's Dental Dictionary, 2nd edition. © 2008 Elsevier, Inc available at http://medical-dictionary.thefreedictionary.com/thyroid+gland

[117] Delbridge L. Total thyroidectomy: the evolution of surgical technique ANZ J Surg. 2003 Sep;73(9):761-8

[118] Sanabria A, Carvalho AL, Silver CE, Rinaldo A, Shaha AR, Kowalski LP, Ferlito A. Routine drainage after thyroid surgery--a meta-analysis. J Surg Oncol. 2007 Sep 1;96(3):273-80

[119] Shaha AR Revision thyroid surgery-technical considerations. Otolaryngol Clin North Am. 2008;41(6):1169

[120] Lefevre JH, Tresallet C, Leenhardt L, Jublanc C, Chigot JP, Menegaux F Reoperative surgery for thyroid disease. Langenbecks Arch Surg. 2007;392(6):685

[121] Levin KE, Clark AH, Duh QY, Demeure M, Siperstein AE, Clark OH Reoperative thyroid surgery. Surgery. 1992;111(6):604

[122] Kraim ps JL, Marechaud R, Gineste D, Fieuzal S, Metaye T, Carretier M, Barbier J. Analysis and pre prevention of recurrent goitre. Surg Gynecol Obstet 1993: 176; 319 – 322

[123] Seiler CA, Glaser C, Wagner HE. Thyroid gland surgery in an endemic region. World J Surg 1996: 20:20; 593–597

[124] Prichard RS, Delbridge L. Reoperation for Benign Disease. p95-104. In: Randolph GW. Surgery of the Thyroid and Parathyroid Glands. Second Edition: Elsevier: 2013

[125] Cushieri A, Grace PA, Darzi A, Borley,Rowley DI Chapter 34 Disorders of the Endocrine Gland In Clinical Surgery second edition Blakwell Publishing p441-449

[126] Cayo AK, Yen TW, Misustin SM, Wall K, Wilson SD, Evans DB, Wang TS Predicting the need for calcium and calcitriol supplementation after total thyroidectomy: results of a prospective, randomized study. Surgery. 2012 Dec;152(6):1059-67. Epub 2012 Oct 13

[127] Hayward NJ, Grodski S, Yeung M, Johnson WR, Serpell J. Recurrent laryngeal nerve injury in thyroid surgery: a review. ANZ J Surg. 2013 Jan;83(1-2):15-21

[128] Banerjee S Chapter 3 Ear, Nose and Throat, Head and Neck In Parchment Smith Essential Revision Notes for Intercollegiate MRCS Book 2 PasTest p809-814

[129] Sadler GP, Mihai R. The thyroid gland. Lennard TWJ. A Companion to Specialist Surgical Practice. Endocrine Surgery. Fourth Edition: Saunders: 2009 p39-72

[130] Thomusch O, Machens A, Sekulla C, Ukkat J, Brauckhoff M, Dralle H. The impact of surgical technique on postoperative hypoparathyroidism in bilateral thyroid surgery: a multivariate analysis of 5846 consecutive patients. Surgery. 2003 Feb;133(2):180-5.

[131] Thomusch O, Machens A, Sekulla C, Ukkat J, Lippert H, Gastinger I, Dralle H. Multivariate analysis of risk factors for postoperative complications in benign goiter surgery: prospective multicenter study in Germany. World J Surg. 2000 Nov;24(11): 1335-41

[132] Tait C (2010) Chapter 5 Endocrine Surgery In Parchment Smith Essential Revision Notes for Intercollegiate MRCS Book 2 PasTest p937-953

[133] Dent CE, Harper CM. Hypoparathyroid tetany (following thyroidectomy) apparently resistant to vitamin D. Proc R Soc Med 1958; 51:489

[134] Jones RM, Davidson CM. Thyrotoxicosis and the hungry bone syndrome: a cause of postoperative tetany. J R Coll Surg Edinb 1987; 32:24

[135] Brasier AR, Nussbaum SR. Hungry bone syndrome: clinical and biochemical predictors of its occurrence after parathyroid surgery. Am J Med 1988; 84:654.

[136] Berkoben, M, Quarles D Hungry bone syndrome following parathyroidectomy. Aug, 2012. Up to Date, Editors: Goldfarb S, Sheridan A. Available at http://www.uptodate.com/contents/hungry-bone-syndrome-following-parathyroidectomy

[137] Green MF. The endocrine system. In: Pathy MSJ, editor. Principles and practice of geriatric medicine. 2nd ed. New York:John Wiley & Sons; 1991. p. 1061-122

[138] Jameson L, Weetman A: Disorders of the thyroid gland. Harrison's principles of internal medicine. 15th edition. Edited by Brawnwald E, Fauci A, Kasper D. New York: McGraw-Hill; 2001::2060-2084

[139] Tietgens ST, Leinung MC: Thyroid storm.Med Clin North Am 1995, 79:169-184

[140] Carroll R, Matfin G. Endocrine and metabolic emergencies: thyroid storm. Ther Adv Endocrinol Metab. 2010 Jun;1(3):139-45

[141] Burch HB, Wartofsky L. Life-threatening thyrotoxicosis: thyroid storm. Endocrinol Metab Clin North Am 1993; 22: 263–77

[142] Kandaswamy C, Balasubramanian V.Review of adult tracheomalacia and its relationship with chronic obstructive pulmonary disease. Curr Opin Pulm Med2009;15:113-9

[143] Melliere D, Guterman R, Danis RK. [Substernal goitre. Report of 45 cases (author's transl)]. [Article in French] J Chir (Paris). 1980 Jan;117(1):13-8

[144] McHenry CR, Piotrowski JJ. Thyroidectomy in patients with marked thyroid enlargement: airway management, morbidity, and outcome. Am Surg. 1994 Aug;60(8): 586-91.

[145] Geelhoed GW. Tracheomalacia from compressing goiter: management after thyroidectomy Surgery. 1988 Dec;104(6):1100-8

[146] Randolph GW, Shin JJ, Grillo HC, Mathisen D, Katlic MR, Kamani D, Zurakowski D. The surgical management of goiter: Part II. Surgical treatment and results. Laryngoscope. 2011 Jan;121(1):68-76

Chapter 9

Trophoblastic Hyperthyroidism and Its Perioperative Concerns

Madhuri S. Kurdi

Additional information is available at the end of the chapter

http://dx.doi.org/10.5772/57523

1. Introduction

A moderately built 25-year-old female with a 24-week pregnancy and per-vaginal bleeding is brought to the operation theatre in the wee hours of the morning for suction evacuation. Her medical and surgical histories are unremarkable. She is highly irritable and moderately pale. She has a pulse rate of 156 beats per minute, blood pressure of 110/80 mm of Hg, respiratory rate of 32 breaths per minute and mild pedal oedema. Her haemoglobin level is 8 gm/dl. Her thyroid function tests are markedly deranged showing severe biochemical hyperthyroidism (SerumT_3*– 6.46 mmol/L,* T_4 *– 470 nmol/L and TSH – 0.03 μ IU/ml). The serum β hCG levels are markedly raised. An ultra-sonogram shows signs of a complete molar pregnancy.*

This is a typical presentation of gestational trophoblastic disease with trophoblastic hyperthyroidism.

Gestational trophoblastic disease includes a group of pregnancy-related tumours called trophoblastic tumours. These include hydatidiform mole and choriocarcinoma. Hyperthyroidism is a rare complication of gestational trophoblastic disease. It is called trophoblastic hyperthyroidism.

2. Gestational trophoblastic disease

The abnormal proliferation of trophoblastic tissue in the developing human placenta results in the condition known as Gestational Trophoblastic Neoplasia [1,2]. Gestational Trophoblastic Neoplasia lesions are histologically distinct malignant lesions that include hydatidiform mole, choriocarcinoma, placental site trophoblastic tumour and epithelioid trophoblastic tumour.

Gestational Trophoblastic Neoplasia often arises after molar pregnancy. It can also occur after any gestation including miscarriages and term pregnancies [2].

Gestational trophoblastic disease is a family of diseases that includes complete and partial molar pregnancy also known as hydatidiform mole, locally invasive or Disseminated choriocarcinoma and placental site trophoblastic tumour [3]. Placental site trophoblastic tumour, invasive mole and choriocarcinoma are termed Gestational Trophoblastic Tumours. They are malignant while hydatidiform mole is a benign form of Gestational Trophoblastic Disease [4].

2.1. Classification of gestational trophoblastic disease (FIGO) (International Federation of Gynaecology and Obstetrics) [5]

Hydatidiform mole-

- complete
- partial

Gestational Trophoblastic Neoplasia-

- Invasive mole
- Choriocarcinoma
- Placental site trophoblastic tumor
- Epithelioid trophoblastic tumor

2.2. Hydatidiform mole

It is an abnormal condition of the ovum where there are partly degenerative and partly hyperplastic changes in the young chorionic villi. These result in the formation of clusters of small cysts of varying sizes. Because of its superficial resemblance to hydatid cyst, it is named as hydatidiform mole and the pregnancy associated with it is known as molar pregnancy. It is best regarded as a benign neoplasia of the chorion with malignant potential [6].

Molar pregnancy is common in Oriental countries – Philippines, China, Indonesia, Japan and India as also in Africa and Central and Latin America [6]. The incidence of molar pregnancy has been reported to range between 0.5 and 2 to 2.5 per one thousand pregnancies [7,8,9]. In some Asian countries, the incidence is as high as 1 in 82 pregnancies [1]. The highest incidence is in Philippines being 1 in 80 pregnancies and lowest in European countries, North America,Australia and New Zealand [6,10]. In the United States,hydatidiform moles are observed in approximately 1in 600 therapeutic abortions and 1 in 1000-2000 pregnancies [2,11]. The incidence in India is about 1 in 400 pregnancies [12]. In Nepal, the incidence of gestational trophoblastic disease as per records from different hospitals is 5.1,2.9,2.8and 4.1 per 1000 live births [13].The incidence of hydatidiform mole in the Middle East is 1:60 to 1:500 [14].

Molar pregnancies develop as a result of abnormal fertilisation [6]. Risk factors for developing a molar pregnancy include advanced maternal age, teen age, inadequate nutrition, disturbed maternal immune mechanisms, cytogenetic abnormality, environmental factors and a history of hydatidiform mole [1]. Although most molar pregnancies are sporadic, a familial syndrome of recurrent hydatidiform mole has been described and first reported in 1980, suggesting an autosomal recessive inheritance pattern [15,16].

2.2.1. *Pathology of hydatidiform mole [6]*

Naked eye appearance. (fig 1)

The mass in the uterus is made of multiple chains and clusters of cysts of varying sizes from a pin head to that of a large grape. The embryo and amniotic sac may or may not be seen. Red areas may be seen suggesting haemorrhage in the decidual space [6] (fig 1)

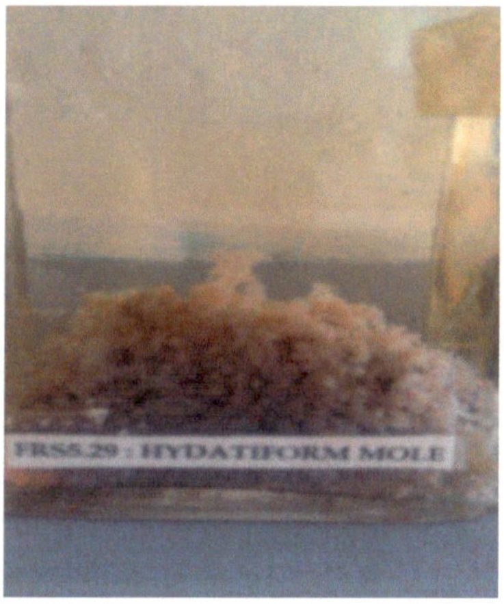

Figure 1. Gross appearance of hydatidiform mole

Microscopic appearance

The villus pattern is distinctly maintained. The vesicles are filled with interstitial fluid that is almost similar to ascitic or oedema fluid but rich in hCG. There are no blood vessels.

2.2.2. *Clinical features of hydatidiform mole*

The traditional presenting features include vaginal bleeding, excessive uterine size, hyperemesis gravidarum, theca lutein cysts and preeclampsia in early pregnancy [17,18]. The clinical presentation has significantly changed in the past years [19].Modern facilities like ultrasonography and serum alpha hCG help early diagnosis even before any signs and symptoms appear [20].

Symptoms: [6]

1. Vaginal bleeding – It may be mixed with fluid from the ruptured cysts giving the appearance of 'white currant in red currant juice'.This is the most common symptom, being present in about 70-90% cases. [19]
2. Lower abdominal pain-This is due to infection, uterine perforation or uterine contractions.
3. Constitutional symptoms – Patient appears sick, has excessive vomiting, breathlessness, thyrotoxic features like tremors, palpitations, anxiety, weight loss and increased appetite.
4. Expulsion of grape-like vesicles per vaginum.

Signs: [6]

1. Signs of early pregnancy.
2. Patient looks very ill.
3. Prominent pallor out of proportion to blood loss.
4. Features of toxaemia (hypertension, oedema and proteinuria) are present in about 50% of cases. Rarely convulsions may occur.
5. Per abdomen –
   a. The size of uterus is more than expected for the period of amenorrhoea.
   b. The uterus feels firm and elastic(doughy) because of the absence of amniotic fluid sac.
   c. Foetal parts are not felt; absence of foetal movements.
   d. Absent foetal heart sounds.
6. Per vaginum-
   a. Internal ballotment cannot be elicited.
   b. Unilateral or bilateral enlarged palpable ovaries are seen in 25-50% of cases.
   c. Vesicles are seen in vaginal discharge.

2.2.3. Investigations and diagnosis

1. Serial quantitative estimation of hCG-The hallmark of diagnosing hydatidiform mole is a positive β-hCG urine assay pregnancy test [18]. High hCG titre in urine diluted up to 1 in 200 to 1 in 500 beyond 100 days of gestation is very suggestive [6]. A retrospective analysis of molar pregnancies reported that 75% of patients present with vaginal bleeding, while 54% presented with enlarged uterus for gestational dates and 100% had excessively elevated β-hCG levels [18]. Qualitative β-hCG urine assays may be misleading in molar pregnancy. There have been reports of false negative both, urine and serum β-hCG pregnancy tests in hydatidiform mole [18].

Christopher and Ladde reported a case of a molar pregnancy presenting with abdominal pain and vaginal spotting with multiple false negative urinary pregnancy tests. The laboratory qualitative urine β-hCG assays were negative. As she was being prepared for transport to the ultrasound suite, she discharged a large, fleshy vesicular mass followed by profuse vaginal bleeding. They attributed this to the fact that qualitative β-hCG assays like sandwich chromatography immunoassays may produce false negative results in a phenomenon known as the high dose hook effect [18].

2. Ultrasonography-The characteristic 'snowstorm appearance' is seen (fig 3).

2.2.4. Types of hydatidiform mole – Molar pregnancies are categorised as complete or partial

Complete moles have diploid karyotype of solely paternal origin [18]. In a complete molar pregnancy, the placenta becomes oedematous secondary to grossly enlarged hydropic chorionic villi and in most cases the foetus, cord and amniotic membranes are absent [1]. The traditional presenting features like vaginal bleeding, excessive uterine size, hyperemesis gravidarum, hyperthyroidism, theca lutein cysts and preeclampsia in early pregnancy are present [17,18]. Patients with a complete molar pregnancy have excessively high levels of serum and urinary hCG resulting from trophoblastic proliferation [1]. hCG serves as a marker for the tumour.The diagnosis is made by ultrasonogram demonstrating a snowstorm appearance without a foetus (fig 3) [7].

Partial moles have triploid karyotype of both maternal and paternal origin. Partial molar pregnancies account for 10% of all hydatidiform moles [1]. In partial mole, there will be some identifiable foetal tissue(fig 2). Sanchez-Ferrer ML et al have described an extremely rare case of a partial hydatidiform mole with a normal fetus [21]. The classic clinical presentation described for complete mole is rare in partial mole and significant hCG level elevation is less common [15].Ultrasonography will not show the classical snow-storm appearance (fig 3). Most often the diagnosis is made upon histological review of curettage specimens [15].

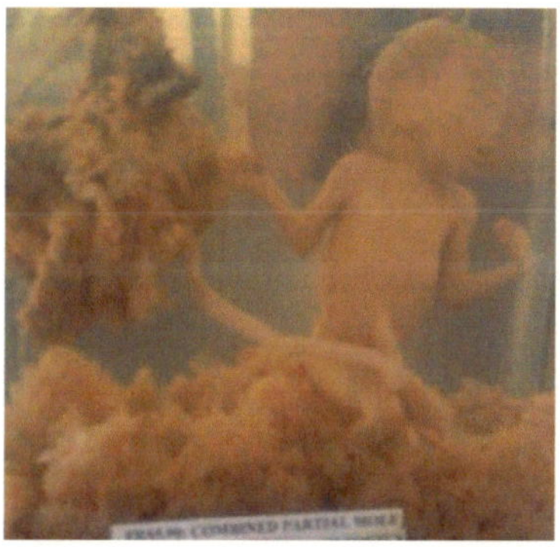

Figure 2. Specimen of partial mole.

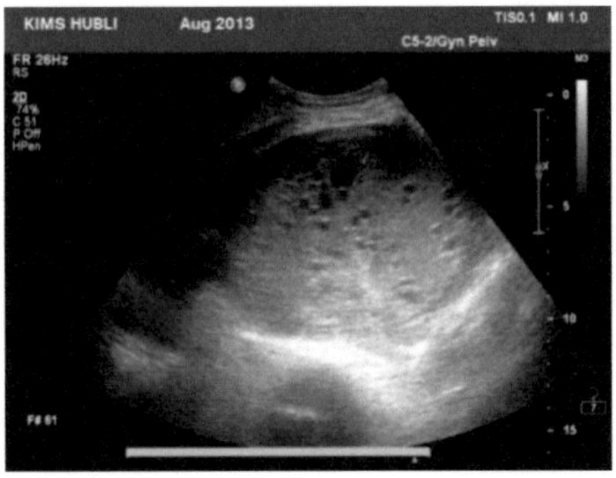

Figure 3. Transabdominal ultrasonogram showing'snowstorm' appearance of a complete mole in the uterus.

2.3. Complications of molar pregnancy

2.3.1. Immediate

Surgical [6]

1. Haemorrhage and shock – due to separation of vesicles or uterine perforation.
2. Sepsis – due to surgery and presence of degenerated vesicles and blood.
3. Uterine perforation – due to perforation by the mole or during surgery.

Medical

Eighty percent of cases of molar pregnancy are uncomplicated and twenty percent are associated with an extensive list of medical complications like hyperthyroidism, severe anaemia, haemorrhage, trophoblastic embolisation and pregnancy induced hypertension, some of which may be of a critical nature [1,12,22].

2.3.2. Late

18-28% of patients with complete mole and 2-4% of patients with partial mole can develop persistent neoplasia or post molar gestational trophoblastic neoplasia [15]. The development of choriocarcinoma following hydatidiform mole ranges from 2-10% [6].

2.4. Management of hydatidiform mole [6]

The principles are:

1. To give adequate supportive therapy to restore blood volume.
2. To evacuate the uterus as soon as diagnosis is made. Complete evacuation of the uterus is made by suction evacuation [1,12]. Hysterotomy is done in case of very low general condition of the patient or profuse vaginal bleeding. Hysterectomy is done in patients having three or more children or if patient's age is more than 35 years.

Suction dilatation and evacuation-Suction dilatation and evacuation is a safe, rapid and effective method for evacuating hydatidiform moles [23,24]. If the patient has already started to expel the mole, the process is hastened by starting an oxytocin drip of 10-20units. The products can then be rapidly evacuated either digitally or with the help of suction cannula [25]. If the process of expulsion of mole has not started, then a definitive plan for uterine evacuation is made. The cervix is dilated gently and slowly [19].If necessary,prostaglandin gels can be introduced into the cervix to promote cervical softening and dilatation [25].Light and careful curettage should be performed following the suction procedure to ensure complete evacuation of the uterine content [19].The use of a bedside ultrasound unit at the time of the procedure will ensure complete evacuation of uterine contents [23].

3. Prophylactic chemotherapy with oral methotrexate for 3 courses of 5 days each.

2.5. Invasive mole

The villus structure is maintained as in hydatidiform mole but the uterine wall may be perforated in multiple areas (fig 4). Distant metastasis can occur via blood stream to lungs, vagina or brain. The treatment is hysterectomy followed by cytotoxic therapy [6].

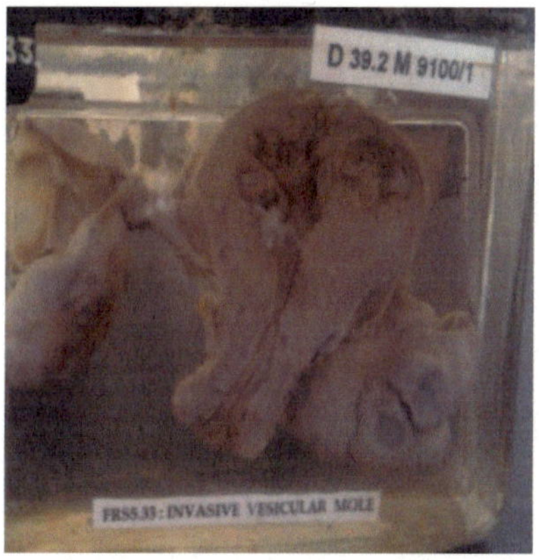

Figure 4. Specimen of an invasive mole

2.6. Choriocarcinoma

The incidence is 1 in 5000 pregnancies in Oriental countries and 1 in 50,000 in Europe and North America. 50% of cases occur after molar pregnancies. The villous pattern of hydatidiform mole is lost here and invasion of uterine wall accompanied by necrosis and haemorrhage is seen.(fig 5) Distant metastases can occur to lungs(70%), anterior vaginal wall(50%), brain(10%) and others [6]. Treatment is done with– [2,6]

1. Cytotoxic drugs.

2. Hysterectomy and cytotoxic drugs.

3. Adjuvant procedures like brain irradiation for cerebral metastasis, craniotomy in cerebral metastasis, hepatic resection to control bleeding from hepatic metastasis and vaginal packing for bleeding from vagina.

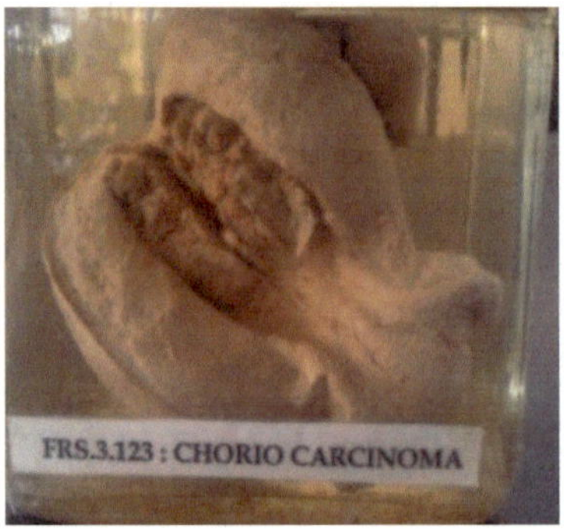

Figure 5. Specimen of choriocarcinoma of the uterus

2.7. Cytotoxic drugs in Gestational Trophoblastic Neoplasias [2]

Gestational Trophoblastic Neoplasias are highly responsive to chemotherapy. Early stage Gestational Trophoblastic Neoplasia is often cured with single agent chemotherapy. Advanced stage requires multiple agent combination regimens. EMACO (Etoposide, Methotrexate, Actinomycin-D, Cyclophosphamide and Vincristine) is the most commonly used regimen for stage IV tumours. MAC regimen with Methotrexate,Actinomycin-D and Cyclophosphamide is also used.

3. Relationship between hCG and thyroid

hCG is a placental glycoprotein. Its levels are high in the first trimester of pregnancy. It shares some structural similarity with TSH [26,27] (fig6). It is composed of alpha and beta subunits, non covalently linked. The alpha subunit is identical to that found in TSH. It consists of a 92 aminoacid chain containing two nitrogen linked oligosaccharide side chains [3]. The beta subunit of hCG consists of 145 aminoacid residues with two N linked and four O linked oligosaccharides. The beta subunit of TSH is composed of 112 residues and one N linked oligosaccharide [28]. TSH and hCG thus share a molecular mimicry and have similar effects on the thyroid [29]. Nonetheless, hCG receptors share 45% homology with the TSH receptors [3].

Several data indicate that hCG is a weak human thyrotropin [30]. In 1967, Burger reported that impure, commercial hCG had thyroid stimulating activity in a mouse bioassay [31]. Bioassays in mice, rats, chicks show that hCG stimulates iodine uptake, activates adenylate cyclase and increases DNA synthesis in cultured rat thyroid cells [32]. It also activates the TSH receptor. But the relative potency of hCG for the TSH receptor is 4000 times less than TSH [3]. It has

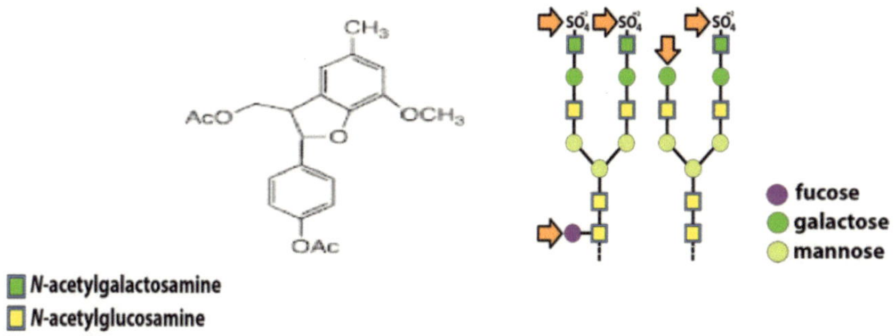

Figure 6. hCG molecular structure and major pituitary TSH glycoforms

been calculated that hCG contains approximately 1/4000th of the thyrotropic activity of human TSH. In bioassays, hCG is only about 1/10000th as potent as human TSH during normal pregnancy [33]. High circulating levels of hCG with their TSH like activity in the first trimester of pregnancy may result in a slightly low TSH and an increase in free T_4 concentration. hCG may stimulate maternal T_4 secretion [34]. It is estimated that an increment of hCG of 10,000UL^{-1} results in an increase of free T_4 of 0.6pmolL^{-1} and a decrease in TSH of 0.1mUL^{-1} [35].Braunstein and Hershman reported that there was an inverse relationship between TSH and hCG at about 10-12 weeks of pregnancy, the time of peak hCG levels [36]. Harada showed an increase of free T_4 and free T_3 associated with the peak hCG [37,38].Serum TSH levels particularly between 7 and 12 weeks of gestation fall to a nadir and present a mirror image with peak hCG values.(fig 7) The lower normal TSH limits in first trimester is approximately 0.03-0.08 mIUL^{-1} secondary to the thyrotropic activity of hCG [7].

Highly purified standard hCG has only trivial TSH like activity [39,40]. Certain fractions of hCG have greater TSH like activity than others [35]. The thyrotropic activity of hCG is influenced by the number and structure of its oligosaccharide side chains. Deglycosylation and partial desialation (removal of sialic acid) of β subunit of hCG enhances its thyrotropic potency in rat thyroid cells [41]. Nevertheless, the circulating hCG patterns are different at various stages of gestation [42]. HCG with reduced sialic acid content is increased in pregnant patients with hyperthyroidism [40]. Partially desialated hCG has the greatest TSH like activity and is often increased in molar pregnancy [35].

The development of hyperthyroidism due to hCG is largely influenced by the level of hCG. Clinically measurable changes in thyroid hormone concentration are only likely if hCG levels are around 50,000-70,000 mIUL^{-1} or more [35]. Extremely high levels are required for the development of clinical hyperthyroidism. Case studies have indicated that, serum levels of hCG of >100,000 mIUL^{-1} are usually needed to produce clinical evidence of thyrotoxicosis [3]. Such high levels are seen in conditions like hyperplacentosis, hyperemesis gravidarum, gestational trophoblastic disease, multiple pregnancy and hyper reaction-luteinalis [7]. These conditions are associated with the clinical entity known as 'transient non autoimmune hyperthyroidism in early pregnancy' wherein hCG is the main mediator of hyperthyroidism [7].

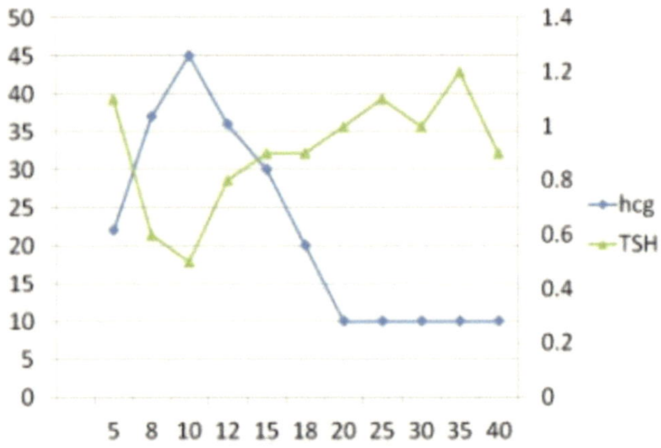

Figure 7. The pattern of serum TSH and HCG changes are shown as a function of gestation age. Between 8 and 14 weeks gestation, changes in serum hCG and TSH are mirror images of each other, and there is a significant negative correlation between the individual TSH (nadir) and peak hCG levels.

4. Epidemiology of hyperthyroidism in gestational trophoblastic disease

Concomitant biochemical thyroid disease in patients with gestational trophoblastic disease is relatively common [3]. Although hyperthyroidism has been reported more frequently in women with a hydatidiform mole than in those with choriocarcinoma, there have been many reports of hyperthyroidism in women with choriocarcinoma as well as a few men with testicular tumours [28].

The prevalence of hyperthyroidism in patients with hydatidiform mole and choriocarcinoma has been reported to be as high as 25-64% [28]. Hyperthyroidism develops in 5-10% cases of molar pregnancy and an incidence up to 30% is reported in India [43]. The prevalence of hyperthyroidism during complete molar pregnancy is as high as 7% [43]. In a study, 30 of 52 patients with gestational trophoblastic neoplasia were found to be thyrotoxic. The New England Trophoblastic Disease Centre estimated that 20% of women with complete moles have hyperthyroidism [28]. But in the same centre, between 1988 and 1993, none of 74 patients with complete mole demonstrated evidence of hyperthyroidism [15].Biochemical hyperthyroidism has been reported in a patient with a dichorionic pregnancy with one viable foetus and a hydatidiform mole [44].

Clinical hyperthyroidism is found in approximately 5% of women with a hydatidiform mole [26]. Clinical thyrotoxicosis is rare in molar pregnancy [45]. Clinical thyrotoxicosis is even more rare in patients with partial mole. The first such case was reported in 2008 [46].Rarely the thyroid stimulation can have potentially life threatening consequences [3]. The prevalence of thyrotoxicosis in patients with trophoblastic tumors was reported to be close to 50% in some older studies [7,47]. But nowadays with the ability of early detection of the disease, the incidence is much lower.

http://dx.doi.org/10.5772/57523

5. Aetiology of hyperthyroidism in molar pregnancy

Historically, the first association between hyperthyroidism and a product of the trophoblast was noted in patients with trophoblastic tumours [28]. In 1971, Hirshman and Higgins reported two case of severe hyperthyroidism in patients with hydatidiform mole and demonstrated for the first time thyrotropic activity in molar tissue [48]. This stimulator differed biologically and immunologically from the other three human stimulators i.e. pituitary thyrotropin, chorionic thyrotropin found in normal pregnancies and the LATS in Grave's disease [7]. They speculated that an excessive amount of the extracted molar stimulator was responsible for the hyperthyroidism in both people [7].Hyperthyroidism in patients with molar pregnancy is thought to occur as a manifestation of excessive levels of circulating hCG which has a weak intrinsic thyroid stimulating activity, or from a thyrotropin like substance released from the mole [1,33,43].

Extremely high levels of hCG are typically required for the development of clinical hyperthyroidism as the relative potency of hCG for the TSH receptor is relatively low [3].HCG levels always exceed 300 IUml-1 in patients with hyperthyroidism caused by trophoblastic disease [41]. The hCG levels are particularly high at 10-14 weeks of gestation in trophoblastic disease [44]. In gestational trophoblastic disease, high levels of hCG cause activation of the thyrotropin receptor and stimulate supraphysiological secretion of thyroid hormone [44]. The level of thyroid stimulation is directly proportional to the hCG concentration [3]. Lemon et al studying thyroid function in trophoblastic diseases reported a high correlation between levels of hCG and TSH measured by radio-immunoassay secondary to cross-sensitivity of TSH and hCG with the antibody they used [49]. None of their patients were clinically hyperthyroid and there was poor correlation between hCG and T3 or T4 levels although high levels of thyroid hormone occurred only at hCG levels greater than 100,000mIU/ml. Basic isoforms of hCG with high bioactivity-immunoactivity ratio may be responsible for hyperthyroidism in some patients with trophoblastic disease [28]. Nevertheless, the hCG molecule from women with trophoblastic diseases has been found to display enhanced thyrotropic activity [50].

Some studies have however, revealed no significant relationship between elevation of serum hCG and abnormally high values of free thyroxine index in patient with trophoblastic tumors. These studies suggest that a substance distinct from hCG and elaborated by the gestational trophoblastic tissue is responsible for thyrotoxicosis observed in patients with trophoblastic tumours.The molar thyrotropin existing in the serum of patients with a hydatidiform mole differs from hCG by its larger molecular size and the duration of action, which is longer [33,43,51].

6. Spectrum of biochemical abnormalities in trophoblastic hyperthyroidism

1. The level of thyroid stimulation is directly proportional to hCG concentration and hence the severity of clinical hyperthyroidism reflects the hCG level in gestational trophoblas-

tic disease. In patients with molar hyperthyroidism, serum hCG levels usually exceed 300U/ml and always exceed 100 U/ml. Patients with clinical evidence of thyrotoxicosis may have serum levels of hCG of >100,000 mIU/L. However, some patients with trophoblastic tumors with very high serum hCG levels do not manifest hyperthyroidism [3,28].

2. In patients with molar pregnancy, evidence for pronounced hypersecretion of T_4 is present. Hence, elevated serum free T_4 & T_3 levels are found [47].

3. A pattern of high values of serum protein bound iodine(PBI) and serum tri-iodothyronine reaction(T3test)and relatively low values of serum cholesterol have been seen in most patients with hydatidiform mole [52].

4. Pronounced increase in urinary P/C ratio occurs in patients with molar pregnancy suggesting that they are hypermetabolic [47].

5. Dowling, Ingbar and Freinket were the first to note the occurrence of striking abnormalities in several aspects of thyroid economy in patients with molar pregnancy. They found marked increases in serum PBI, $PB^{131}I$, butanol-extractable ^{131}I, thyroidal ^{131}I uptake and absolute iodine uptake(AIU) in the patients [53]

6. In some cases, even when serum free T_4 and T_3 concentrations were only slightly elevated, serum TSH concentrations were low and serum TSH responses to TRH were low [28].

7. Several patients of trophoblastic tumors demonstrated thyroid hyperfunction or marked increases in serum PBI but failed to display signs or symptoms of frank thyrotoxicosis [47].

7. Comparison of trophoblastic hyperthyroidism with other types of hyperthyroidism and with the thyroid economy of normal pregnancy [28,47]

1. Patients with trophoblastic hyperthyroidism have higher serum T4/T3 ratiosthan patients with Grave's hyperthyroidism.

2. Thyroid stimulating immunoglobulin is not detectable in trophoblastic hyperthyroidism unlike Grave's Disease.

3. Several of the changes in certain aspects of thyroid economy which occur in molar pregnancy resemble superficially those seen in normal pregnancy. These include the increase in thyroidal ^{131}I uptake and serum $PB^{131}I$; inpatients with molar pregnancy, however, these indices tend to be more markedly increased.Values for serum PBI and T_4 concentration in molar pregnancy are usually much greater than in normal pregnancy.

4. In patients with the usual varieties of hyperthyroidism, the absolute concentration of free T_4 in serum is usually quite elevated as a result of increase in both: the total concentration of T_4 in serum and the free proportion. In patients with molar pregnancy, a smaller increase in concentration of free T_4 is generally seen since the proportion of free T_4 is subnormal.

5. Trophoblastic tumours secrete less oestrogen than normal placental tissue so that the increase in serum thyroxine-binding globulin (TBG) concentration is less in molar pregnancy than in normal pregnancy.

8. Some biochemical case profiles of trophoblastic hyperthyroidism

There is a spectrum of thyroid function abnormalities in gestational trophoblastic neoplasias and thyroid function in an individual patient is determined by the relative influence of the thyroid stimulator, nonthyroidal illnesses and the pregnancy [54].

1. In a study of the thyroid status of 27 African patients with gestational trophoblastic neoplasia, 15 patients were found to be biochemically hyperthyroid. Of the 15 patients, 9 were clinically thyrotoxic. It was found that when serum levels of hCG reached a level of about $0.1x10^6$IU/L, 13 of 16 patients were biochemically hyperthyroid; at serum levels of $0.3x10^6$IU/L of hCG, most patients were clinically thyrotoxic. T_4 was invariably raised in these patients but the T_3:T_4 ratios tended to be low(0.015 ± 0.005);rT_3:T_3 ratios were high and TSH levels were not raised [55].

2. In 7 patients with metastatic trophoblastic disease, there was laboratory evidence of increased thyroid function but clinical hyperthyroidism was either not present or minimal and thyroid gland size was normal. There was uniform elevation of 24 hour radioiodine uptake, serum PBI, BMR and the serum cholesterol was depressed [56].

3. In a study on 47 patients with hydatidiform mole, only 1 was found to be clinically hyperthyroid, although 10 had serum total thyroxine values exceeding those found in normal pregnancy(8 to 17 μ gm/dl). Among 34 patients in whom free thyroxine indices could be calculated, 18 had elevated values for the free thyroxine index(>10.6), and 9 had elevated values for total thyroxine and free thyroxineindex [57].

4. An ^{131}I –tracer test performed in a patient with molar pregnancy indicated a very high thyroidal ^{131}I uptake, conversion ratio and thyroidal ^{131}I secretion rate [58].

5. Studies on 11 patients were done before and after removal of a molar pregnancy. Before evacuation of the mole, all patients demonstrated moderately to greatly elevated values for thyroidal ^{131}I uptake, absolute iodine uptake and serum protein bound ^{131}I. Values for serum PBI and serum thyroxine (T_4) concentration were consistently increased averaging more than twice found in normal pregnancy. The maximum binding capacity of the T_4-binding globulin(TBG) was variably affected and ranged between the values found in normal controls and those found in the normal pregnancy. Values for the absolute of free T_4 in the serum were only moderately elevated since the proportion of free T_4 was moderately low, although not as low as in normal pregnancy [47].

9. Clinical presentation of hyperthyroidism in gestational trophoblastic disease

Hyperthyroidism has been reported as a complication of complete mole and persistent trophoblastic disease, both metastatic and non metastatic [41]. Trophoblastic hyperthyroidism has a widely divergent clinical pattern. Clinical hyperthyroidism is usually seen in patients with extremely high levels of hCG [30]. The clinical scenario may vary from absence of symptoms to thyroid storm [41,59]. Hyperthyroidism presents clinically as a physiological state dominated by an increased metabolic rate.Myocardial contractility, heart rate, stroke volume and ventricular size increase. Peripheral vascular resistance decreases in skin and muscle The typical clinical findings include fatigue, weight loss, nervousness, excessive sweating, heat intolerance, hyperactivity, tremor, weakness, hyperdynamic precordium, diarrhoea, increased appetite, incapacitation [27], muscle weakness, tachycardia, minimal or no enlargement of thyroid gland. Ophthalmopathy is not observed in this condition [41]. Cardiomyopathy is seen. Reflexes become hyper-reactive. [27].

Mild to moderate hyperthyroidism may be difficult to diagnose clinically during pregnancy since normal parturients may experience symptoms such as heat intolerance, tachycardia, emotional instability and vomiting. A resting tachycardia not slowed by the Valsalva manoeuvre is a strong indication of hyperthyroidism [60]. Several patients develop supraventricular tachycardia and pulmonary oedema. The nausea, vomiting and toxaemia of pregnancy that occur commonly in molar gestation may obscure the features of hyperthyroidism [28].

The development of biochemical and clinical thyrotoxicosis in patients with choriocarcinoma depends upon the duration of the choriocarcinoma and the level of hCG [61]. In choriocarcinoma, the symptoms of metastasis to pelvis, lung, liver and brain may dominate the clinical picture. There may be laboratory evidence of increased thyroid function without clinically overt hyperthyroidism just as in hydatidiform mole [28].

During emergency surgery, the cardiovascular clinical manifestations of hyperthyroidism like tachycardia can often be missed because they may be attributed to hypovolaemia [59].

10. Management of trophoblastic hyperthyroidism

Surgical removal of the hydatidiform mole in a hyperthyroid patient rapidly cures the hyperthyroidism and should be performed as soon as possible [43,59]. Therapy of hyperthyroidism is not indicated in the vast majority of cases, since evacuation of the mole or chemotherapy in the management of choriocarcinoma, removing high levels of hCG, cures the hyperthyroidism. In those cases of severe symptoms, Lugol's solution, intravenous iodine and β blocking agents are indicated [7]. Therapy with potassium iodide given orally or sodium iodide given intravenously(1 gm q8 hourly) will rapidly reduce serum free T4 and T3 levels. Propranolol and other beta-adrenergic antagonist drugs are helpful to control tachycardia and other symptoms of sympathetic activation. Supportive measures such as fluid and electrolyte replacement should be done as needed [28].

When hyperthyroidism occurs in the context of choriocarcinoma, case reports have demonstrated that the biomarkers of choriocarcinoma and thyroid function parallel the regression and subsequent relapse of the tumor [3]. Several women with metastatic choriocarcinoma and hyperthyroidism have achieved complete remission with chemotherapy. In the thyrotoxic patient with choriocarcinoma, the hyperthyroidism should be treated by any of the usual medical therapies [28]. The hyperthyroidism status secondary to molar disease rapidly resolves after evacuation while that secondary to choriocarcinoma takes a longer time to resolve [41].

Moskovitz JB and Bond MC reported the successful management of a case of thyroid storm in a 17year old patient. She presented to a community hospital's emergency department with history of palpitations and tachycardia since one week. Beta blockers and calcium channel blockers were administered. The tachycardia partially responded. She was then referred to a tertiary centre for evaluation. There the diagnosis of molar pregnancy was made using ultrasonogram and thyroid storm was diagnosed. She was given intensive care support, treated with β-blockers and propylthiouracil. Surgical evacuation of molar pregnancy was done and her symptoms soon resolved [62].

Walkington et al reported a case of a 21 year old woman who presented 2 months after a right salphingectomy for a ruptured ectopic pregnancy. She was breathless at rest, agitated and had a resting tachycardia. Pelvis ultrasound and MRI showed a mass near right ovary. She was diagnosed with choriocarcinoma with no evidence of metastasis. Serum hCG was $1.176x10^6 IUL^{-1}$. Thyroid functions showed her to be hyperthyroid with TSH <0.03 $mIUL^{-1}$, free T_4=73$pmolL^{-1}$ and free T_3=21.6$pmolL^{-1}$. She was commenced on carbimazole and propranolol. Her serum hCG and TFT measurements were as follows (table 1). Her TFTs normalised in parallel with the fall in serum hCG. She was slowly weaned off her anti-thyroid treatment and she became biochemically euthyroid at commencement of her third cycle of chemotherapy [3].

Day	HCG ($IU\ l^{-1}$)	TSH($mIU\ l^{-1}$)	FT_4($pmol\ l^{-1}$)	Carbimazole
0	791711	<0.03	73	40mgOD
7	156420	<0.03	15.2	40mgOD
21	19986	0.15	16.1	20mgOD
42	333	0.83	12.2	Stop

Abbreviations: FT4=free T4; HCG=human chorionic gonadotrophin; OD=once daily; TFT=thyroid function tests; TSH=thyroid stimulating hormone

Table 1. Summary of serial HCG and TFT measurements

11. Perioperative management of trophoblastic hyperthyroidism

20% of cases of trophoblastic hyperthyroidism can develop severe perioperative complications like high output cardiac failure secondary to thyrotoxicosis, thyroid storm, embolisation of pulmonary arteries by trophoblastic materials, hypovolaemia, disseminated intravascular coagulation, pulmonary oedema secondary to severe anaemia and acute pulmonary distress secondary to any of these problems. They may require intensive care support [1]. Hence the perioperative management and optimisation of hyperthyroid state prior to surgical evacuation of the mole is very important [59].The perioperative management of hyperthyroidism focuses on the control of sympathetic activity so that cardiovascular side-effects are not manifested [51].

11.1. Preoperative preparation

Preoperative optimisation with anti-thyroid and chemotherapeutic drugs is imperative to reduce perioperative morbidity [59]. Every anaesthesiologist should be well aware of the critical nature of perioperative complications that can be associated with a molar pregnancy. A detailed pre-anaesthesia work up, preoperative optimisation of the patients' thyroid and volume status, planning and conducting anaesthesia carefully and being prepared for advanced perioperative management are a must [63].

Preoperative evaluation of these patients should be based on history, physical examination and laboratory testing [64]. The patient must be admitted to an intensive care unit preoperatively. Blood count, electrolytes, blood gases, thyroid, hepatic, renal functions, β-hCG and chest radiogram should be carefully evaluated [51]. Treatment has to be individualised. The patient can be prepared for surgery with oral propylthiouracil (50-100mg qid), propranolol (20mg tid), intravenous glucocorticoids and sodium iodide [27]. Some cases may require only beta blockers whereas others may require in addition antithyroid drugs. Some may not require any treatment if the hyperthyroidism is only biochemical and asymptomatic [41]. Dehydration and anaemia if present should be corrected [25].

The diagnosis of hyperthyroidism in molar pregnancy is often made in semi-urgent conditions. Hence rapid stabilisation of the disease before surgery becomes important [45]. If there is no time to make the patient pharmacologically euthyroid, intravenous administration of iodine and β-adrenergic receptor blockers for emergency treatment of hyperthyroidism may be advisable [65]. These drugs, however, may be hazardous in patients who have heart failure or pulmonary complications [64]. The role of plasmapheresis for the rapid hormonal control in the preoperative period has been described. The use of plasmapheresis for the first time in the treatment of hyperthyroidism is reported in the 1970s. Erbil et al reported the use of plasmapheresis in a patient with severe hyperthyroidism due to hydatidiform mole for the rapid control of hormonal levels [66]. A case of successful rapid preoperative preparation by 3-4 sittings of plasmapheresis of a patient with secondary hyperthyroidism due to molar pregnancy has been described [67]. A study conducted by Ozbey et al concluded that plasmapheresis is a treatment option to be considered only when anti-thyroid drugs are contraindicated [68].

11.2. Anaesthetic management

Sedation, monitored anaesthesia care, TIVA, general anaesthesia and spinal anaesthesia are the various anaesthetic techniques that can be adopted for a case of evacuation of molar pregnancy [1,22,25,63]. Beta blockers for attenuation of sympathetic activity, emergency drugs like lidocaine for ventricular arrhythmias, steroids and hypotensive agents like sodium nitroprusside should be kept ready [69]. For patients with thyrotoxicosis due to molar pregnancy, it is recommended that placement of invasive monitors like central venous pressure be considered before induction of anaesthesia [1].

General anaesthesia may be the preferred technique in hypotensive bleeding patients scheduled for emergency evacuation. Uterine relaxation caused by inhaled anaesthetics may however increase blood loss [69]. Hence inhaled anaesthetics with known tocolytic qualities such as halothane, enflurane and isoflurane should be used in lower concentrations [64]. A nitrous oxide, opioid, muscle relaxant technique may also be preferred [51,64]. The safe use of sevoflurane at 2.5 % concentrations has been reported by some authors without increasing the chances of bleeding due to uterine relaxation [51].Drugs that minimally affect the cardiovascular system are the most rational choice in these patients [69]. Adequate premedication is important to decrease unnecessary catecholamine release [69]. The anaesthesiologist should avoid the administration of medications that stimulate the sympathetic nervous system and should achieve an adequate depth of anaesthesia prior to surgical stimulation [69]. Medications associated with tachycardia should be avoided e.g. atropine, ketamine.

In stable patients, spinal anaesthesia is preferable [69]. It can be used because

a. It is probably safe in patients with thyrotoxicosis.

b. It has favourable nontocolytic pharmacological properties.

c. It has preferable effects on the pulmonary system.

d. The sympathetic blockade associated with a regional technique may be desirable.

e. It is associated with a decrease in heart rate and blood pressure during surgery.

f. One can diagnose complications like thyroid storm at an earlier stage than when the patient is sedated or under GA by maintaining the patients consciousness [64,69].

Intravenous fluids and blood must be administered judiciously as these patients have a propensity to develop pulmonary oedema. Blood replacement may be required to treat bleeding. Diuretics may be given intermittently [51].

Successful use of total intravenous anaesthesia (TIVA) has been reported for evacuation of molar pregnancy with hyperthyroidism. E. Erturk et al reported the anaesthetic management of a 25 year old woman having a hydatidiform mole with hyperthyroidism using TIVA technique with propofol, remifentanil and esmolol infusion for controlling sympathetic hyperactivity during surgery [26].

11.3. Postoperative care

Postoperatively, intensive care management may be indicated because most of the cardiopulmonary complications develop in the postoperative period [64]. Mechanical ventilatory support must be provided if necessary. Treatment of thyroid storm, if it occurs, includes general supportive measures plus the administration of glucocorticoids, propylthiouracil, sodium iodideand propranolol [27].

Solak M and Akturk G reported the successful perioperative management of a case of trophoblastic hyperthyroidism. A 22 year old woman, in her third month of pregnancy, presented for emergency evacuation. She had a history of vaginal bleeding and signs of hyperthyroidism like tremor, palpitation, sweating and tachycardia for three weeks. Examination revealed an arterial blood pressure of 140/70 mm of Hg, a heart rate ranging from 110 to 130 beats per minute, a small thyroid nodule and signs of hydatidiform mole in sonography and computerised tomography. Studies of thyroid function were obtained: free triiodothyronine – 8.50pgml^{-1} (normal range 3.05-5.35 pgml^{-1}) and free thyroxine – 5.56ngdl^{-1} (normal range 0.71-1.85 ngdl^{-1}). Serum β-hCG was 961.96 mIUml^{-1} (normal range 0-5 mIUml^{-1}). Serum thyroid stimulating hormone levels were within normal limits. The patient appeared apprehensive, pale and shivering. She was administered intramusculardiazepam 5 mg 45 minutes preoperatively. Arterial blood pressure came down to 110/70 mm of Hg and there was sinus tachycardia (130 beats per minute). Spinal anaesthesia with 4 ml of 0.5% bupivacaine was administered at L_{3-4} level. She lost 1000 – 1500 ml of blood intraoperatively and received approximately 100 ml of whole blood. She was haemodynamically stable throughout the surgery which lasted for 30 minutes. Serum free T_4 values were 4.13 and 1.25 ngml^{-1} on the 7th and 14th post-operative days respectively. She became euthyroid few weeks after evacuation of the mole [64].

Puneet Khanna, Anil Kumar and Maya Dehran reported the successful perioperative management of a 44 year old female with hydatidiform mole. She had a history of irregular menstrual cycles since three months. Preoperatively she appeared anxious, afebrile with a pulse rate of 116 per minute, blood pressure of 120/80 mm of Hg and a respiratory rate of 20 per minute. The height of uterus was 14 weeks on per abdominal examination. Haemoglobin was 13.1gms%. Thyroid function tests revealed TSH=0.03IU/ml(0.03-5-5), T_3=221IU/ml(70-200) and T_4=14IU/ml(4.5-12.5). Ultra-sonogram of the abdomen showed signs of an invasive hydatidiform mole. β-hCG levels were raised to 8,35,300mIUL^{-1}. She was put on tab. neomercazole 15 mgTDS, tab. propranolol 20 mgBD, Lugol's iodine 4 drops TDS and inj. dexamethasone 2mg 6th hourly.She was also started on chemotherapy with methotrexate on alternate days and three cycles were given. Her β-hCG levels and thyroid functions were closely monitored. She was posted for total abdominal hysterectomy and bilateral salphingo-oophorectomy but was postponed due to persistent tachycardia reflecting an uncontrolled hyperthyroid state. The dose and frequency of tab. propranolol was increased to 40mg 6th hourly. After three weeks her hyperthyroid state was partly optimised($T_4$9.94IU/ml and $T_3$0.014IU/ml) and she was accepted for the planned procedure. Tab.diazepam 5mg was given on the night before and on the day of surgery. Patient was given combined spinal epidural block in L_{3-4} space. Intravenous sedation was given with midazolam and fentanyl. Intravenous dexamethasone was also given. Tabs.neomercazole, propranolol, amlodipine and dexamethasone were continued post-operatively and Lugol's iodine was stopped. Epidural analgesia with morphine was provided postoperatively and on 3rd post-operative day thyroid function test started showing improvement. On the 10th post-operative day, both β-hCG levels and thyroid function tests normalised [59].

Laurent V and co-authors reported a case of successful perioperative management of a Senegalese patient with hydatidiform mole. The patient had serum hCG levels of 900,000 IU. She was clinically hyperthyroid with raised T_4 and T_3 levels but a very low TSH concentration. She was given *propranolol and carbimazole for 2 days. After that suction curettage was performed under general anaesthesia. Propranolol was again administered 6 hours after surgery. Thyroid function tests returned to normal levels two weeks after mole removal and serum hCG concentrations closely paralleled those of free thyroxine [45].*

12. Complications of hyperthyroidism in molar pregnancy

The two most serious maternal complications of untreated hyperthyroidism are heart failure, being more common and thyroid storm [70]

12.1. Heart failure

High output cardiac failure secondary to the thyrotoxicosis can occur in the perioperative period [43]. High output heart failure is caused by the myocardial effects of thyroxine. Pulmonary hypertension which is correlated with untreated or inadequately controlled hyperthyroidism can result in heart failure and pulmonary oedema [70]. Haemodynamic problems like tachycardia, hypertension,increase in total blood volume,decrease in systemic vascular resistance and increased cardiac output can result in cardiac decompensation and arrhythmias [69]. Symptoms of high output cardiac failure include breathlessness at rest or on exertion, exercise intolerance, fatigue, fluid retention and signs like tachycardia,tachypnea,raised jugular venous pressure, pulmonary rales,pleural effusion, peripheral oedema and warm peripheries due to peripheral vasodilatation. Cardiac ultra-sound may show preserved left ventricular ejection fraction [71].

Management of high output cardiac failure includes [72,73]

- Correction of the underlying hyperthyroidism.
- Carbimazole to alleviate thyrotoxicosis.
- Diuretics like frusemide to reverse the volume overload.
- Beta adrenoceptor blockers like esmolol and propranolol in particular to alleviate the symptoms of hyperthyroidism and to control the heart rate.A cautious trial of ultrashort acting beta blockers like esmolol can be done with invasive monitoring to detect the occurrence of depressed myocardial contractility.
- Amiodarone to treat atrial fibrillation if present.
- Digoxin to slow down ventricular response rate in atrial fibrillation.

12.2. Thyrotoxicosis and thyroid storm

Thyroid storm occurs perioperatively in patients who have received either incomplete or no treatment for the pre-existing hyperthyroidism [43,74]. Thyroid storm can lead to high output cardiac failure [12].Cases of thyroid storm occurring in the intraoperative period have been reported [75]. Severe thyrotoxicosis can occur even after surgical evacuation of the mole

[76].Thyroid storm is a clinical diagnosis with manifestions like hyperpyrexia, severe dehydration, tachycardia,tachypnoea, diaphoresis, diarrhoea, atrial fibrillation, extreme anxiety, altered consciousness and haemodynamic instability leading to cardiovascular collapse [27,69]. Treatment of thyroid storm includes cooling blankets, intravenous hydration, glucose and electrolyte replacement, oxygen, glucocorticoids like dexamethasone or hydrocortisone intravenously, anti-thyroid drugs like oral/rectal propylthiouracil, methimazole, iodine in the form of intravenous sodium iodide or oral Lugol's iodine, β blockers like propranolol or esmolol, plasma exchange, dantrolene and B-complex multivitamins [27].

12.3. Mortality and pulmonary morbidity

Few cases of mortality after surgical evacuation in patients with molar pregnancy have been described [63,12] and some of them were hyperthyroid [63,77]. Respiratory complications including pulmonary oedema and acute respiratory distress syndrome (ARDS) were observed in these cases [63,77]. Few authors have also reported successful intensive treatment of ARDS occurring in hyperthyroid patients with molar pregnancy [74].

Severe thyrotoxicosis has been reported after commencing treatment for gestational trophoblastic disease. A 53-year-old woman developed profound cardiovascular instability one day after surgical evacuation of a complete hydatidiform mole. She was not known to have pre-existing thyroid disease but investigations confirmed thyrotoxicosis [76]

Carrasco C and Cotoras J reported an interesting case of molar pregnancy with complications of hyperthyroidism. An 18 year old woman was admitted with a history of four days of cardiac failure with acute pulmonary oedema, high blood pressure, left ventricular dilatation and moderate to severe systolic dysfunction. Twenty four hours after admission she had a miscarriage expelling a mole. The diagnosis of hyperthyroidism caused by a mole and early preeclampsia was confirmed and the patient was managed with diuretics and dopamine. Symptoms abated. Thyroid function tests, cardiac function and size returned to normal values [78].

Hershman JM and Higgins HP reported a case of a 29 year old, 4 months pregnant Italian woman. She came complaining of shortness of breath, extreme fatigue, nervousness and heat intolerance. Since the past one week she had severe nausea and vomiting and vaginal spotting. On examination, she appeared anxious with soft, warm skin, fine hair and sweaty palms. The pulse rate was 110 per minute and regular, the blood pressure was 150/60 mm of Hg. The thyroid gland was slightly enlarged. Grade 2 ejection murmur was heard over the pulmonary area and a ventricular gallop was heard over the apex. The peripheral pulses were bounding. Ultrasonography showed signs of a molar pregnancy. The protein bound iodine(PBI)level was 22.7 mμg, serum thyroxine-iodine was 18mμg/100ml, 24 hour uptake of radioactive iodine was 75% and serum free thyroxine was raised: 14.8 mμg/100ml (normal 3-5mμg / 100 ml). Carbimazole 60mg per day was started. On the evening of the 7th day, supraventricular tachycardia suddenly developed and acute pulmonary oedema ensued shortly. She was treated with nasal oxygen, digoxin, ouabain and diuretics. A plasmapheresis was performed and packed red cells were transfused. The next day, there was a rapid tachycardia but no evidence of congestive heart failure. On the 8th day, a total abdominal hysterectomy was performed. Two further episodes of pulmonary oedema treated successfully with digoxin, occurred on the first and third post-operative days. She improved *markedly. Tachycardia came back to normal; radio iodine uptake and PBI came back to normal by 14 days [48].*

An unusual case of a 13 year old Caucasian patient with a complete hydatidiform mole was reported wherein during anaesthesia induction, she presented symptoms compatible with a thyrotoxic crisis. The patient had complaints of amenorrhoea, abdominal pain and vaginal bleeding. She was tachypnoeic, tachycardic, hypertensive, pale and dehydrated. Her haemoglobin was 9.9gm/dl, serum TSH was 0.009mIU/ml (normal 0.35 – 5.5). HCG levels were higher than 400,000 IU/L. She underwent chest, abdominal and pelvic CT scanning with iodinated contrast and was scheduled to undergo a uterine curettage. General anaesthesia was administered via intravenous induction with fentanyl, propofol, endotracheal intubation and muscle relaxation with atracurium. After oro-tracheal intubation, she developed sinus tachycardia (170 beats per minute), hypertension (160/120 mm of Hg), hypercarbia (52 mm of Hg) and acute pulmonary oedema. She was diagnosed to be in a thyrotoxic crisis. She was treated with intravenous esmolol and sodium nitroprusside 75μg/kg/min respectively with satisfactory response and transferred to the ICU and managed there till she became haemodynamically stable. The use of iodinated substances can trigger thyrotoxic crisis (Jod-Basedow phenomenon) and in this case, the iodinated contrast used to perform scan preoperatively could have contributed to the development of thyrotoxic crisis [79].

13. Conclusions

Trophoblastic tumors are associated with biochemical and clinical hyperthyroidism. Hence measurement of thyroid function in patients with gestational trophoblastic disease is important. Thyroid function normalises rapidly with treatment of the underlying gestational trophoblastic disease and consequent fall in hCG levels. Treatment of gestational trophoblastic disease includes surgical evacuation or chemotherapy. Hydatidiform mole with hyperthyroidism is a perioperative challenge. All patients should be stabilised with β-blockers and antithyroid medications prior to induction of anaesthesia for surgical evacuation. Vigilant monitoring and intensive care should be done perioperatively to watch for the occurrence of cardiopulmonary complications or thyroid storm.

Acknowledgements

The author wishes to express her heartfelt thanks to Dr. Kaushic Theerth, Dr. Radhika Deva of the department of Anaesthesiology, Dr. Venkatesh K V of the department of Obstetrics and Gynaecology, Dr. Jagadish Sutagatti and Dr. Gurunandini Achar of the department of Radiodiagnosis, Professor and Head of the department of Pathology Dr. Sujata Giriyan, Karnataka Institute of Medical Sciences, Hubli for their generous help in literature search and technical aspects of writing this chapter.

Author details

Madhuri S. Kurdi*

Address all correspondence to: drmadhuri_kurdi@yahoo.com

Department of Anaesthesiology and Critical Care, Karnataka Institute Of Medical Sciences (KIMS) Hubli, Karnataka, India

References

[1] Celeski D, Micho J, Walters L. Anesthetic implications of a partial molar pregnancy and associated complications. AANAJ 2001; 69:49-53.

[2] Taymaa May, Goldstein DP, Berkowitz Ross S. Current chemotherapeutic management of patients with gestational trophoblastic neoplasia. Chemotherapy Research and Practice 2011. Available from http://dx.doi.org/10.1155/2011/806256.

[3] Walkington L, Webster J, Hancock BW, Everard J, Coleman RE. Hyperthyroidism and human chorionic gonadotropin production in gestational trophoblastic disease. British Journal of Cancer 2011; 104:1665-9.

[4] Newlands ES, Bower M, Fisher RA, Paradinas FJ. Management of placental site trophoblastic tumors. J Reprod Med 1998;43:53-59.

[5] Cunningham Gary F, Leveno Kenneth J, Bloom Stoven L, Hauth John C, Rouse DJ, Spong CY. Gestational trophoblastic diseases. In: Alyssa Fried, Karen Davis, editors. William's Obstetrics. 23rd ed. USA:McGraw Hill Companies; 2010. p257-265.

[6] Dutta DC. Haemorrhage in early pregnancy. In: Hiralal Konar, editor. Textbook of Obstetrics. 7th ed. Kolkata: New Central Book Agency; 2011 p158-199.

[7] Goldman AM, Mestman JH. Transient non-autoimmune hyperthyroidism of early pregnancy. Journal of Thyroid Research 2011; Available from http://dx.doi.org/10.4061/2011/142413.

[8] Atrash HK, Hogue CJ, Grimes DA. Epidemiology of hydatidiform mole during early gestation. Am J Obstet Gynecol 1986; 154:906-9.

[9] Smith H O. Gestational trophoblastic disease epidemiology and trends. Clin Obstet Gynecol 2003;46: 541-56.

[10] Heidarpour M, Khanahmadi M. Diagnostic value of P63 in differentiating normal gestation from molar pregnancy. J Res Med Sci 2013;462-6.

[11] Steigrad SJ. Epidemiology of gestational trophoblastic diseases. Best Pract Res Clin Obstet Gynaecol 2003;17:837-847.

[12] Bhatia S, Naithani Udita, Chhetty YK, Prasad Narendra, Jagtap RS, Agrawal I. Case report – Acute pulmonary edema after evacuation of molar pregnancy. Anaesthesia, Pain and Intensive Care 2011; 15(2):114-117. Available from http://www.apicareonline.com

[13] Thepa K, Shreshtha M, Sharma S, Pandey S. Trend of complete hydatidiform mole. J Nepal Med Assoc 2010;49:10-3.

[14] Padubidri V, AnandEla. Gestational trophoblastic diseases. In: Textbook of Obstetrics. 1st ed New Delhi: B. I. publications private limited; 2006. p88-96.

[15] Garner EIO, Goldstein DP, Feltmate CM, Berkowitz RS. Gestational trophoblastic disease. Clinical Obstetrics and Gynecology 2007; 50(1):112-22.

[16] Fisher RA, Hodges MD, Newlands ES. Familial recurrent hydatidiform mole: a review. J Reprod Med 2004; 49:595-601.

[17] Soto-Wright Valena, Bernstein Marilyn, Goldstein Donald Peter, Berkowitz RS. The changing clinical presentation of complete molar pregnancy. Obstet and Gynecol 1995; 86(5):775-9.

[18] Hunter Christopher L, Ladde Jay. Molar pregnancy with false negative β-hCG urine in the emergency department. West J Emerg Med 2011; 12(2):213-5.

[19] Riadh B et al. Clinical analysis and management of gestational trophoblastic diseases. A 90 cases study. Int Journal of Biomedical Sciences 2009;5(4):321-325.

[20] Koirala A, Khatiwada P, Giri A, Kandel P, Regmi M, Upreti D. The demographics of molar pregnancies in BPKIHS. Kathmandu Univ Med J 2011; 36(4): 298-300.

[21] Sanchez-Ferrer ML et al. Partial mole with a diploid fetus: Case study and literature review. Fetal Diagn Ther 2009; 25(3):34-8.

[22] Chantigan RC, Chantigan PD. Problems of early pregnancy. In: Chestnut DM, editor. Obstetric Anaesthesia Principles and Practice. 3rd ed. St Louis:Mosby;2004,p241-54.

[23] Hanna R K, Soper J T. The role of surgery and radiation therapy in the management of gestational trophoblastic disease. Oncologist 2010;15(6)593-600.

[24] Soper J T. Role of surgery and radiation therapy in the management of gestational trophoblastic disease. Best Pract Res Clin Obstet Gynaecol 2003;17:943-957.

[25] DaftaryShirish N, Chakravarti Sudip. Gestational trophoblastic disease. In: Manual of Obstetrics 2nd ed. New Delhi: Elsevier ; 2005. p 252-59.

[26] Erturk E, Bostan H, Geze S, Saracoglu S, Erciyes N, Eroglu A. Total intravenous anaesthesia for evacuation of a hydatidiform mole and termination of pregnancy in a patient with thyrotoxicosis. Int J Obstet Anesth 2007; 16(4):363-6.

[27] Wissler RN. Endocrine disorders. In: Chestnut DH. (ed) Obstetric Anaesthesia Principles and Practice. 3rd ed. Philadelphia Elsevier Mosby 2004:744-9.

[28] Goodwin Thomas M, Hershman JM. Hyperthyroidism due to inappropriate production of human chorionic gonadotropin. Clinical Obstetrics and Gynecology 1997; 40(1):32-44.

[29] Fisher PM, Hancock BW. Gestational trophoblastic diseases and their treatment. Cancer Treat Rev 1997; 23:1-16.

[30] Rajan R. Thyroid and reproduction. In: Postgraduate Reproductive Endocrinology 4th ed. New Delhi: Jaypee Brothers Medical Publishers (P) ltd; 1997 p145-7.

[31] Burger A. Studies on a thyroid stimulating factor in urinary chorionic gonadotropin preparations. Acta Endocrinol (Copen) 1967; 55: 587-599.

[32] Hershman JM. "Physiological and pathological aspects of the effects of human chorionic gonadotropin on the thyroid". Best practice and research: Clinical Endocrinology and Metabolism 2004; 18(2):249-265.

[33] Hershman JM. Role of human chorionic gonadotropin as a thyroid stimulator. J Clin Endocrinol Metab 1992; 74:258-9.

[34] Zaman Maseehuz. Management of thyroid disorders in pregnancy. Pakistan Journal of Radiology 2008; 18(1):09-11.

[35] Girling Joanna. Thyroid disease and pregnancy. In: Michael de Swiet, editor. Medical Disorders in Obstetric Practice 4th ed. UK: Blackwell Science Ltd; 2002 p415-38.

[36] Braunstein GD, Hershman JM. Comparison of serum pituitary thyrotropin and chorionic gonadotropin concentrations throughout pregnancy. J Clin Endocrinol Metab 1976; 42:1123-26.

[37] Hershman JM. The role of human chorionic gonadotropin as a thyroid stimulator in normal pregnancy. J Clin Endocrinol Metab 2008; 93(9):3305 –6.

[38] Harada A, Hershman JM, Reed AW, Braunstein GD, Dignam WJ, Derzkoc, Friedman S, Jewelenicz R, Pekary AF. Comparison of thyroid stimulators and thyroid hormone concentrations in the sera of thyroid hormone concentrations in the sera of pregnant women. J Clin Endocrinol Metab 1979; 48:793-97.

[39] Yamazaki K, Sato K, Shizumek Kanaji Y, Ito Y, Obara T, Nakagawa T, Koizumi T, Nishimura R. Potent thyrotropic activity of human chorionic gonadotropin variants in terms of I125 incorporation and de novo synthesized thyroid hormone release in human thyroid follicles. J Clin Endocrinol Metab 1995; 80:473.

[40] Leon Sproff, Robert H Glass, Nathan G Kase. Reproduction and the thyroid. In: Charles Mitchel, editor. Clinical Gynaecologic Endocrinology and Infertility 6th ed. USA: Lippincott Williams and Wilkins; 1999 p821-8.

[41] Padmanabhan LD, Mhaskar R, Mhaskar A, Vallikad E. Trophoblastic hyperthyroidism. JAPI 2003; 51:1011-13.

[42] Ballabio M, Poshychinda M, Ekins RP. Pregnancy induced changes in thyroid function: role of human chorionic gonadotropin as putative regulator of maternal thyroid. J Clin Endocrinol Metab 1991; 73(4):824-31.

[43] Dave N, Fernandes S, Ambi U, Iyer H. hydatidiform mole with hyperthyroidism – perioperative challenges. J Obstet Gynecol India 2009; 59:356-7.Hershman JM, Higgins HP. Hydatidiform mole – a cause of clinical hyperthyroidism. The New England Journal of Medicine 1971; 284(11):573-7.

[44] Hughes Katherine, Campbell Alastair, Cooper Sarah, Sandeep Thekkepat, Adamson K. Thyrotoxicosis complicating molar pregnancy. Endocrine Abstracts 2007; 13:326.

[45] Laurent V, Besson L, Doussin JF, Rondelet B, Banssillon V. Hyperthyroidism induced by molar pregnancy. Ann Fr Anesth Reanim 1993; 12(4):424-7.

[46] Chiniwala NU,Wolf PD, Bruno CP, Kaur S, Spector H, Yacono K. Thyroid storm caused by a partial Hydatidiform mole. Thyroid 2008;18(4):479-81.

[47] Galton VA, Ingbar SH, Jimenez FJ, Hershman JM. Alterations in thyroid hormone economy in patients with hydatidiform mole. The Journal of Clinical Investigations 1971; 50:1345-54.

[48] Hershman JM, Higgins HP. Hydatidiform mole-a cause of clinical hyperthyroidism. The New England Journal of Medicine 1971;284(11):573-7.

[49] Lemon M et al. Thyroid function in trophoblastic disease. Br J Obstet Gynecol 1987; 11:1084-8.

[50] Kato K, Mostafa MH, Mann K, Schindler AE, Hoermann R. The human chorionic gonadotropin molecule from patients with trophoblastic diseases has a high thyrotropic activity but is less active in the ovary. Gynecol Endocrinol 2004; 18(5):269-77.

[51] Erol DD, Serhan CA, Ihsan U. Preoperative preparation and general anaesthesia administration with sevoflurane in a patient who develops thyrotoxicosis and cardiogenic dysfunction due to a hydatidiform mole. The Internet Journal of Anesthesiology 2004; Available from:http://www.ispub.com/journal/the_internet_journal_of_anesthesiology/archive/volume_8_number_1_12.html

[52] Bruun T, Kristoffersen K. Thyroid function during pregnancy with special reference to hydatidiform mole and hyperemesis. Acta Endocrinol (Copenh) 1978; 88(2):383-9.

[53] Dowling JT, Ingbar SH, Freinkel N. Iodine metabolism in hydatidiform mole and choriocarcinoma. The Journal of Clinical Endocrinology and Metabolism 1960; 20(1): 1-12.

[54] Desai RK, Norman RJ, Jialal I, Joubert SM. Spectrum of thyroid function abnormalities in gestational trophoblastic neoplasia. Clin Endocrinol (Oxf) 1988; 29(6):583-92.

[55] Norman RJ, Green-Thompson RW, Jialal I, Soutter WP, Pillay NL, Joubert SM. Hyperthyroidism in gestational trophoblastic neoplasia. Clin Endocrinol (Oxf) 1981; 15(4):395-401.

[56] Odell WD, Bates RW, Rivlin RS, Lipsett MB, Hertz RB. Increased thyroid function without clinical hyperthyroidism in patients with choriocarcinoma. J Clin Endocrinol Metab 1963; 23: 658-664.

[57] Amir SM, Osathanondh R, Berkowitz RS, Goldstein DP. Human chorionic gonadotropin and thyroid function in patients with hydatidiform mole. Am J Obstet Gynecol 1984; 150(6):723-8.

[58] Kock H, von Kessel H, Stolte L, von Leusden H. Thyroid function in molar pregnancy. J Clin Endocrinol Metab 1966; 26:1128-1134.

[59] Khanna P, Kumar A, Dehran M. Gestational trophoblastic disease with hyperthyroidism: Anesthetic management. J Obstet Anaesth Crit Care 2012; 2(1):31-3.

[60] Halpern SH. Anaesthesia for Caesarean Section in patients with uncontrolled hyperthyroidism Can J Anaesth 1989; 36(4):454-9.

[61] Morley JE, Jacobson RJ, Melamed J, Hershman JM. Choriocarcinoma as a cause of thyrotoxicosis. Am J Med 1976; 60(7):1036-40.

[62] Moskovitz JB, Bond MC. Molar pregnancy induced thyroid storm. The Journal of Emergency Medicine 2010; 38(5):e71-e76.

[63] Kurdi MS. Hydatidiform mole: A sour encounter with a grapy case. Indian J Anaesth 2011; 55:171-3.

[64] Solak M, Akturk G. Spinal anaesthesia in a patient with hyperthyroidism due to hydatidiform mole. Anesth Analg 1993; 77:851-2.

[65] Soutter WP, Norman R, Green-Thompson RW. The treatment of choriocarcinoma causing severe thyrotoxicosis. Br J Obstet Gynecol 1981; 88(9):938-43.

[66] Erbil Y et al. Severe hyperthyroidism requiring therapeutic plasmapheresis in a patient with hydatidiform mole. Gynecol Endocrinol 2006; 22(7):402-4.

[67] Azezli Adil, Bayraktaroglu Taner, Topuz Sanet, Kalayoglu-Besisik Sevgi. Hyperthyroidism in molar pregnancy: rapid preoperative preparation by plasmapheresis and complete improvement after evacuation. Transfus Apher Sci 2007; 36(1): 87-9.

[68] Ozbey N, Kalayoglu-Besisik S, Gul N, Bozbora A, Sencer E, Molevalilar S. Therapeutic plasmapheresis in patients with severe hyperthyroidism in whom antithyroid drugs are contraindicated. Int J Clin Pract 2004; 58(6):554-8.

[69] Lynch EP. Endocrine disease. In: Andre Van Zundert, Gerard W Ostheimer, editors. Pain Relief and Anaesthesia in Obstetrics 1st ed. New York: Churchill Livingstone; 1996 p605-48.

[70] Yang Ming-Jie, Cheng Ming-Huei. Pregnancy complicated with pulmonary oedema due to hyperthyroidism. J Chin Med Assoc 2005; 68(7):336-338.

[71] Mehta P A, Dubrey SW. High output heart failure. QJM 2009;102(4):235-41.

[72] Panagoulis C, Halapas A, Chariatis E, Driva P, Matsakas E. Hyperthyroidism and the heart. Hellenic J Cardiol 2008;49:169-175.

[73] Choudhury R P, Mac Dernot J. Heart failure in thyrotoxicosis, an approach to management. Br J Clin Pharmacol 1998; 46(5):421-24.

[74] Malyer RH, Trivedi TH, Padhiyar NN, Moulick ND, Yeolekar ME. ARDS in a case of vesicular with secondary hyperthyroidism. J Assoc Physicians India 2004; 52:992-3.

[75] Kim JM, Arakawa K, McCann V. Severe hyperthyroidism associated with hydatidiform mole. Anaesthesiology 1976;44(5):445-48.

[76] Struthmann L, Gunthner Biller M, Bergaver F, Friese K, Mylovas I. Complete hydatidiform mole in a perimenopausal woman with a subsequent severe thyrotoxicosis. Arch Gynecol Obstet 2009; 279(3):411-3.

[77] Huberman RP, Fon GT, Bein ME. Benign molar pregnancies: pulmonary complications. Am J Roentgenol 1982; 138:71-74.

[78] Carrasco C, Cotoras J. Gestational hyperthyroidism: a case associated to molar pregnancy. Rev Med Chil 2001; 129(3):303-6.

[79] Carlos Edvardo David de Almeida, Erick Freitas Curi, Carlos Roberto David de Almeida, Denise Fernandes Vieira. Thyrotoxic crisis associated with gestational trophoblastic disease. Rev Bras Anesthesiol 2011; 61(5):604-609.